Pediatric and Adult MRI Atlas of Bone Marrow

Hakan Ilaslan • Murali Sundaram

Pediatric and Adult MRI Atlas of Bone Marrow

Normal Appearances, Variants and Diffuse Disease States

Springer

Hakan Ilaslan
Cleveland Clinic Lerner College of Medicine
Cleveland Clinic Department of Radiology
Cleveland, OH
USA

Murali Sundaram
Cleveland Clinic Lerner College of Medicine
Cleveland Clinic Department of Radiology
Cleveland, OH
USA

ISBN 978-3-662-56844-6 ISBN 978-3-642-02740-6 (eBook)
DOI 10.1007/978-3-642-02740-6

Springer Heidelberg New York Dordrecht London

Softcover reprint of the hardcover 1st edition 2016

Printed on acid-free paper

Springer-Verlag GmbH Berlin Heidelberg is part of Springer Science+Business Media (www.springer.com)

Dedicated to my parents Elif and Mustafa Ilaslan for the emphases of their children's education and support of all their every endeavors; this is a small thank you.

Hakan Ilaslan

Dedicated to the memory of Gautam and for Aparna and Priya, in enduring gratitude.

Murali Sundaram

Foreword

Old maps often use the term "terra incognita" for regions that have not been explored, documented, or mapped. Cartographers have sometimes presumed that these "unknown lands" are home to fantastic, imaginary creatures, quite different from what is found in the known world.

Until relatively recently, the bone marrow was "terra incognita" for radiologists because with the exception of a few regions of cancellous bone, its contents were not visible to medical imaging. No radiographic, ultrasound, or even CT methods could reveal the composition and regional variations of the marrow.

MRI has started to shed some light into the black box of the bone marrow, although as the reader of this book will learn, our ability to discriminate among conditions by imaging alone remains limited.

In recent years, we have learned that all three of the major constituents of marrow – cancellous bone, fat, and the hematopoietic cell lines – are much more complicated than previously thought. Cancellous bone is now known to have a very complex relationship between structure and function. Often called "trabecular bone," it is now clear that it only sometimes takes the form of "trabeculae."

Marrow fat (and somatic fat as well) has recently taken center stage in a whole host of metabolic conditions, some of these are physiological and some pathological. For example, it now appears that fat plays an important role in insulin metabolism and cardiovascular disease.

The cellular elements are the most complex of all, being comprised of a host of different cell types, as well as their precursors.

MRI, for all its obvious complexity and sophistication, is still a rather limited tool to investigate this complexity, being mostly confined to images based upon T1 and T2 relaxivity, as well as gadolinium perfusion. It is amazing how well we are able to do by using these relatively simple tools, combined with a bit of anatomy and physiology!

That said, in my experience unexpected findings in the bone marrow are a frequent cause of diagnostic uncertainty and sometimes outright error among residents and practicing radiologists. They will benefit from this book.

Evaluation of bone marrow is difficult because of the dynamic nature of the organ. It varies from one anatomical location to another, may demonstrate substantial differences between individuals, and changes continuously throughout life both in normal physiological states and as a response to disease.

The atlas format is particularly well suited to this subject because it allows the authors to show many examples, spanning the spectrum of normal and abnormal states. They have drawn upon their vast clinical experience to provide many illustrations of each normal and pathological state.

The illustrations of marrow vascularity are particularly beautiful. There are excellent examples of the bone marrow in fetal MRI and many fine illustrations of age-related developmental changes in the extremities.

For those who are less familiar with bone marrow imaging, this book can be read in the conventional way – text first followed by images. For those more experienced, an interesting approach is to look at images first, form an impression, and then look to the text for answers and explanations.

However one chooses to interact with this book, there is much to learn. This book fills an important niche and will be much appreciated by the radiology community.

Daniel I Rosenthal, MD
Professor of Radiology
Harvard University
Cambridge, MA, USA

Vice Chair of Radiology
Massachusetts General Hospital
Boston, MA, USA

Contents

Contributors

Hakan Ilaslan, MD Associate Professor of Radiology, Cleveland Clinic Lerner College of Medicine, Staff Radiologist, Cleveland Clinic Department of Radiology, Cleveland, OH, USA

S. Pinar Karakas-Rothey, MD Department of Diagnostic Imaging, University of California San Francisco Benioff Children's Hospital at Oakland, Oakland, CA, USA

Kambiz Motamedi, MD Professor of Radiology, University of California Los Angeles, Staff Radiologist, Department of Radiology, Ronald Reagan UCLA Medical Center, Los Angeles, CA, USA

Kathleen Ruchalski, MD Assistant Professor of Radiology, University of California Los Angeles, Department of Radiology, Ronald Reagan UCLA Medical Center, Los Angeles, CA, USA

Leanne L. Seeger, MD Professor of Radiology, University of California Los Angeles, Staff Radiologist, Department of Radiology, Ronald Reagan UCLA Medical Center, Los Angeles, CA, USA

Murali Sundaram, MD Professor of Radiology, Cleveland Clinic Lerner College of Medicine, Staff Radiologist, Cleveland Clinic Department of Radiology, Cleveland, OH, USA

1 Normal Bone Marrow: In Utero Through the Adult Years

S. Pinar Karakas-Rothey and Hakan Ilaslan

1.1 Hematopoiesis

Hematopoiesis, the formation of blood cells, commences and is confined to the yolk sac of the fetus for the first 6 weeks. Between the sixth and twentieth weeks of age, the reticuloendothelial system, the liver and spleen, take over the process of blood cell formation [1]. From the sixteenth week, hematopoiesis commences in the bone marrow coinciding with the development of bone cavities [1, 2]. From then on, bone marrow remains the primary site for hematopoiesis. With advancing years, the number of sites and volume of hematopoietic bone marrow progressively decreases.

1.2 Development of Bone and Bone Marrow

The skeletal system develops from primitive mesenchymal cells that are precursors of membranous bone or cartilage. The cranium and facial bones are formed directly from the mesenchyme by intramembranous ossification. The skull base, long bones, clavicles, and vertebral column develop by endochondral ossification from cartilaginous models [3]. The long bones develop by means of longitudinal and spherical growth. Longitudinal growth is provided by the primary epiphysis with the newly developed bone layered in the metaphysis [3]. The spherical growth is provided by intramembranous bone deposition from the surrounding periosteum and perichondrium. The secondary physis surrounding the secondary ossification center is responsible for its spherical growth [3].

In infants, the hematopoietic (red) marrow is composed of almost equal amounts of blood cell precursors and fat cells and supplied by a rich vascular network. The yellow marrow is primarily formed by fat cells and has a sparse blood supply. The red marrow fat cells may contain slightly greater concentrations of unsaturated fatty acids, but otherwise there is no significant difference between red and yellow marrow fat cells [4]. The normal sequential transformation of bone marrow is appreciated earlier on magnetic resonance imaging (MRI) than on histologic studies due to the higher sensitivity of MRI in demonstrating small amounts of scattered fat [3, 5].

H. Ilaslan, M. Sundaram, *Pediatric and Adult MRI Atlas of Bone Marrow: Normal Appearances, Variants and Diffuse Disease States*, DOI 10.1007/978-3-642-02740-6_1

1.3 Anatomy and Physiology

Bone marrow is one of the largest and most important organs of the body with a weight of approximately 3000 g in adult men and 2600 g in adult women [4]. The osseous component of marrow comprises cancellous bone which is within the confines of the cortex. Cancellous bone is formed by primary and bridging secondary trabecula and provides both architectural support and a mineral depot. Furthermore, cancellous bone is the site of osteoblastic, osteoclastic, and osteocytic activity. The vascular system of marrow is complex with an arterial supply largely from the nutrient artery that penetrates to the center of the medullary cavity (Fig. 1.1a). Ascending and descending branches of the nutrient artery run parallel to the long axis of bone (Fig. 1.1b, c). Branches from the nutrient artery enter the endosteal surface of the cortex and coalesce with vessels of periosteal origin (Fig. 1.1d). These transosteal vessels widen to form sinusoids as they enter the endosteal surface of the cortex (Fig. 1.1d). The sinusoidal system forms a very extensive anastomosing complex among adipocytes of the bone marrow. The sinusoidal system drains into the central venous sinus of the medullary canal, which then exits through the nutrient foramen alongside the artery. Red marrow shows a slightly higher degree of enhancement on postcontrast MRI in comparison to fatty marrow due to its rich blood supply (Fig. 1.2). Nerves of the bone marrow follow a course similar to the arterial supply and are composed of abundant sympathetic and afferent nerve fibers [6]. Sympathetic fibers are thought to help modulate release of marrow cells [7]. Cellular marrow refers to all stages of erythrocytic, leukocytic, and thrombocytic evolution along with the reticuloendothelial system cells and adipocytes. Adipocytes are a major component of bone marrow. When hematopoiesis decreases, the adipocytes increase their volume and number, whereas during increased hematopoietic activity, the fat cells atrophy. Lymph nodules are present in human bone marrow although true lymphatic vessels have never been demonstrated [8]. The red or cellular marrow is hematopoietically active, producing red blood cells (RBCs), white blood cells (WBCs), and platelet precursors. Yellow marrow is composed of fat cells and considered hematopoietically inactive. These two types of marrow differ in their respective chemical compositions resulting in different signal characteristics on MRI. Recognition of these differences is important to understand physiological and pathological MRI appearances of the bone marrow. In infants and young children, red marrow consists of approximately 40 % water, 40 % fat, and 20 % protein [9]. As the individual ages, the fatty elements of hematopoietic marrow increase, and by age 70 years, red marrow is composed of approximately 60 % fat, 30 % water, and 10 % protein [9]. These differences in composition of red marrow are reflected on MRI appearances in different age groups (Fig. 1.3). Yellow marrow has a more stable composition throughout different age groups with approximately 80 % fat, 15 % water, and 5 % protein [4].

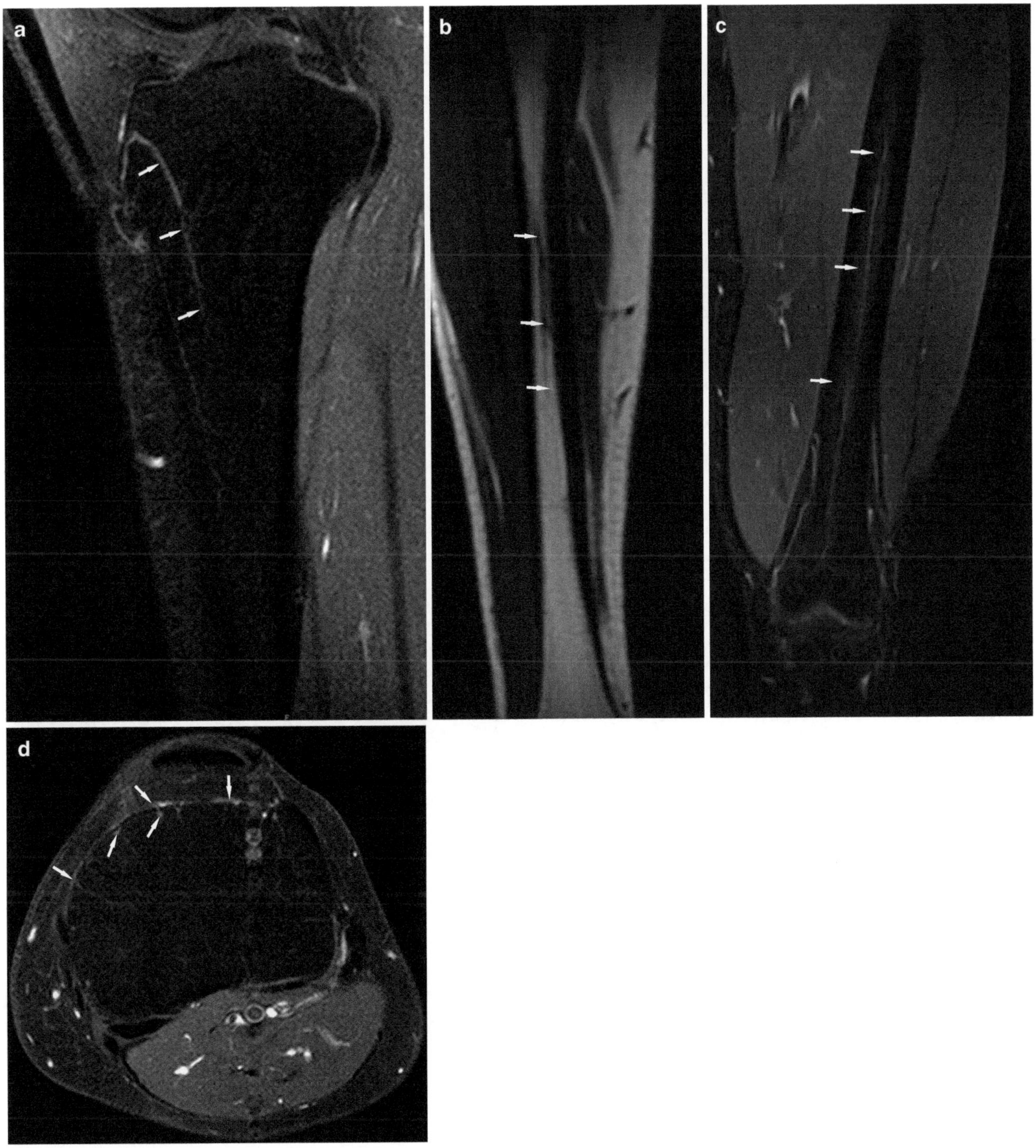

Fig. 1.1 Sagittal proton density-weighted image of the proximal tibia (**a**) shows nutrient artery penetrating the medullary cavity (*arrows*). Coronal T1-weighted image of the tibia (**b**) and coronal T2-weighted image of the femur (**c**) show nutrient artery running parallel to the long axis of these bones (*arrows*). Axial proton density-weighted image of the proximal tibia (**d**) shows branches of the nutrient artery that enter the endosteal surface of the cortex and communicate with periosteal vessels (*arrows*)

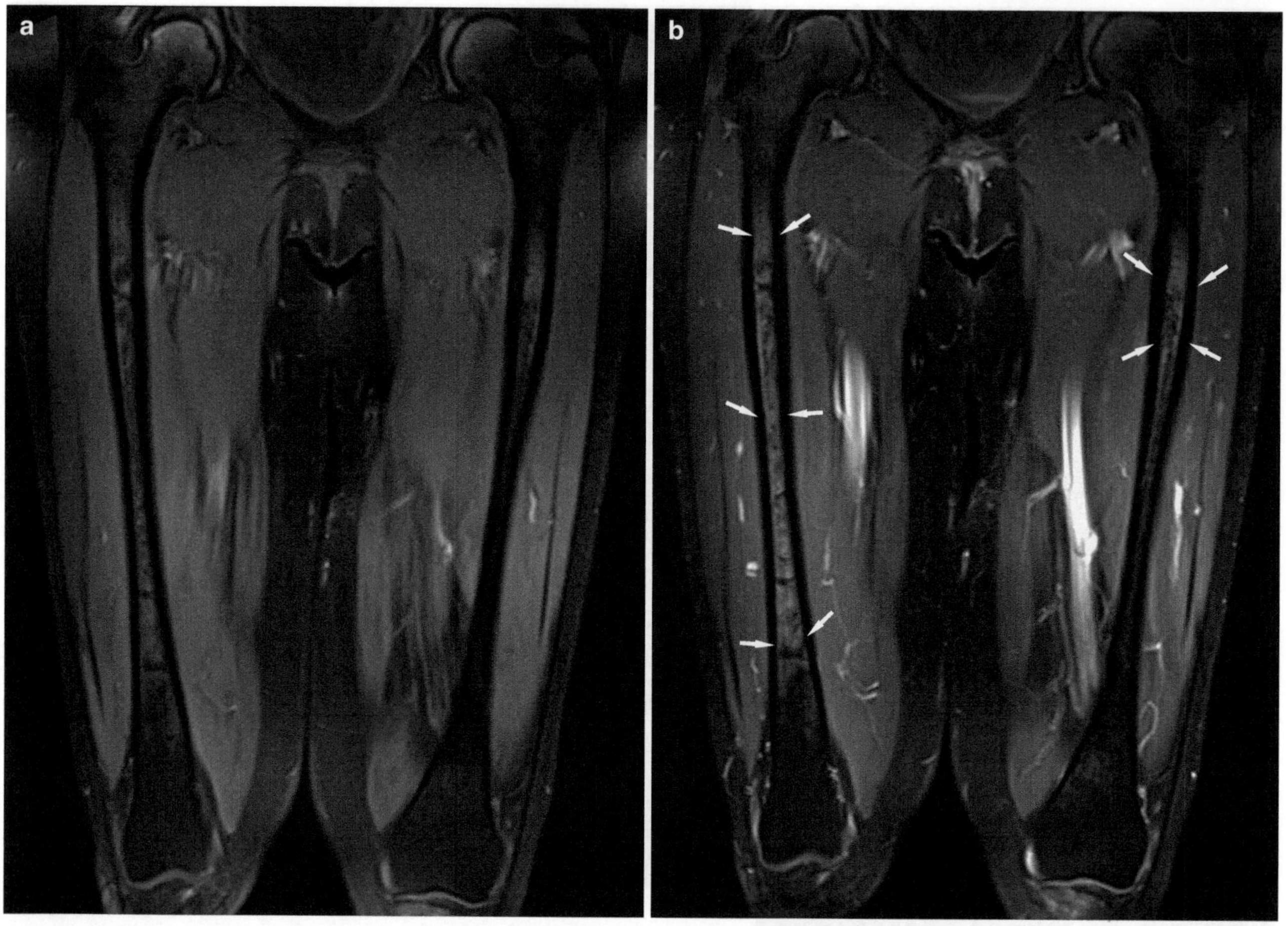

Fig. 1.2 Coronal precontrast T1-weighted fat-suppressed image of bilateral thighs shows red marrow in bilateral femoral diaphysis (**a**). After the administration of intravenous contrast, a subtle enhancement of bone marrow is noted (**b**), corresponding to areas of red marrow seen in the precontrast image (*arrows*)

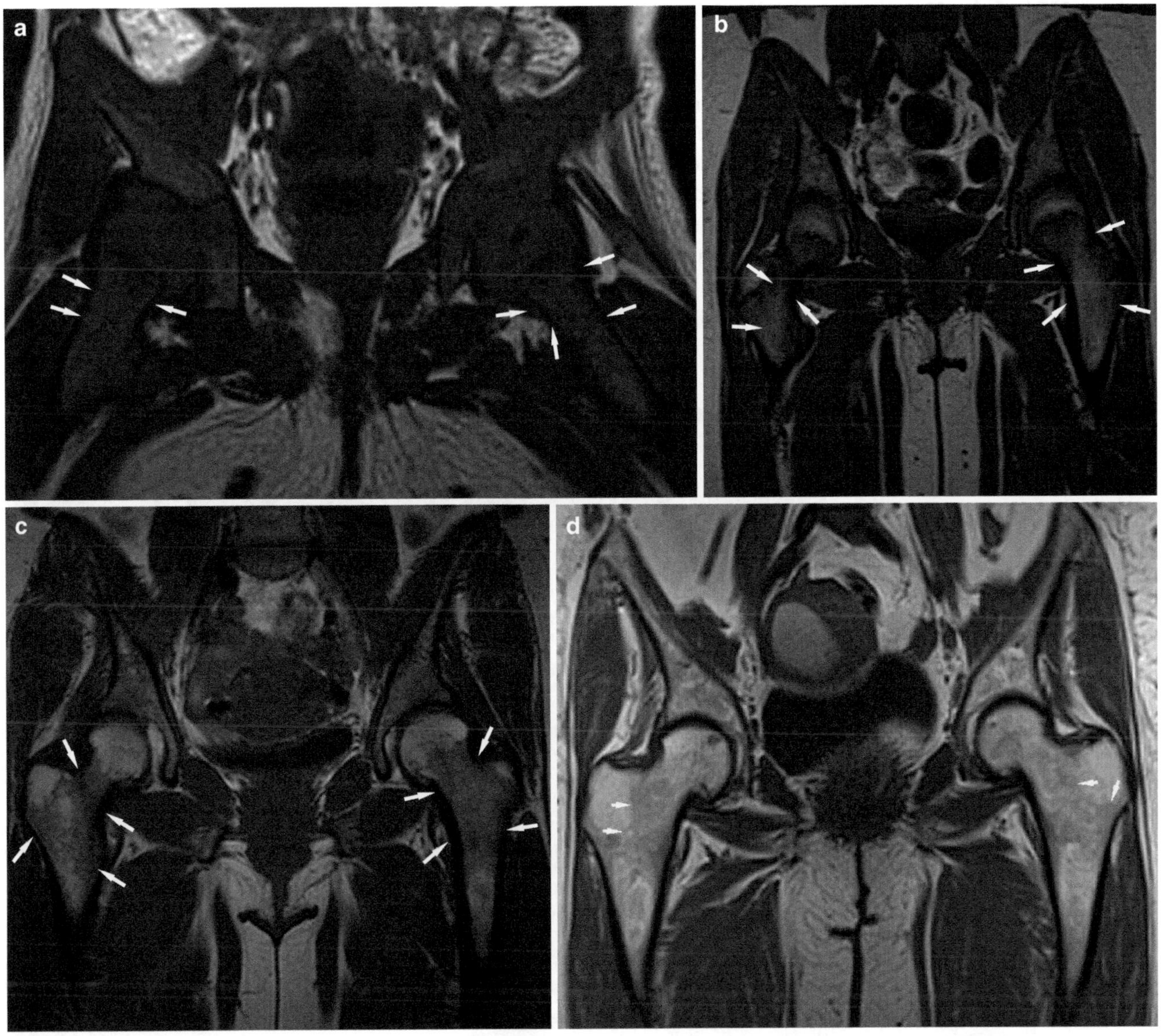

Fig. 1.3 Coronal T1-weighted images of the pelvis in different ages. A 6-month-old girl (**a**), an 8-year-old girl (**b**), a 45-year-old woman (**c**), and an 88-year-old woman (**d**) all show varying degrees of red marrow (*arrows*). Note the changing hyperintensity of red marrow correlating with the ages of individuals, which reflects the increase in fatty elements within hematopoietic marrow

1.4 MRI of the Normal Appendicular Skeleton

In the second trimester of pregnancy, the long bone shafts of the fetus have small medullary cavities and thick cortices giving an overall low T1 and T2 signal intensity due to a large ossified component of bone and a tiny marrow cavity which may be difficult to visualize [2] (Fig. 1.4). Later, the marrow spaces progressively expand, and the bones start to reflect the entirely hematopoietic pattern of marrow typical for a newborn (Figs. 1.5, 1.6, 1.7, and 1.8). Cartilaginous apophyses and epiphyses do not show this change (Fig. 1.8b). During the neonatal period, the signal intensity of hematopoietic marrow is hyperintense on T2 and isointense or hypointense to that of normal skeletal muscle on T1-weighted images, reflecting the higher percentage of cellular marrow with abundance of water and hemosiderin [9–11] (Fig. 1.8a). Following the neonatal period, if T1 marrow signal intensity is found to be lower than that of normal skeletal muscle, this should alert the interpreter to a pathological marrow state (Fig. 1.9). There are no statistically significant differences in epiphyseal marrow conversion between boys and girls [5, 11, 12].

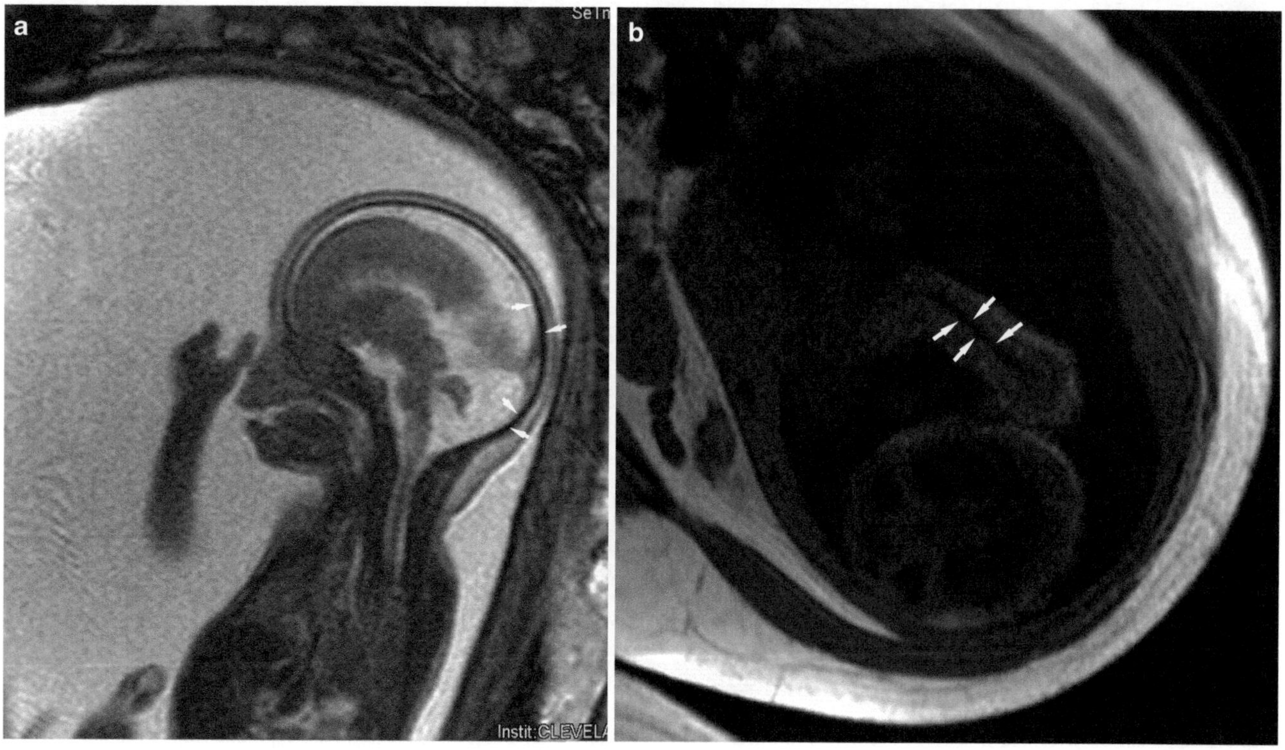

Fig. 1.4 MRI in a 20-week-old fetus. Images obtained using TrueFISP technique (true fast imaging with steady-state precession) show prominent cortices (*arrows*) without appreciable bone marrow about the skull (**a**) and humerus (**b**)

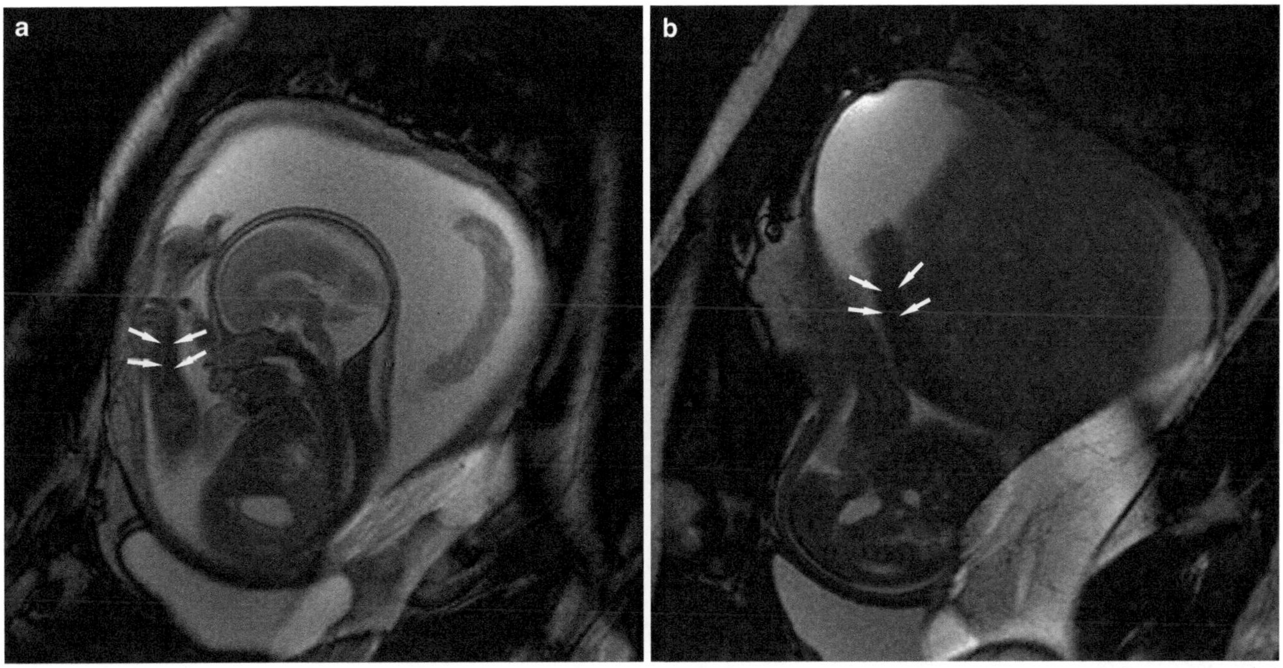

Fig. 1.5 MRI in a 25-week-old fetus. Images obtained using TrueFISP technique show subtle bone marrow signal (*arrows*) about femur (**a**) and forearm (**b**)

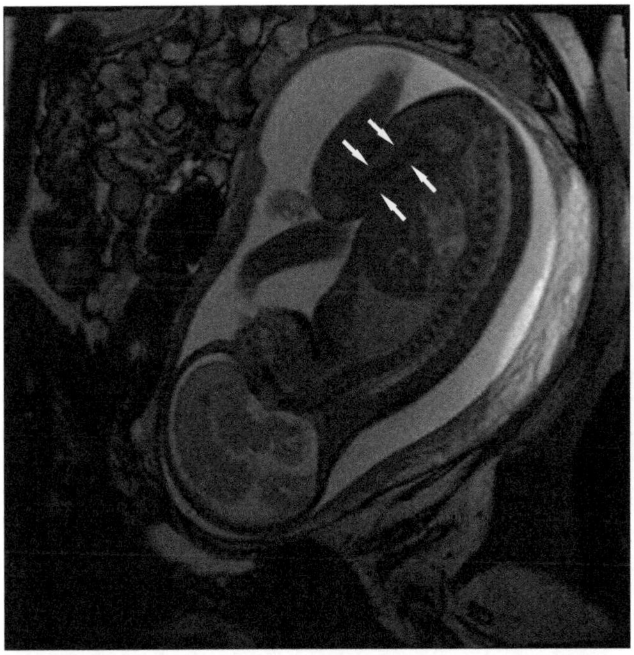

Fig. 1.6 MRI in a 28-week, 2-day-old fetus. Images obtained using TrueFISP technique show obvious bone marrow signal (*arrows*) about the femur

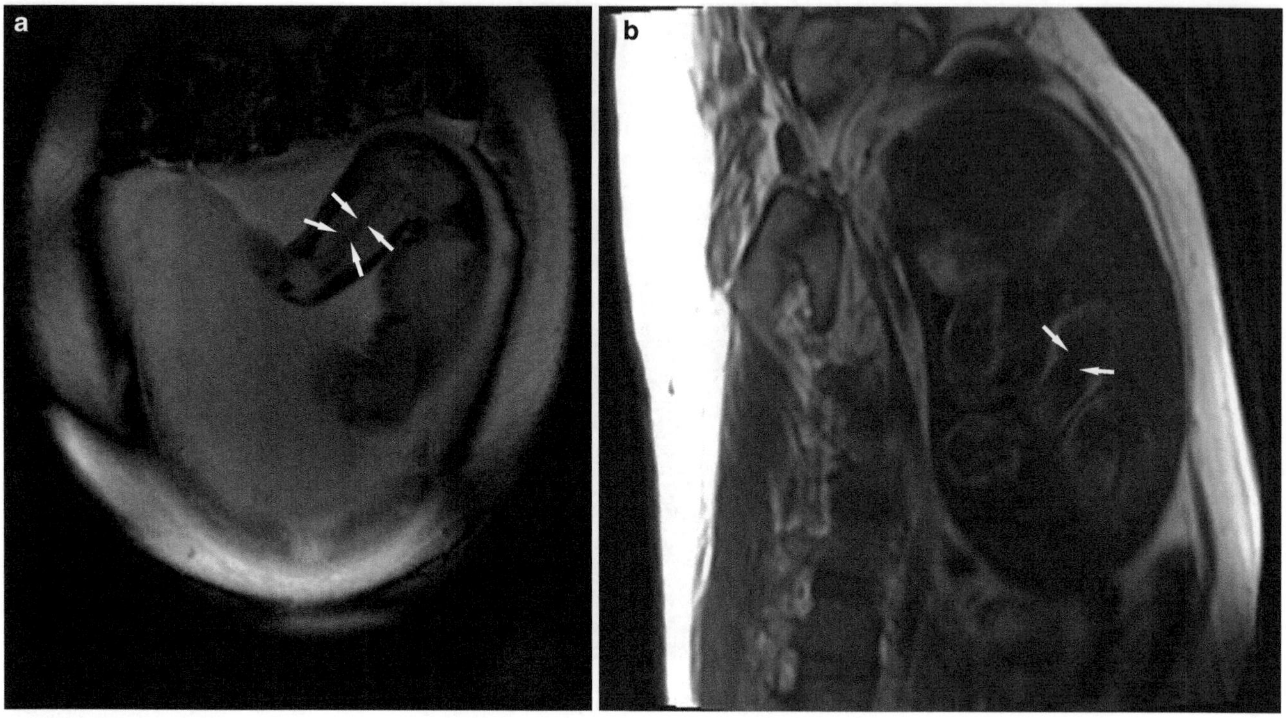

Fig. 1.7 MRI in a 33-week, 2-day-old fetus. Humeral bone marrow signal (*arrows*) is visualized on images obtained using TrueFISP technique (**a**) and T1-weighted image (**b**)

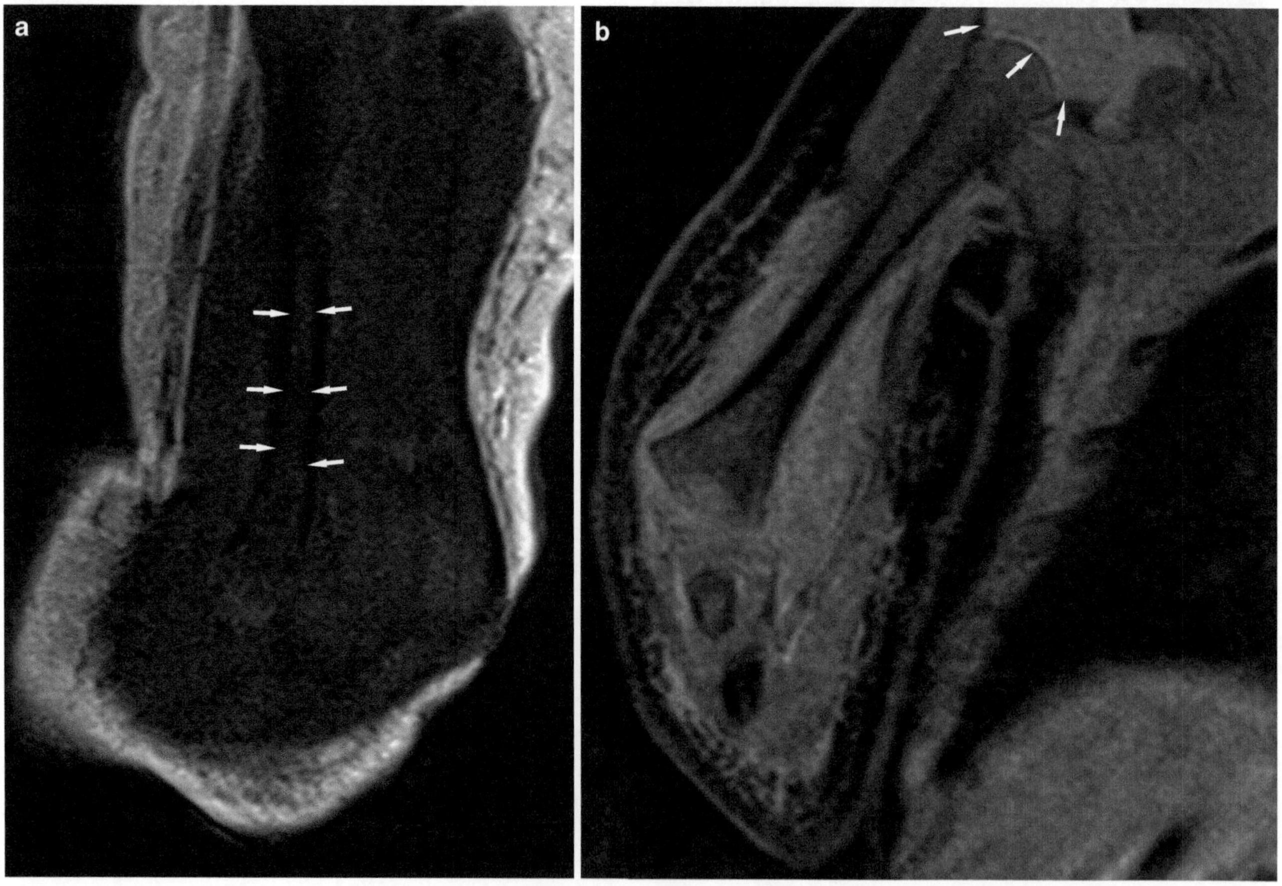

Fig. 1.8 MRI in a 2-day-old neonate. Prominent red marrow signal is noted in the humeral shaft with signal intensity (*arrows*) isointense to adjacent skeletal muscle on T1-weighted coronal image (**a**). Bone marrow appears slightly hyperintense on T2-weighted coronal image (**b**). Note the more hyperintense signal in the cartilaginous proximal humeral epiphysis

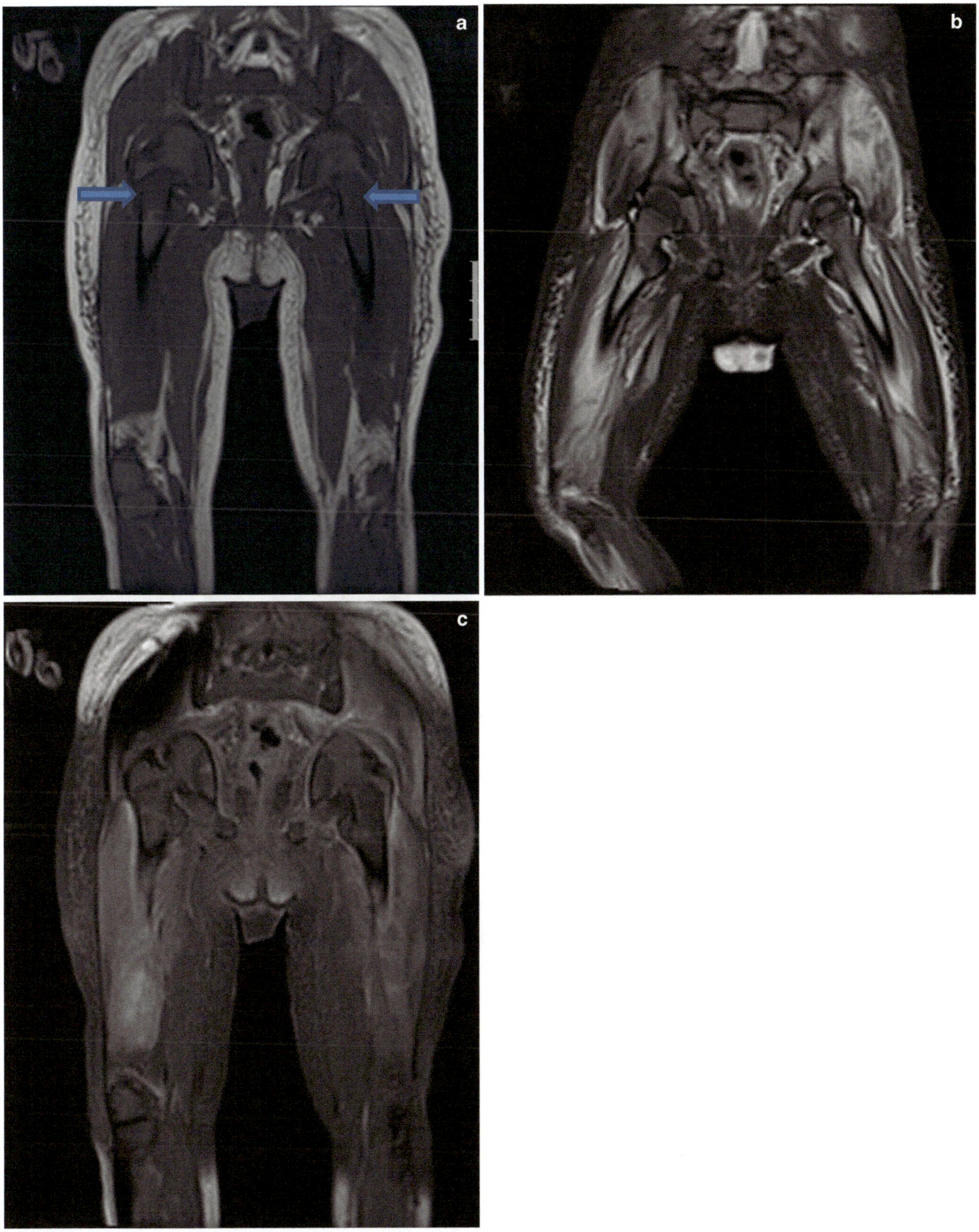

Fig. 1.9 A 2-year-old boy presented with difficulty in walking. MRI of the pelvis and thighs demonstrates symmetrical abnormal bone marrow signal in pelvis and femurs. On T1-weighted images (**a**), the bone marrow signal is lower than that of adjacent skeletal muscle, suggestive of an infiltrative pathologic marrow state (*arrows*). T2-weighted fat-suppressed (**b**) image shows hyperintense marrow signal and muscle edema. Mild diffuse bone marrow and muscle enhancement is noted on postcontrast T1-weighted fat-suppressed image (**c**). A biopsy revealed acute lymphoid leukemia

In the early months of life, the cartilaginous epiphyses have higher signal intensity than the metaphysis (Fig. 1.8) on both T1- and T2-weighted sequences. The epiphyseal cartilage ossifies by means of endochondral ossification and initially contains dense trabecula and hematopoietic marrow that is hypointense to the surrounding cartilage [12–15]. After a brief period, usually in 6 months, epiphyses convert to yellow marrow [10, 12] (Fig. 1.10). After the conversion, apophyses and epiphyses contain the greatest concentration of fat within each bone and appear isointense to subcutaneous fat on all pulse sequences [10] (Fig. 1.11). Occasionally, patches or islands of red marrow persist in apophyses and epiphyses in adults particularly about the proximal femur and humerus [19] (Figs. 1.12 and 1.13) although diffuse involvement is not considered normal and typically is seen in significant chronic anemic states such as the hereditary hemoglobinopathies.

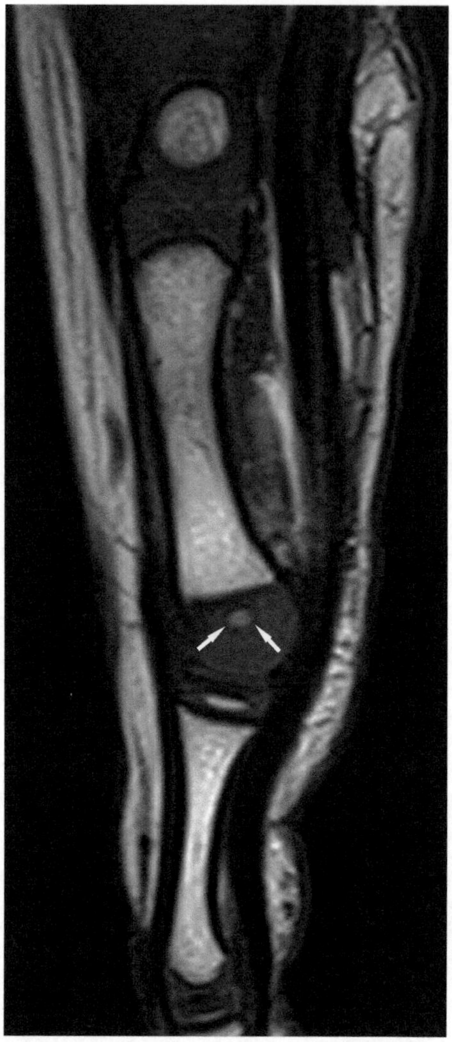

Fig. 1.10 A 3-year-old boy. Sagittal T1-weighted image of the foot shows a focus of fatty marrow formation within cartilaginous epiphyses of the metatarsal proximally and distally (*arrows*)

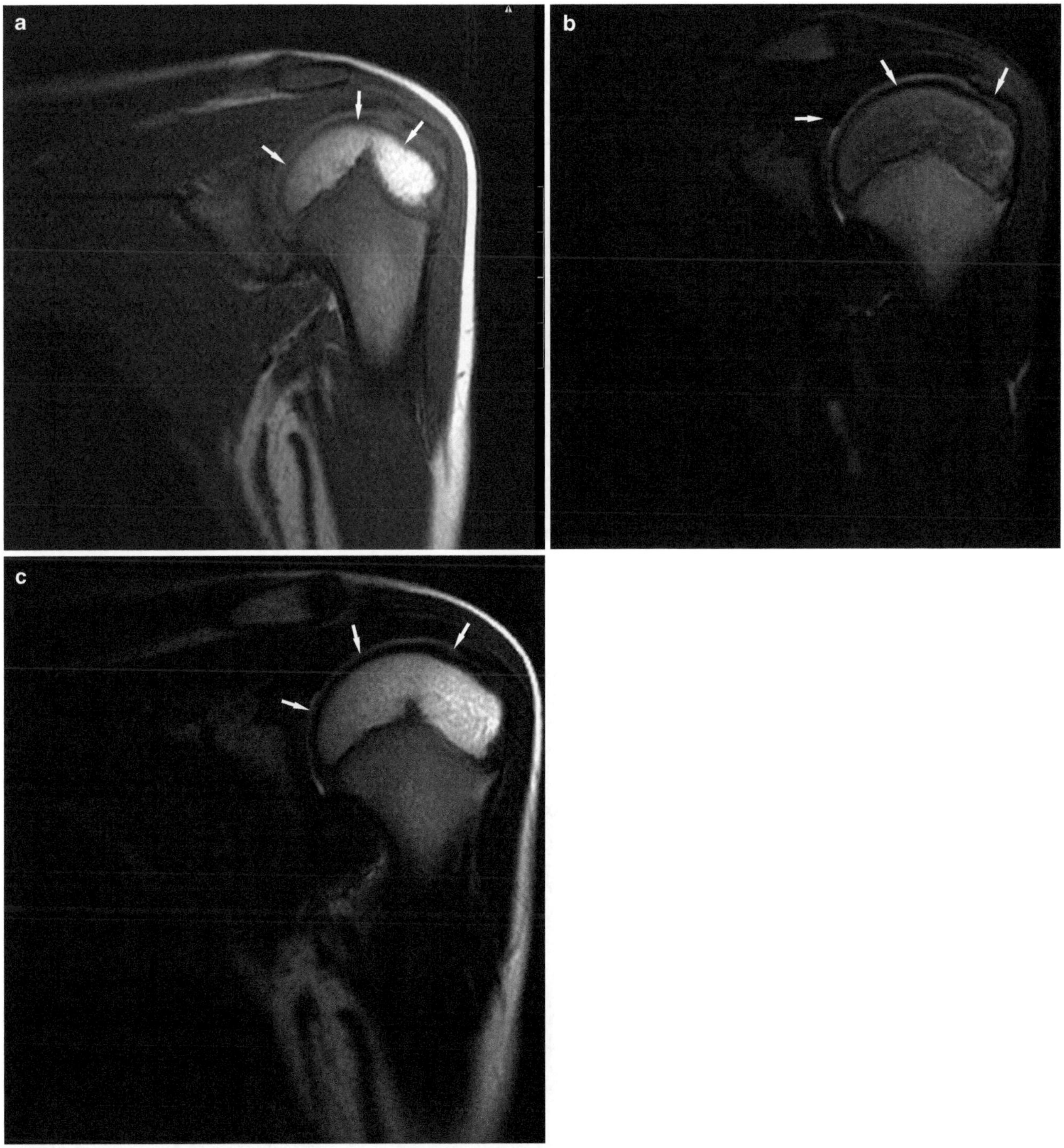

Fig. 1.11 An 8-year-old boy. Coronal T1-weighted (**a**), T2-weighted fat-suppressed (**b**), and T2-weighted nonfat-suppressed (**c**) images of the left shoulder demonstrate homogeneous fatty signal within the humeral head apophysis and epiphysis (*arrows*). Red marrow is noted in the humeral metaphysis and visualized glenoid

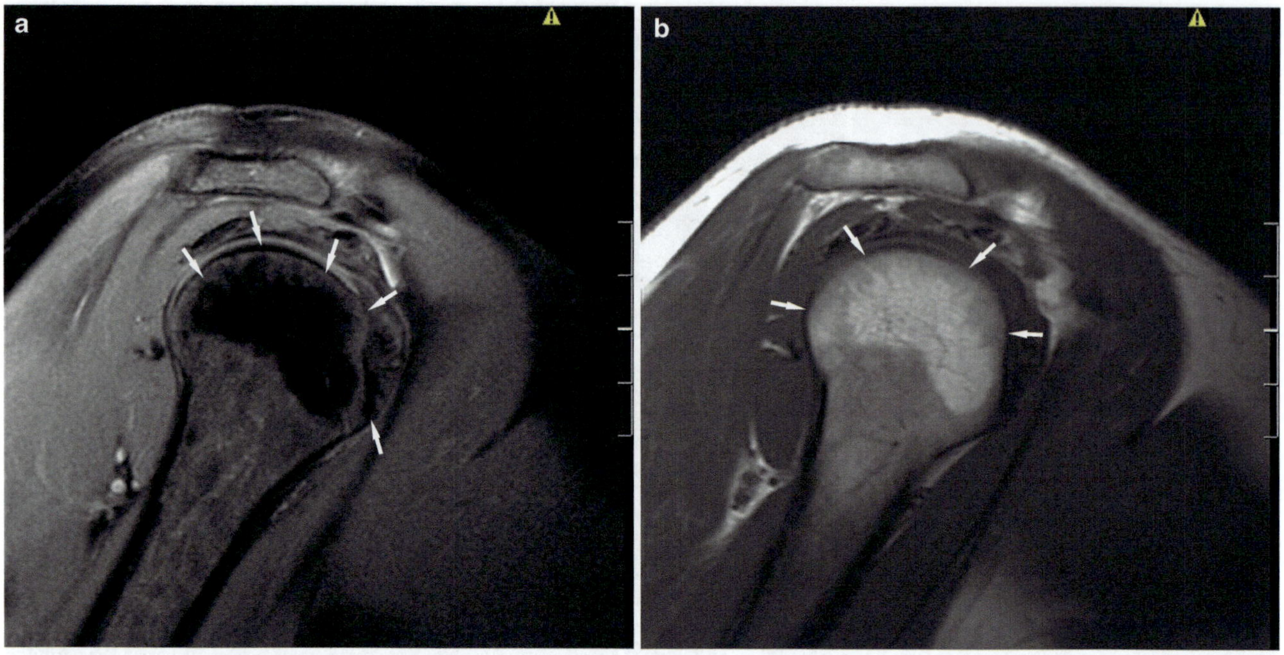

Fig. 1.12 A 28-year-old man. Sagittal T1-weighted (**a**) and T2-weighted fat-suppressed (**b**) images of the shoulder demonstrate subtle red marrow signal in the epiphysis (*arrows*)

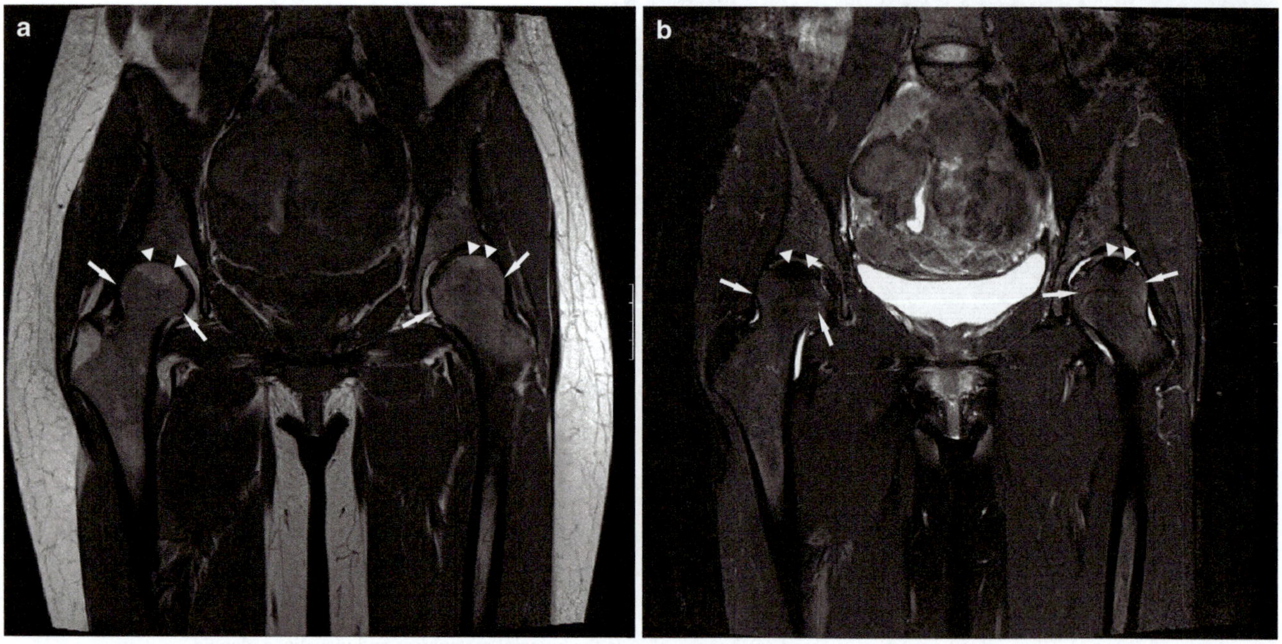

Fig. 1.13 A 37-year-old woman. Coronal T1-weighted (**a**) and T2-weighted fat-suppressed (**b**) images of the pelvis demonstrate foci of red marrow signal in the proximal femoral epiphysis bilaterally (*arrows*) with some preservation of fatty signal (*arrowheads*)

Fig. 1.14 Coronal T1-weighted images of hands in various age groups demonstrating evolution of bone marrow changes. Prominent red marrow hypointense to skeletal muscle is noted in the metacarpals and phalanges of a newborn (2 days old) (**a**). Minimal residual red marrow signal is noted in the metacarpals and phalanges of a 10-month-old boy (**b**) and a 13-month-old girl (**c**) (*arrows*). Completely fatty bone marrow of all carpals, metacarpals, and phalanges is noted in a 5-year-old boy (**d**), a 7-year-old boy (**e**), a 13-year-old boy (**f**), and an 18-year-old man (**g**). Note the evolution of cartilaginous epiphyses and growth plates

Metadiaphyseal bone marrow evolves by changing its composition from predominantly cellular hematopoietic marrow to fatty marrow starting shortly after birth. The locations of marrow conversion progress from periphery to central commencing in the terminal phalanges of the hands and feet. By the age of 1 year, the marrow of the hands and feet is entirely composed of fatty marrow [15, 16] (Figs. 1.14 and 1.15). Individual long bone marrow conversion also progresses from central to peripheral and from diaphysis to distal metaphysis and then to proximal metaphysis with a variable symmetry and rate that is influenced by the type and location of bone, age, sex, and the health of the individual. The final segments of the appendicular skeleton to convert are the proximal humeral and femoral metaphyses. Islands or foci of red marrow are usually seen in these locations in varying amounts during adulthood and should not be mistaken for disease.

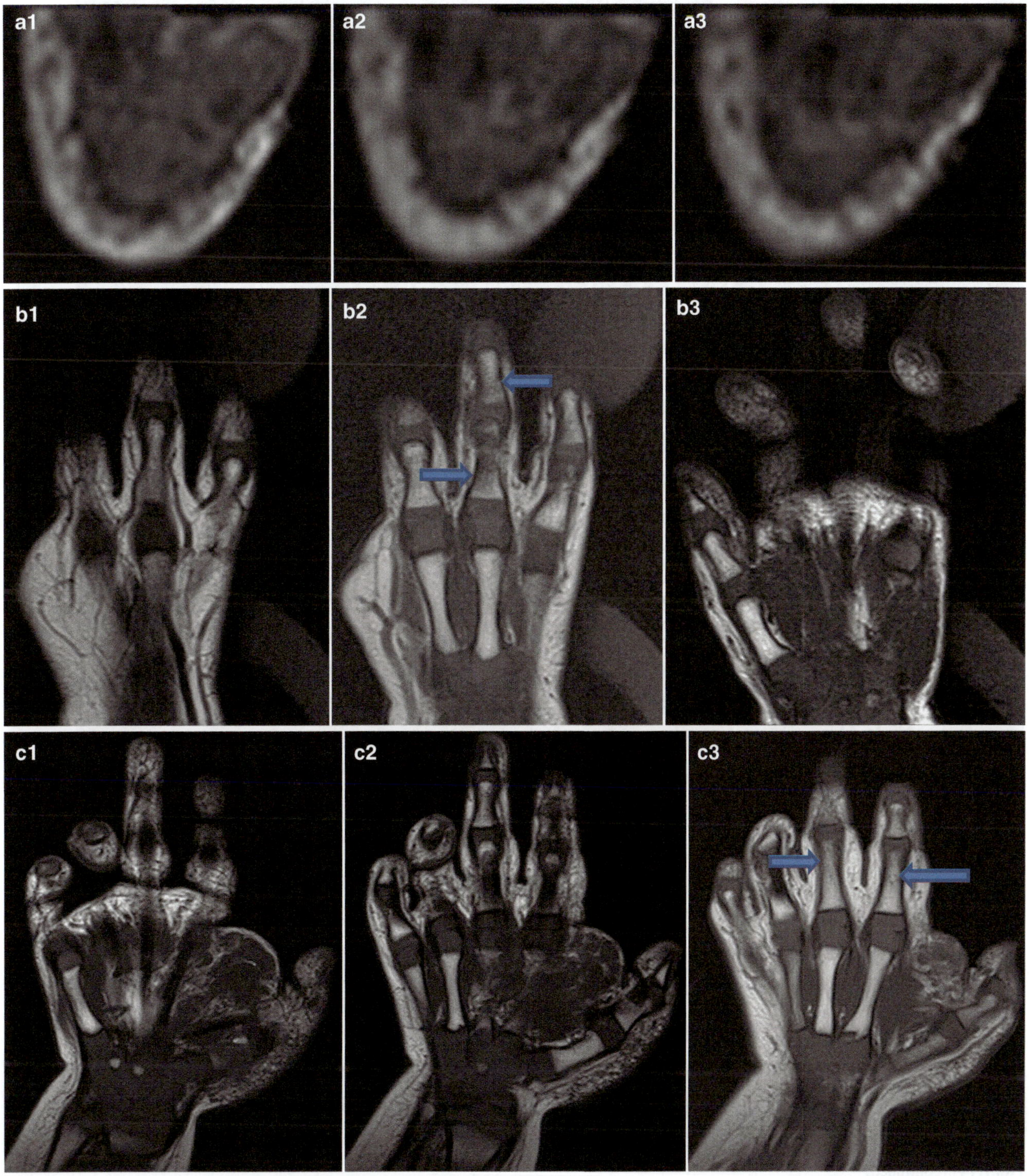

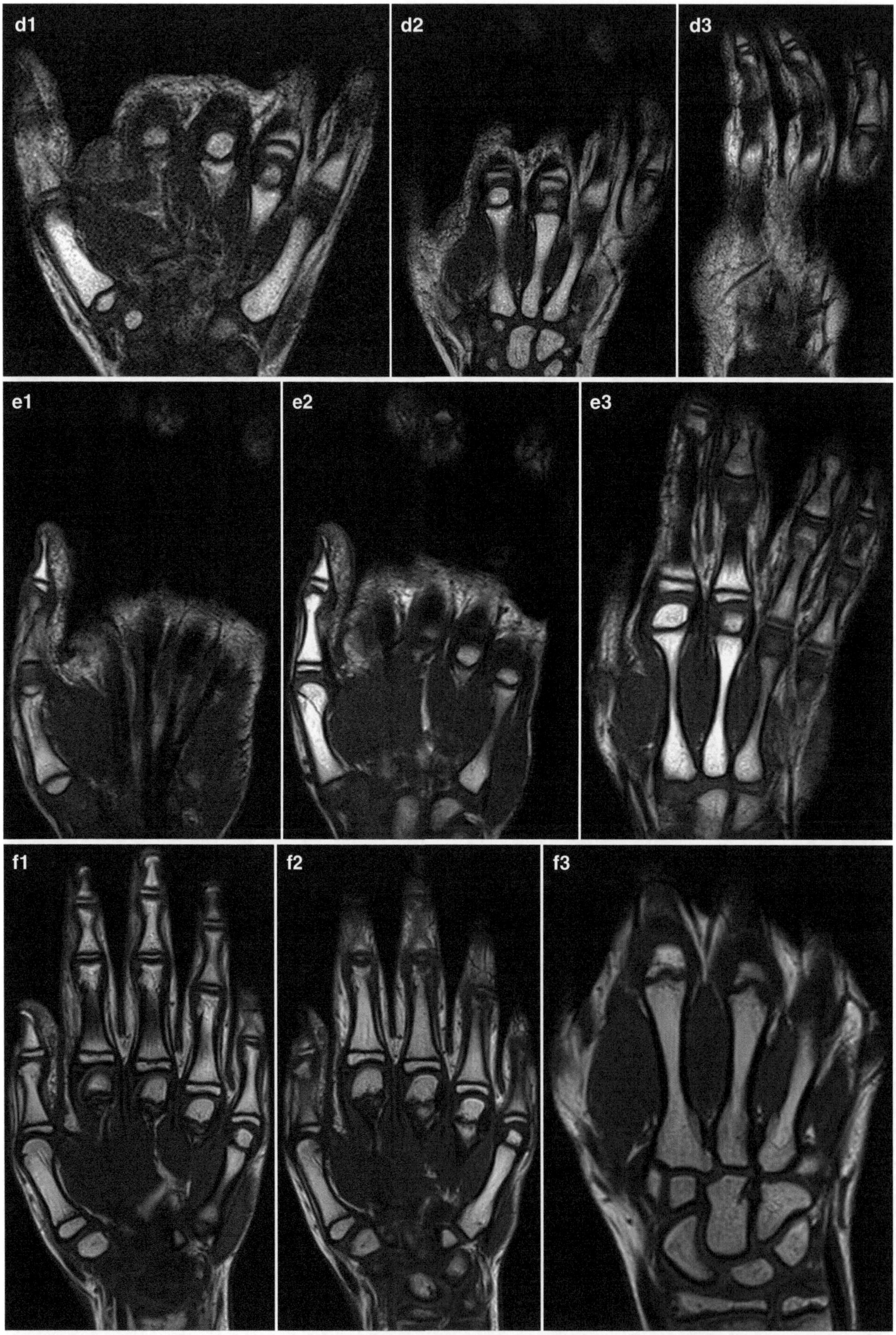

Fig. 1.14 (continued)

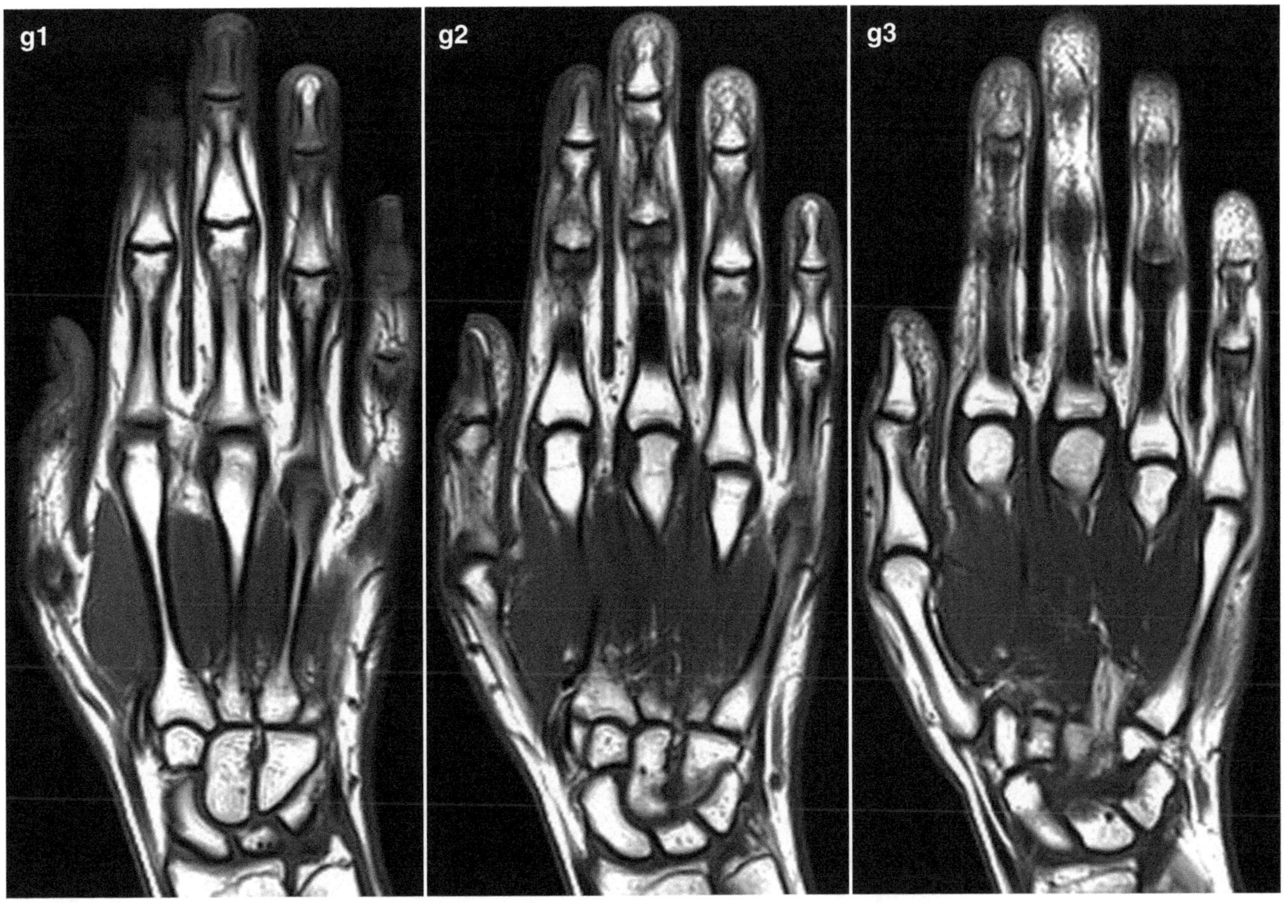

Fig. 1.14 (continued)

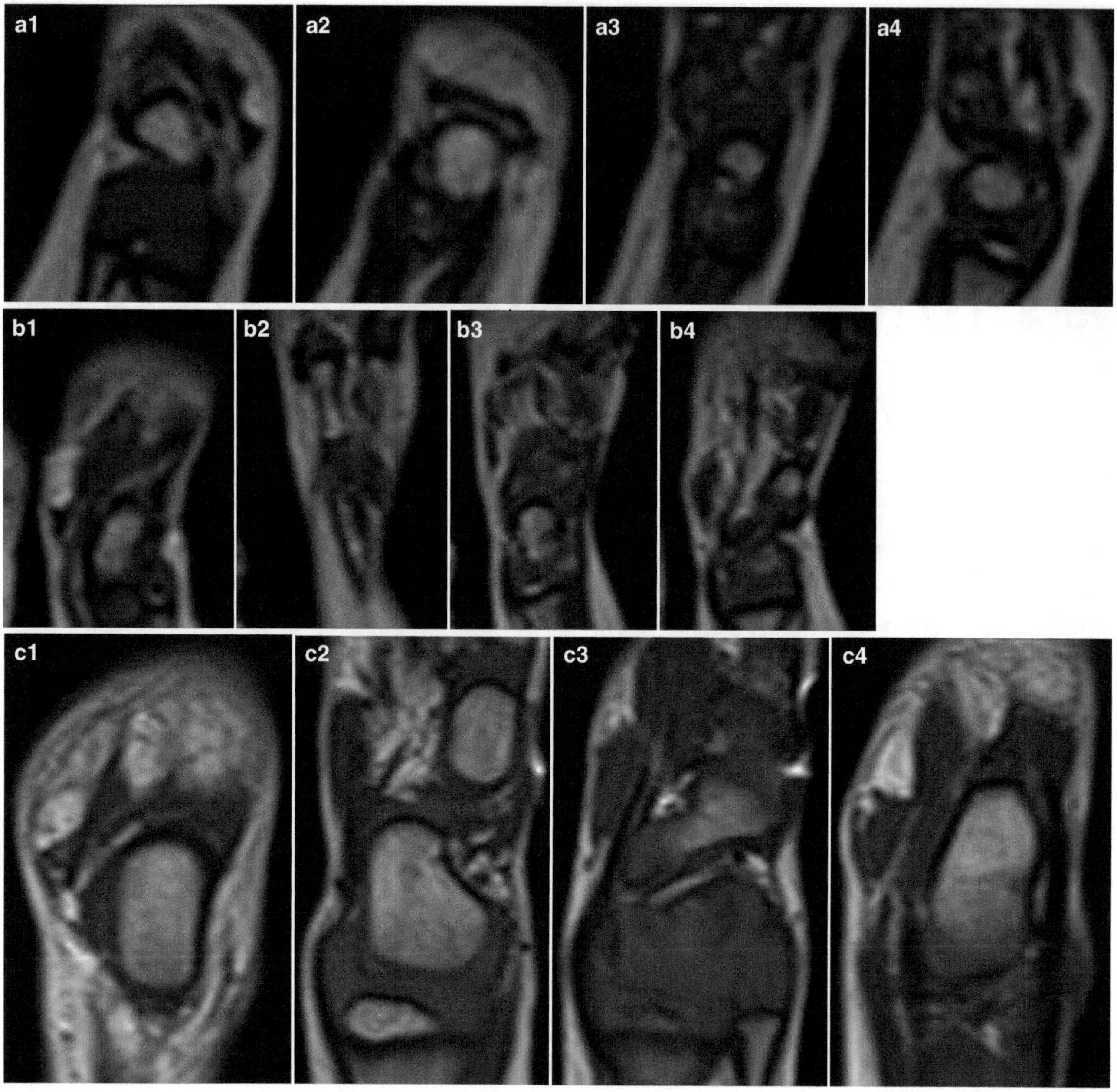

Fig. 1.15 Coronal T1-weighted images of hind feet in various age groups demonstrating evolution of bone marrow changes. Completely fatty bone marrow of all tarsals and metatarsals is noted in a 11-month-old girl (**a**), a 17-month-old girl (**b**), a 21-month-old boy (**c**), a 5-year-old girl (**d**), a 9-year-old girl (**e**), and 12-year-old girl (**f**)

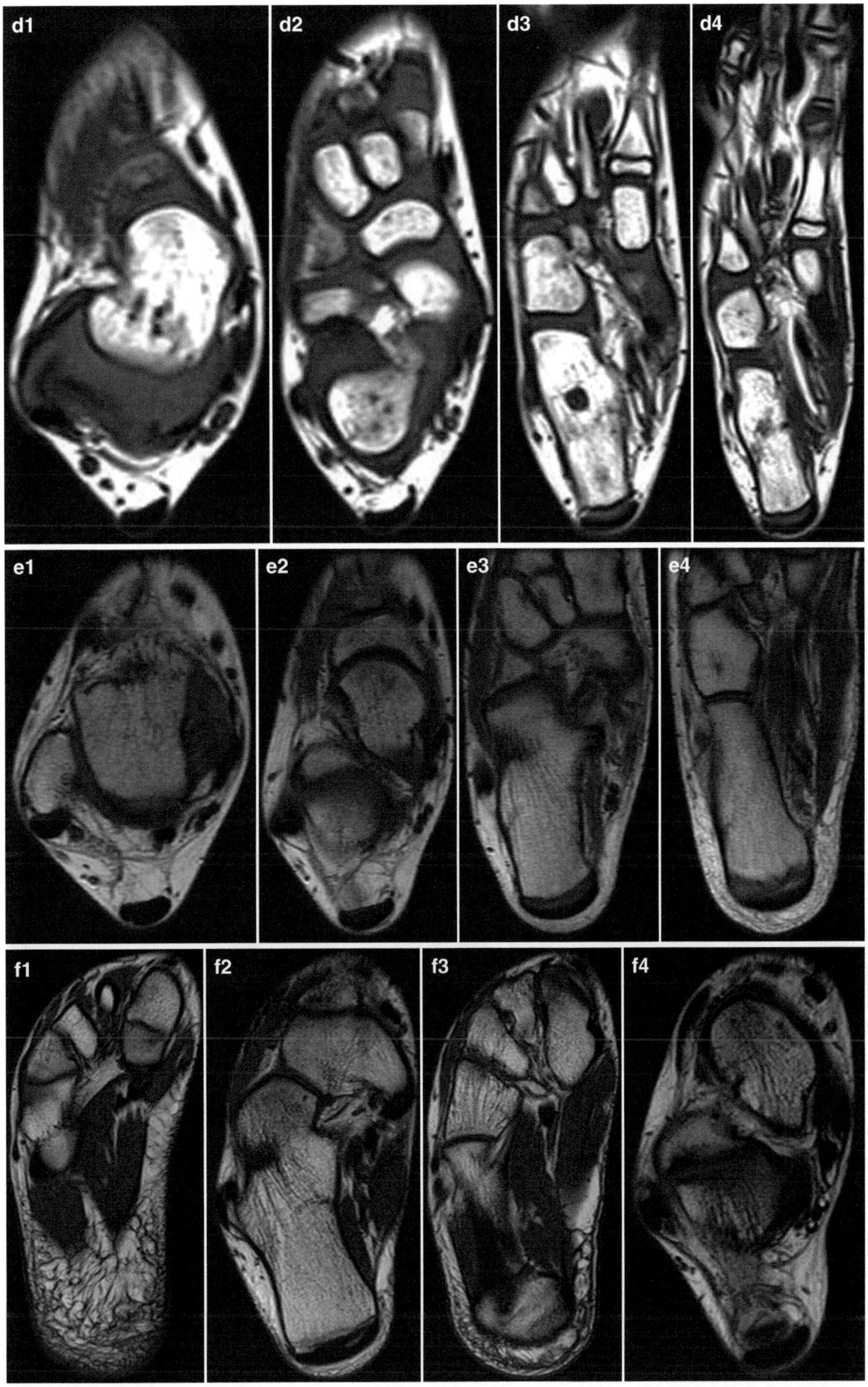

Fig. 1.15 (continued)

Normal anatomical structures and red marrow patterns can simulate marrow lesions if one is not aware of their fairly characteristic and predictable appearance. In skeletally immature individuals, patches of metaphyseal red marrow almost always show a flame-shaped configuration with their bases at or adjacent to the physis (Fig. 1.16). They have characteristically straight vertical margins and increased signal intensity relative to muscle on T1- and T2-weighted images [3] (Fig. 1.16). On axial images, the physis usually shows irregular areas of low signal intensity on T1-weighted images and high signal intensity T2-weighted sequences (Fig. 1.17). Physeal fusion is a normal physiologic process of skeletal maturation which starts with a mineralized bridge between the diaphysis and epiphysis and ends with complete replacement of the cartilaginous physis by marrow [17]. The process of physeal closure occurs through different types of union ranging from an initial single narrow perforation of cartilage to multiple initial perforations followed by spread to involve the entire physis. These physeal perforations can be peripheral or central [17]. Each physis may have a different pattern of closure [18]. Most frequently, the process of physeal fusion starts centrally and proceeds centrifugally with small remnants of cartilaginous physis remaining in the periphery [18] as shown on previous MRI studies of the knee [19, 20] (Fig. 1.18). During the process of skeletal maturation, new cartilage is added to the epiphyseal border of the physis that subsequently is mineralized as a form of metaplastic bone, forming the first union between the epiphysis and diaphysis [17]. The formation of these metaplastic bone–neofibrocartilage perforations of the physis may act as tethers to the surrounding bone and may alter localized mechanics [21]. The decrease in relative bone flexibility at these areas during strenuous activity in athletic teenagers may cause localized microtrauma with possible vascular damage and bleeding. This in turn may result in increased signal seen on fluid-sensitive MRI sequences and termed "focal periphyseal edema" (FOPE) zone [21] (Figs. 1.19 and 1.20).

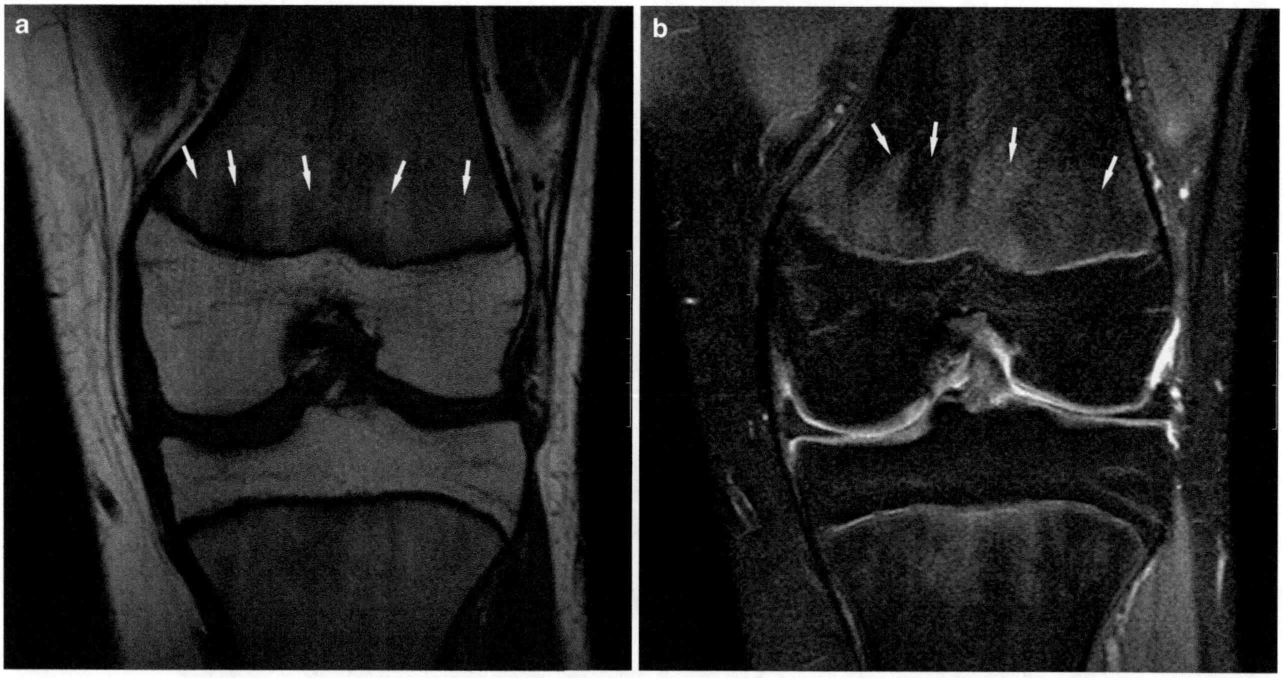

Fig. 1.16 A 16-year-old boy. Coronal T1-weighted (**a**) and T2-weighted (**b**) images of left knee show flame-shaped patches of red marrow abutting growth plate (*arrows*)

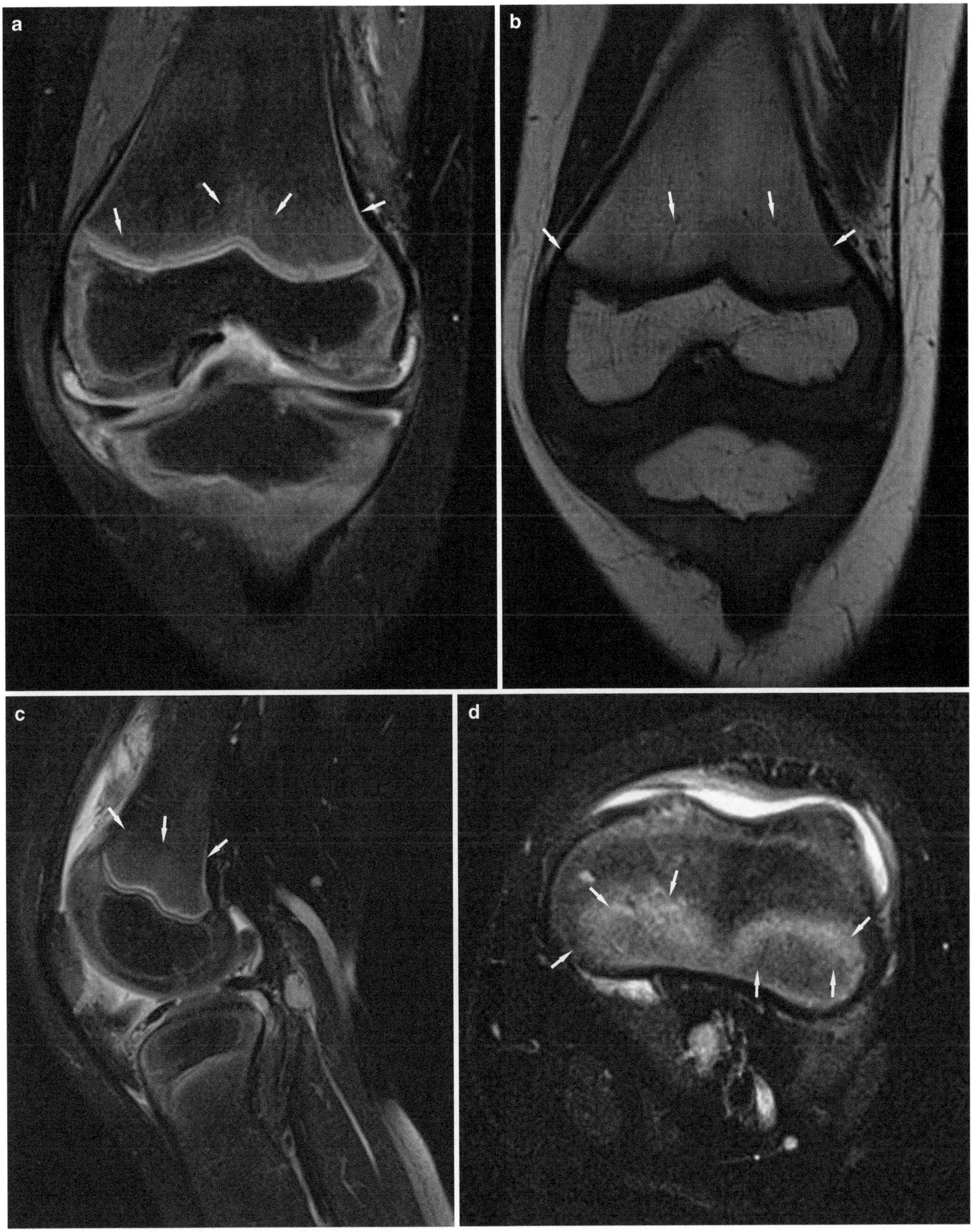

Fig. 1.17 A 7-year-old boy. Coronal T2-weighted (**a**), coronal T1-weighted (**b**), and sagittal T2-weighted (**c**) images show red marrow in the metaphyses abutting the epiphysis (*arrows*) Note the hyperintense signal corresponding to growth plate (*arrows*) on axial T2-weighted image (**d**)

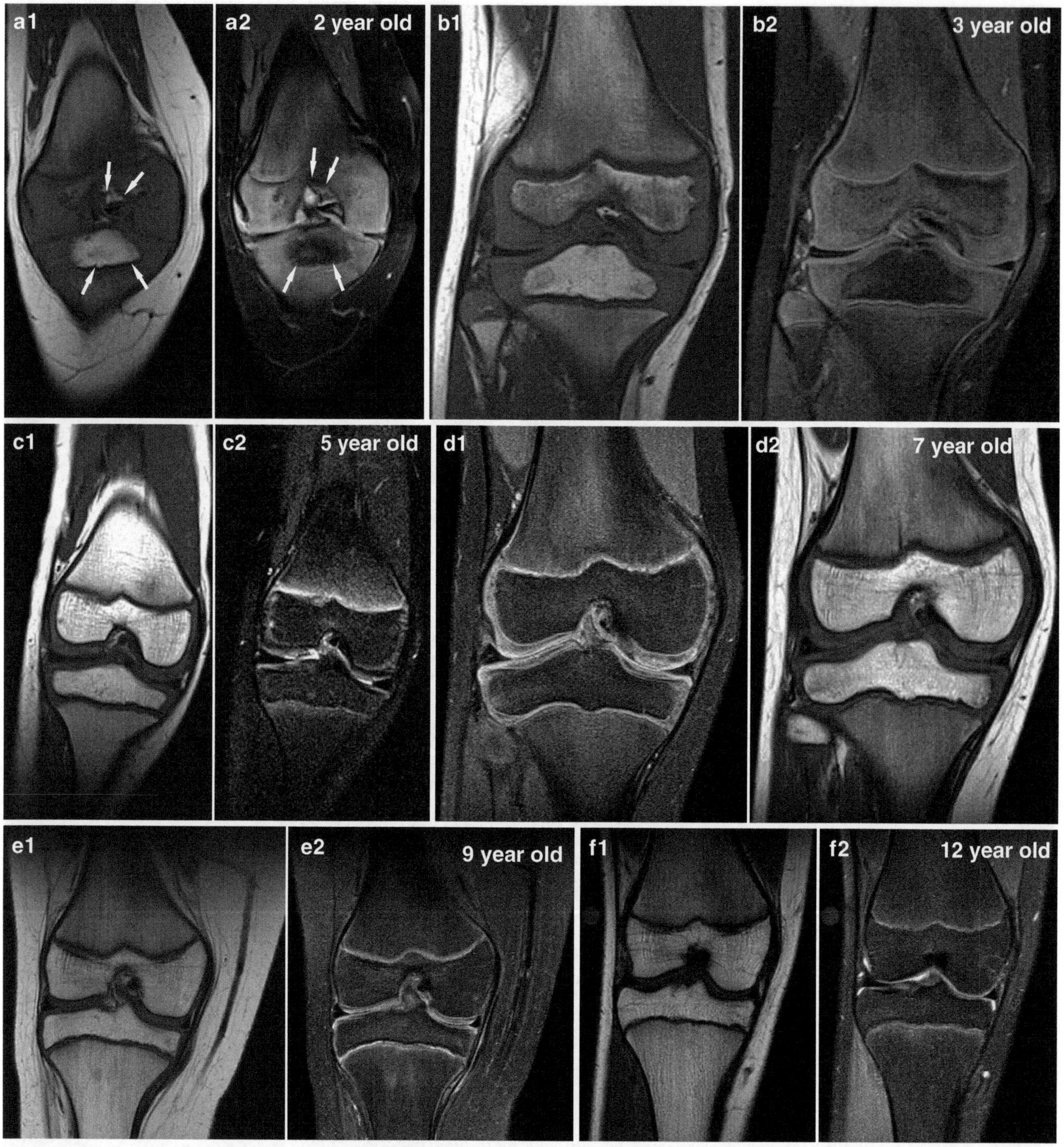

Fig. 1.18 Coronal T1- and T2-weighted images of the knee in various age groups. Largely cartilaginous epiphyses of the distal femur and proximal tibia are noted in a 2-year-old boy (**a1**, **a2**) with small focus of fatty marrow signal centrally (*arrows*). Epiphyses turn into fatty marrow gradually (**b1**, **b2**–**h1**, **h2**) [*Ages on the images*]. In a 14-year-old girl, areas of bridging near the center of the distal femoral epiphysis are seen (**g1**, **g2**) (*arrows*). These areas have disappeared at 1-year follow-up of the same patient, when complete closure of the growth plate is noted (**h1**, **h2**)

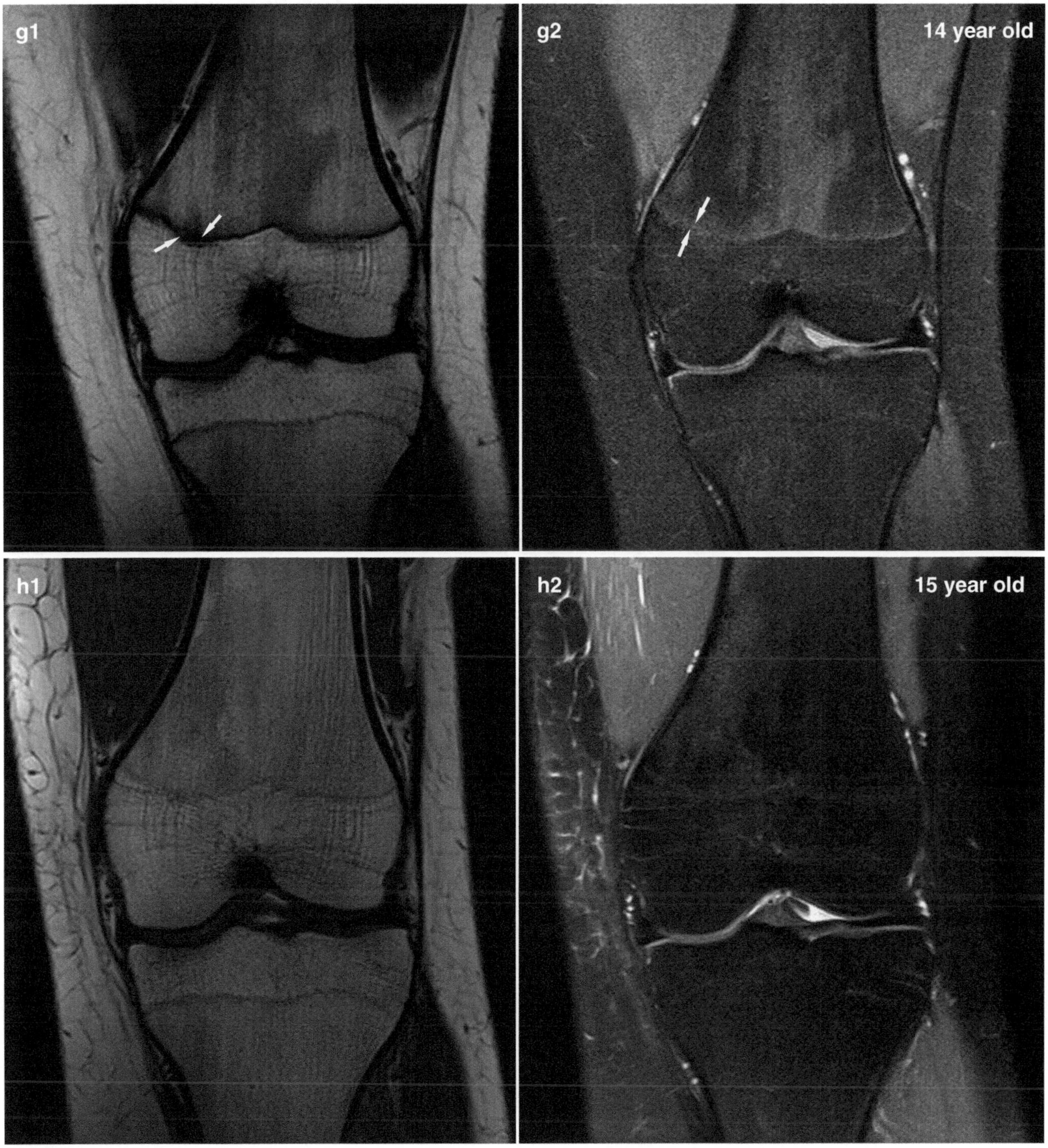

Fig. 1.18 (continued)

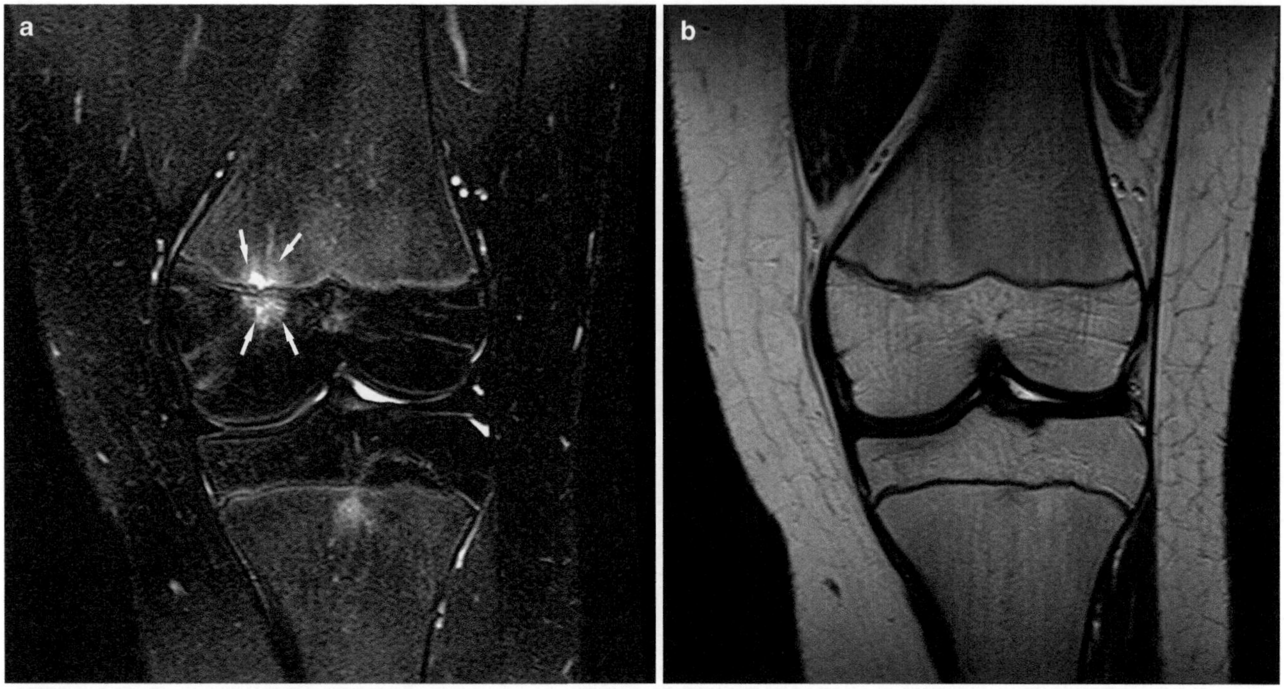

Fig. 1.19 A 11-year-old boy. Coronal T2-weighted (**a**) image shows periphyseal edema-like signal centrally in the proximal tibia and medially in the distal femur (*arrows*) without a corresponding abnormality on T1-weighted coronal image (**b**)

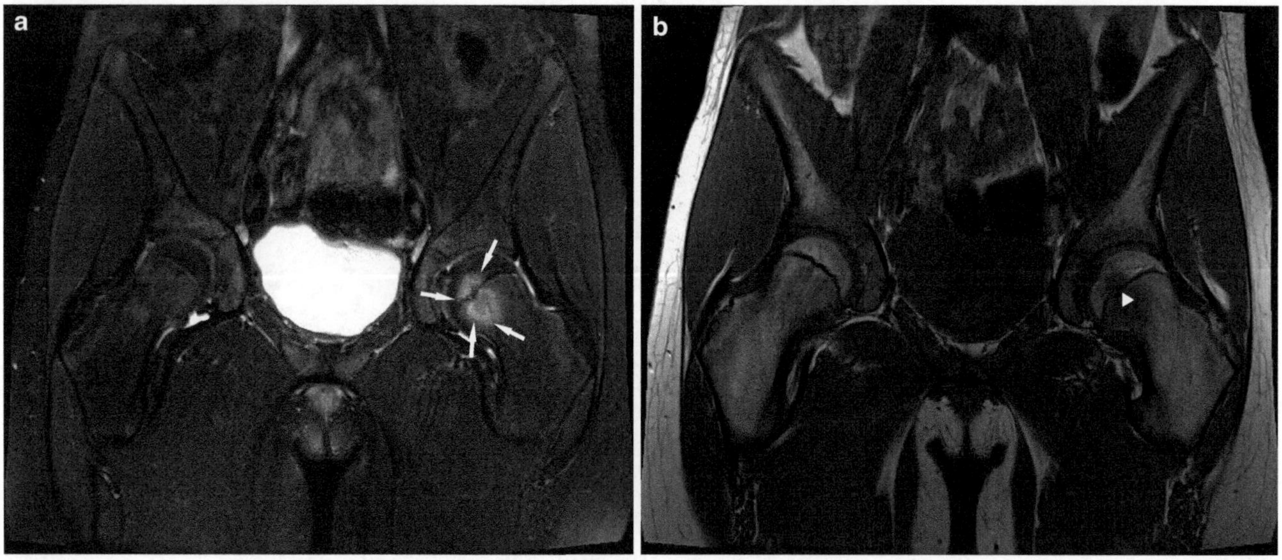

Fig. 1.20 A 12-year-old girl. Coronal T2-weighted fat-suppressed (**a**) image of the pelvis shows marked edema-like signal surrounding the left proximal femoral growth plate centrally (*arrows*). There is mild thickening of the growth plate focally in this area (*arrowhead*) on the corresponding T1-weighted image (**b**)

The distal femur, the trochlea of the elbow, and occasionally the proximal femur may show fragmentation of the epiphysis, but all the fragments of the epiphysis should show normal fatty marrow signal (Fig. 1.21). The speckled appearance of the bones of the hind foot and midfoot may represent focal islands of perivascular red marrow which can occur with altered foot dynamics or immobilization and potentially mimic disease [3, 22] (Fig. 1.22). This can occur in the affected side, the contralateral side, or both.

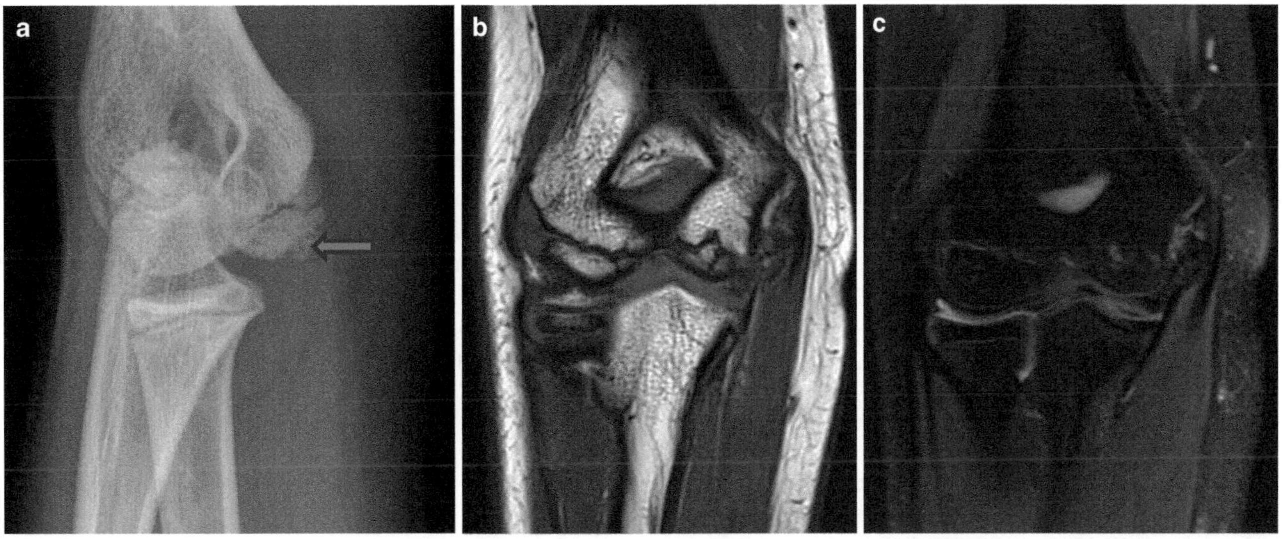

Fig. 1.21 A 13-year-old boy. Oblique radiograph of the right elbow demonstrates fragmented trochlear epiphysis (**a**) (*arrows*). Coronal T1-weighted (**b**) and T2-weighted (**c**) images demonstrate preservation of normal fatty signal within the trochlear epiphysis, consistent with a normal variant

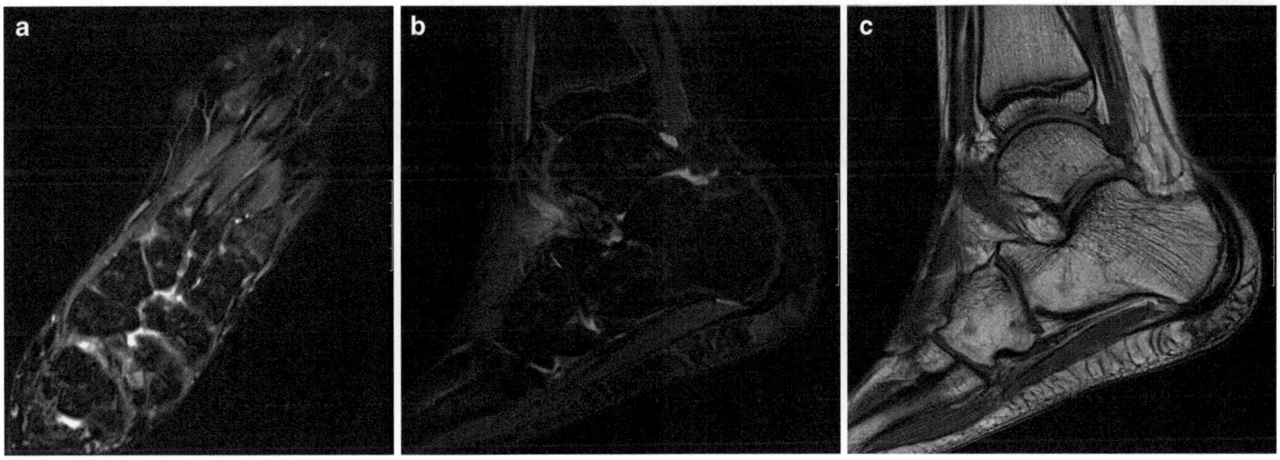

Fig. 1.22 A 16-year-old girl with a 10-day history of ankle sprain and immobilization. T2-weighted fat-suppressed sagittal (**a**) and axial oblique (**b**) images of the right foot demonstrate multiple tiny foci of edema-like signal. There is very subtle corresponding T1-weighted abnormality (**c**). Findings are consistent with disuse-related bone marrow changes

The normal adult human bone marrow is predominantly comprised of adipocytes which show increased signal intensity on both T1- and T2-weighted images similar to subcutaneous fat. The MRI appearance of normal bone marrow largely depends on the relative proportion of hematopoietic cells and adipocytes. Red marrow shows mild to moderate decrease in signal intensity on T1-weighted images, intermediate to low signal intensity on T2-weighted images, and moderate increase in signal intensity on fat-saturated intermediate or T2-weighted images. Red marrow signal is typically hyperintense to adjacent skeletal muscle on T1-weighted images [23]. On T2-weighted and inversion recovery images, there is no internal standard with which marrow signal intensity can be compared; therefore, it is unreliable and inadvisable to assess the bone marrow status and composition solely on the basis of inversion recovery and T2-weighted images. Trabecular bone or mineral matrix provides a supporting framework for the red and yellow marrow elements. On MRI both cortical and trabecular bone produce little or no signal due to the lack of mobile protons; hence, "signal void" is outlined by signal in the adjacent tissues. Trabecular bone being present in greater amounts about the metaphysis and epiphysis is more likely to be visualized and recognized in these locations (Fig. 1.23). It is not unusual to see unique marrow signal appearances at the metadiaphyseal junctions especially in proximal femurs at the subtrochanteric region that create the "pseudolesion" appearance with convex upper contour (Fig. 1.24). This is perhaps related to sudden change in trabecular pattern and should not be mistaken for a lesion (Fig. 1.25). Such appearances are typically symmetric on both sides (Fig. 1.26) although occasionally unilateral changes could be observed (Fig. 1.27) or comparison may not be possible (Fig. 1.28). Similar marrow appearances may also be seen in proximal humeri, below the lesser and greater tuberosities (Fig. 1.29). Some of the proximal humeral bone marrow changes could be due to dissecting reactive cysts from rotator cuff insertion of greater or lesser tuberosities (Fig. 1.30).

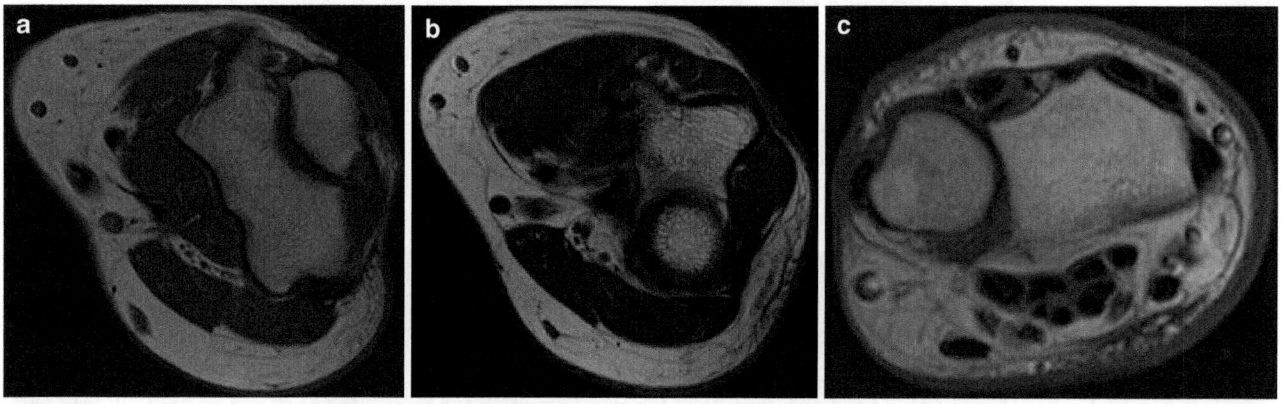

Fig. 1.23 A 48-year-old woman. Axial T1-weighted images through the elbow (**a**, **b**) and distal forearm (**c**) demonstrate a fine meshwork of trabecular structure within the fatty marrow

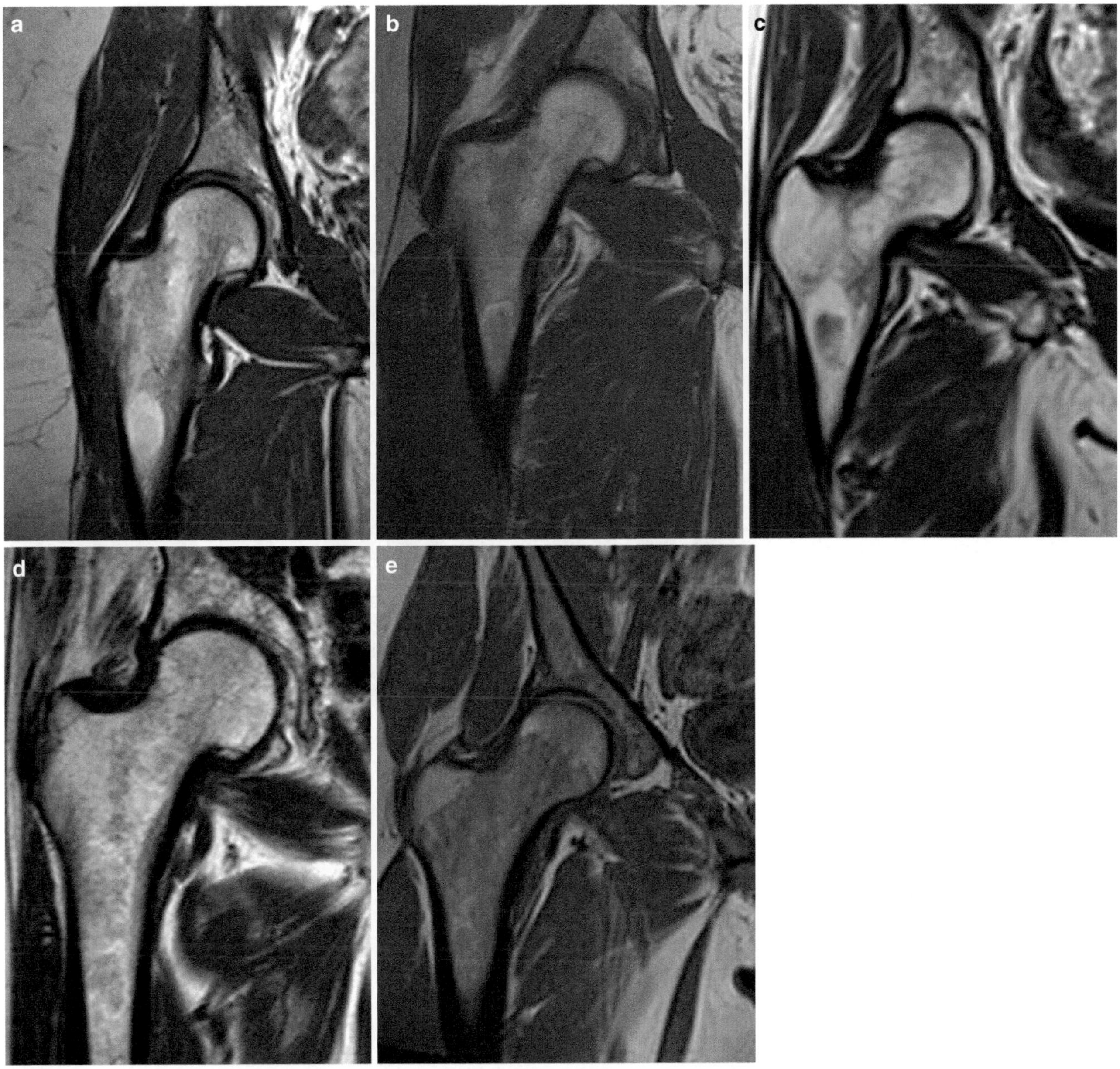

Fig. 1.24 Coronal T1-weighted images through right hip in five different adult individuals showing different patterns of red marrow within proximal femur, some of which simulate a lesion in subtrochanteric area. Fatty signal in subtrochanteric femur is outlined by red marrow in intertrochanteric region (**a**). Red marrow signal in subtrochanteric femur may be outlined by a thin (**b**) or prominent (**c**) rim of fatty signal. Intertrochanteric red marrow may be patchy (**d**) or relatively diffuse (**e**)

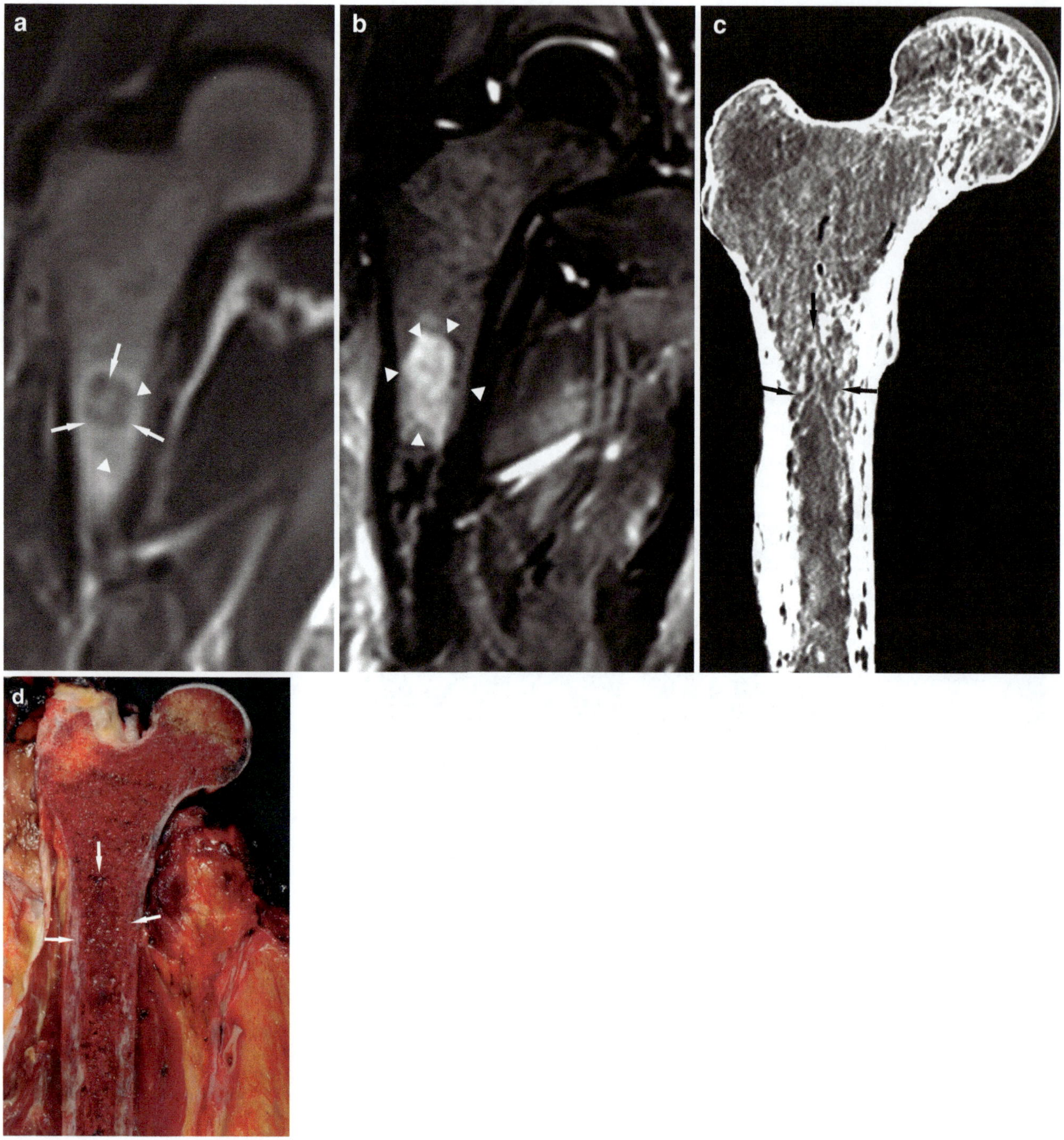

Fig. 1.25 A 57-year-old woman. Coronal T1-weighted (**a**) and STIR (**b**) images of the right hip demonstrate a pseudolesion of red marrow in the subtrochanteric femur (*arrowheads*). Specimen CT with coronal reconstruction (**c**) and gross pathology examination in postmortem examination (**d**) reveals unique dome-shaped trabecular structure of the proximal femur (*arrows*)

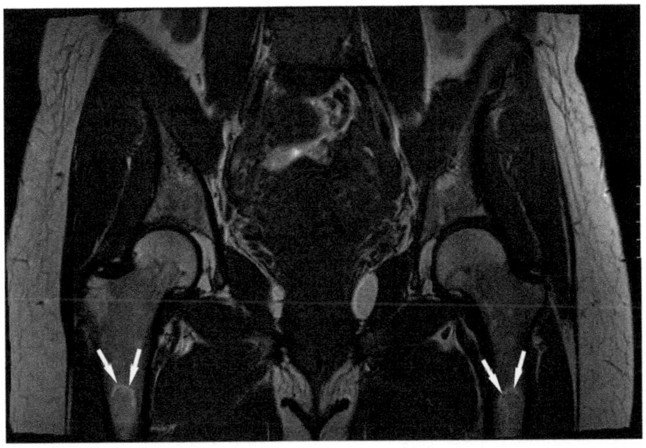

Fig. 1.26 A 37-year-old woman. Coronal T1-weighted image of the pelvis shows typical red marrow in subtrochanteric femora with convex upper surfaces (*arrows*)

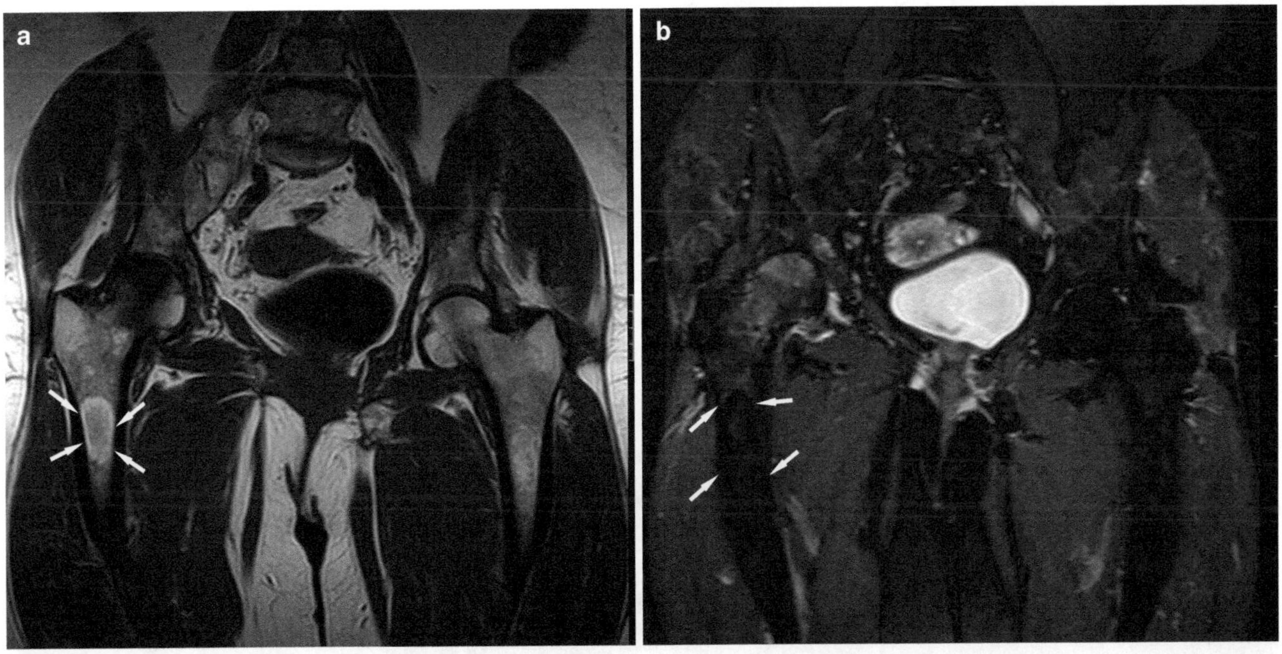

Fig. 1.27 A 63-year-old woman. Coronal T1-weighted (**a**) and STIR (**b**) images of the pelvis show asymmetric appearance of red marrow in subtrochanteric femora, likely due to physiologic response from right hip osteoarthritis and altered mechanics of weight-bearing resulting in increased fatty marrow (*arrows*)

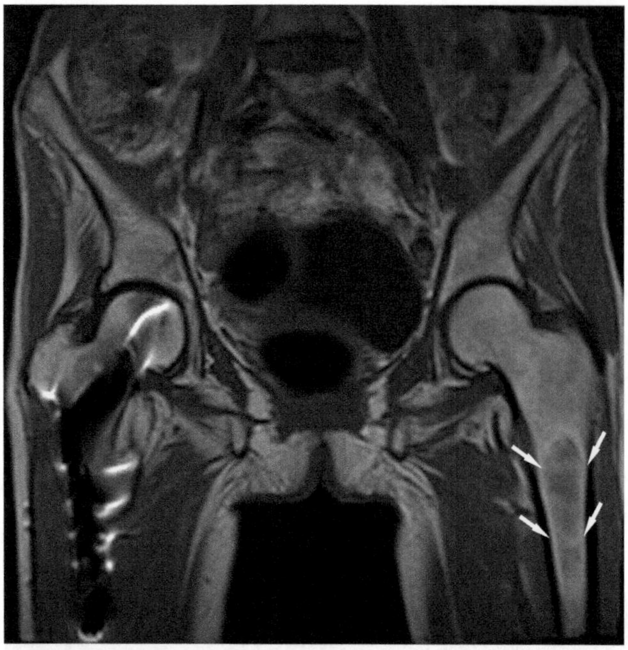

Fig. 1.28 A 67-year-old woman. Coronal T1-weighted image of the pelvis shows prominent red marrow in left subtrochanteric femur (*arrows*). Right femoral marrow is largely obscured by hardware from prior plate–screw fixation

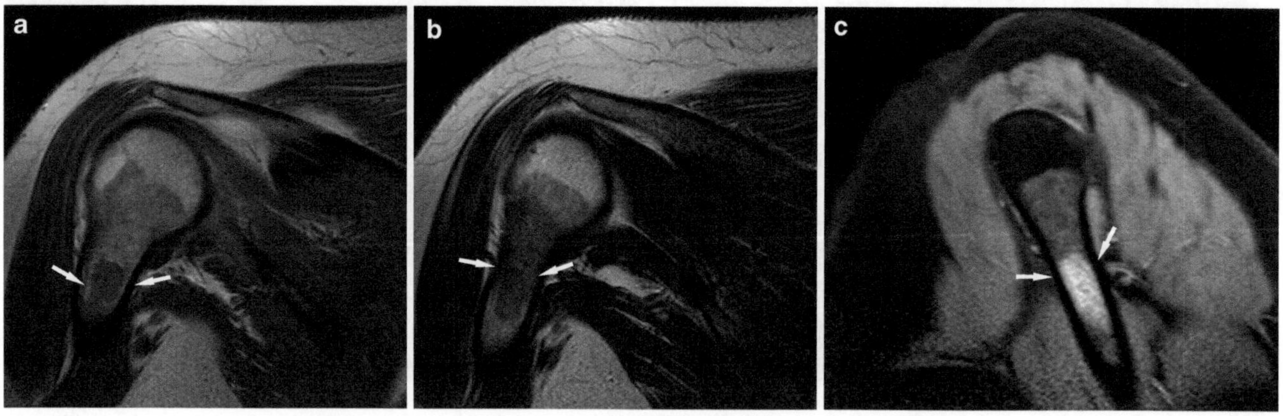

Fig. 1.29 A 37-year-old man. Coronal T1-weighted (**a**), coronal T2-weighted (**b**), and sagittal STIR images (**c**) of the right shoulder demonstrate prominent red marrow signal in the proximal humerus (*arrows*) simulating a lesion

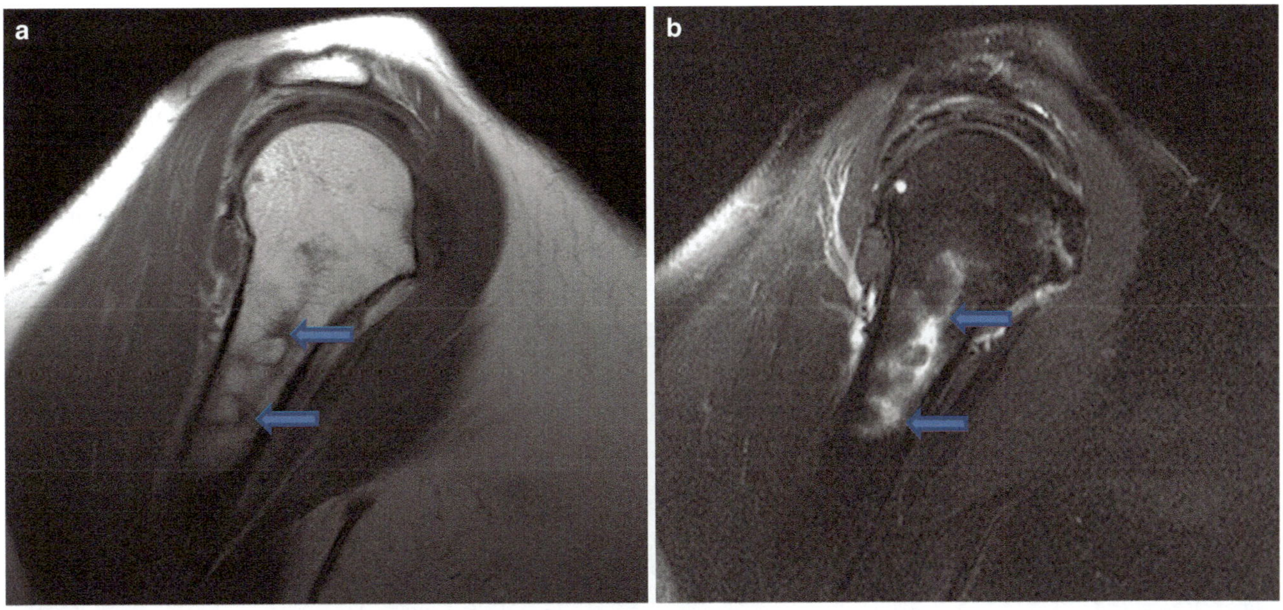

Fig. 1.30 A 38-year-old man. Sagittal T1-weighted (**a**) and T2-weighted (**b**) images from the right shoulder demonstrate abnormal bone marrow signal in the proximal humeral shaft (*arrows*), which appears to extend into the greater tuberosity, consistent with dissecting ganglion cyst from rotator cuff insertion

Normally, there is a variable amount of red marrow interspersed in the background of fatty marrow. It is unusual to see diffuse purely fatty marrow outside the hands and feet without evidence of any interspersed red marrow signal in the absence of prior radiation. This variability in volume and patterns of red marrow distribution sometimes raises concerns in the unwary for marrow-infiltrating neoplasms resulting in unnecessary further investigations and uncertainty. These patterns in the metaphysis, diaphysis, or both are frequently encountered in routine upper and lower extremity joint imaging. Red marrow could present as diffuse (Fig. 1.31), large patches (Fig. 1.32), linear lines running parallel to the cortex (Fig. 1.33), or small nodular areas, each measuring a few millimeters (Fig. 1.34) or a combination of two or more such patterns (Fig. 1.35).

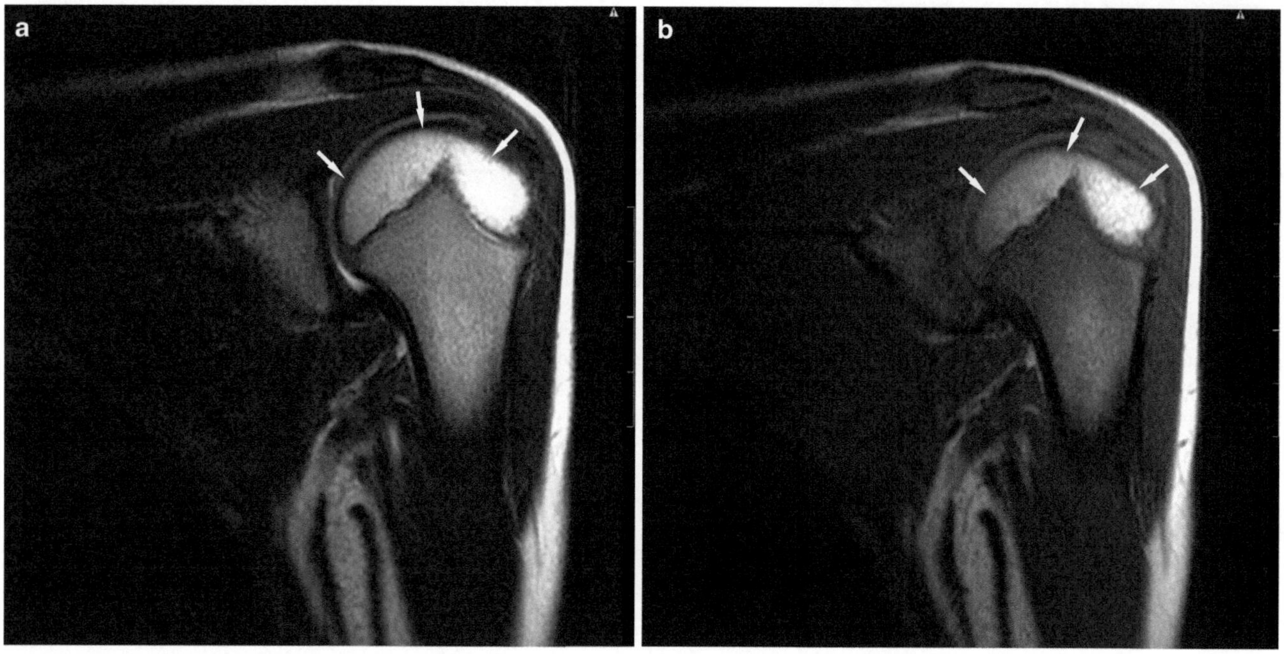

Fig. 1.31 An 8-year-old boy. Coronal T1-weighted (**a**) and T2-weighted (**b**) images show diffuse red marrow in the proximal humeral metadiaphysis and visualized glenoid. Note the fatty marrow in the proximal humeral epiphysis and apophysis (*arrows*)

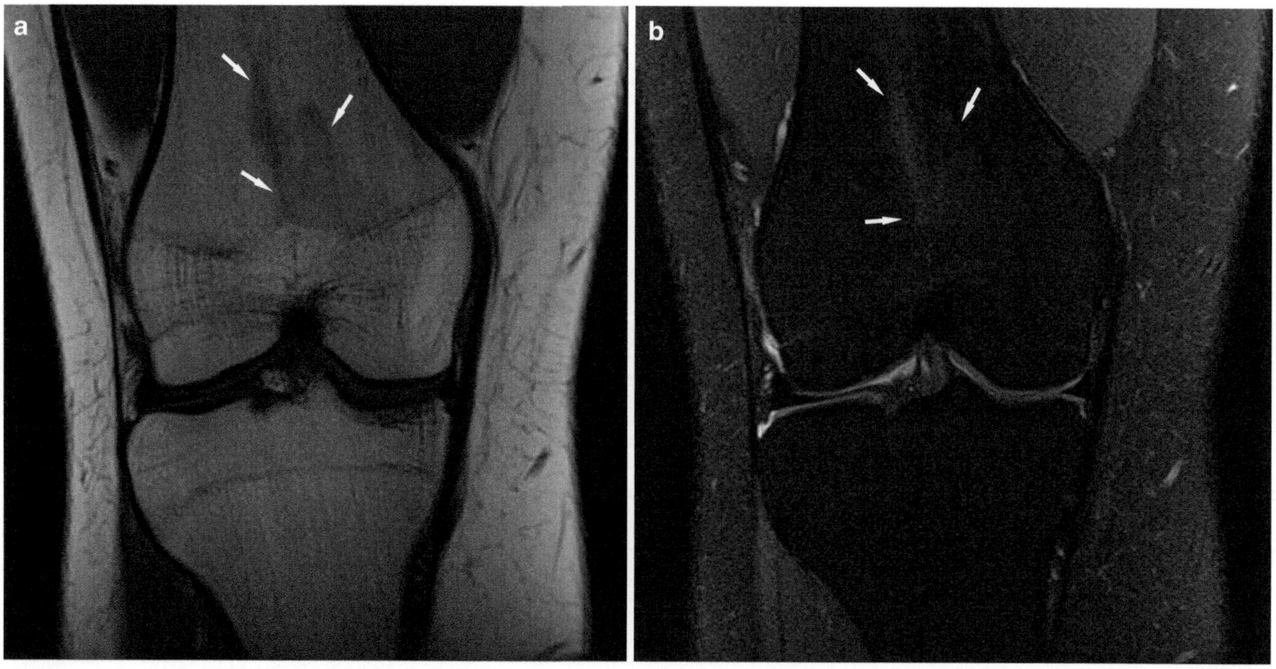

Fig. 1.32 A 27-year-old woman. Coronal T1-weighted (**a**) and T2-weighted (**b**) images of the right knee demonstrate a large area of red marrow in the distal femur (*arrows*)

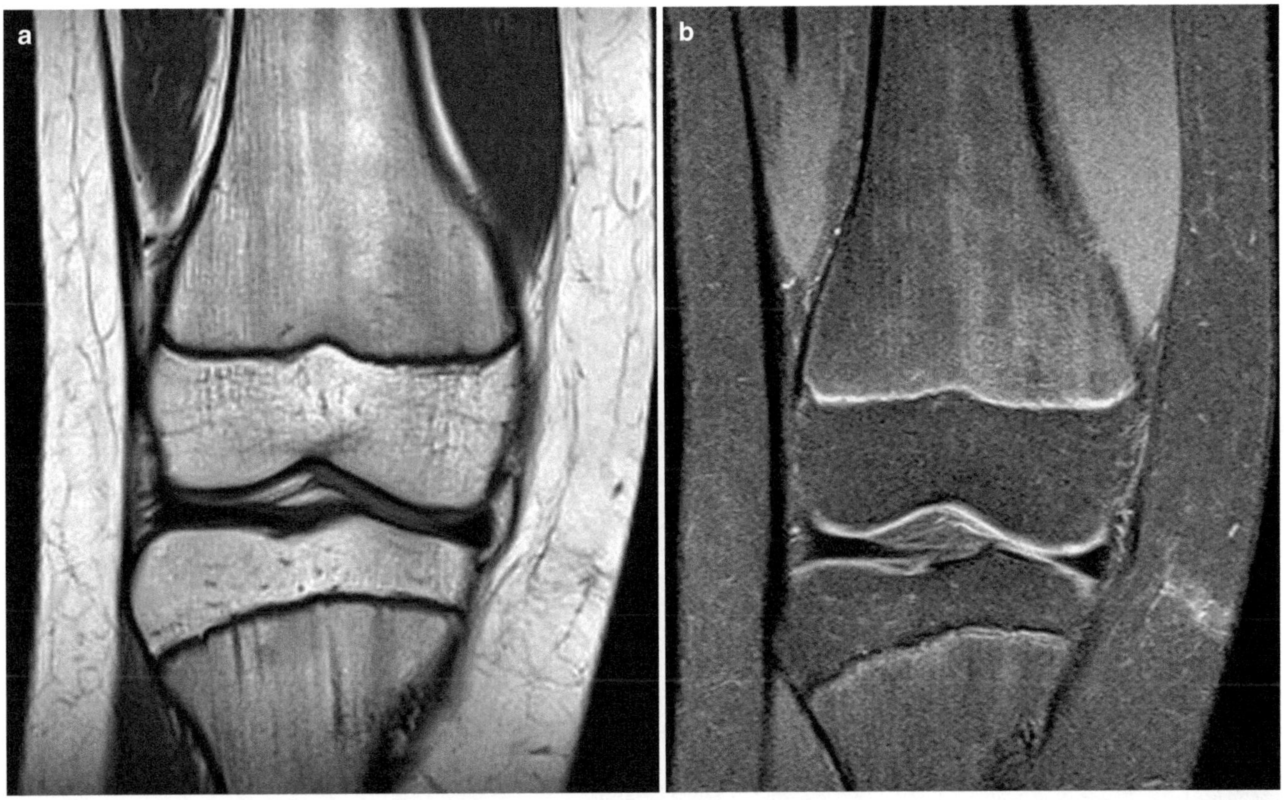

Fig. 1.33 A 19-year-old man. Coronal T1-weighted (**a**) and T2-weighted (**b**) images show red marrow in the distal femur and proximal tibia in the form of linear lines parallel to the cortex

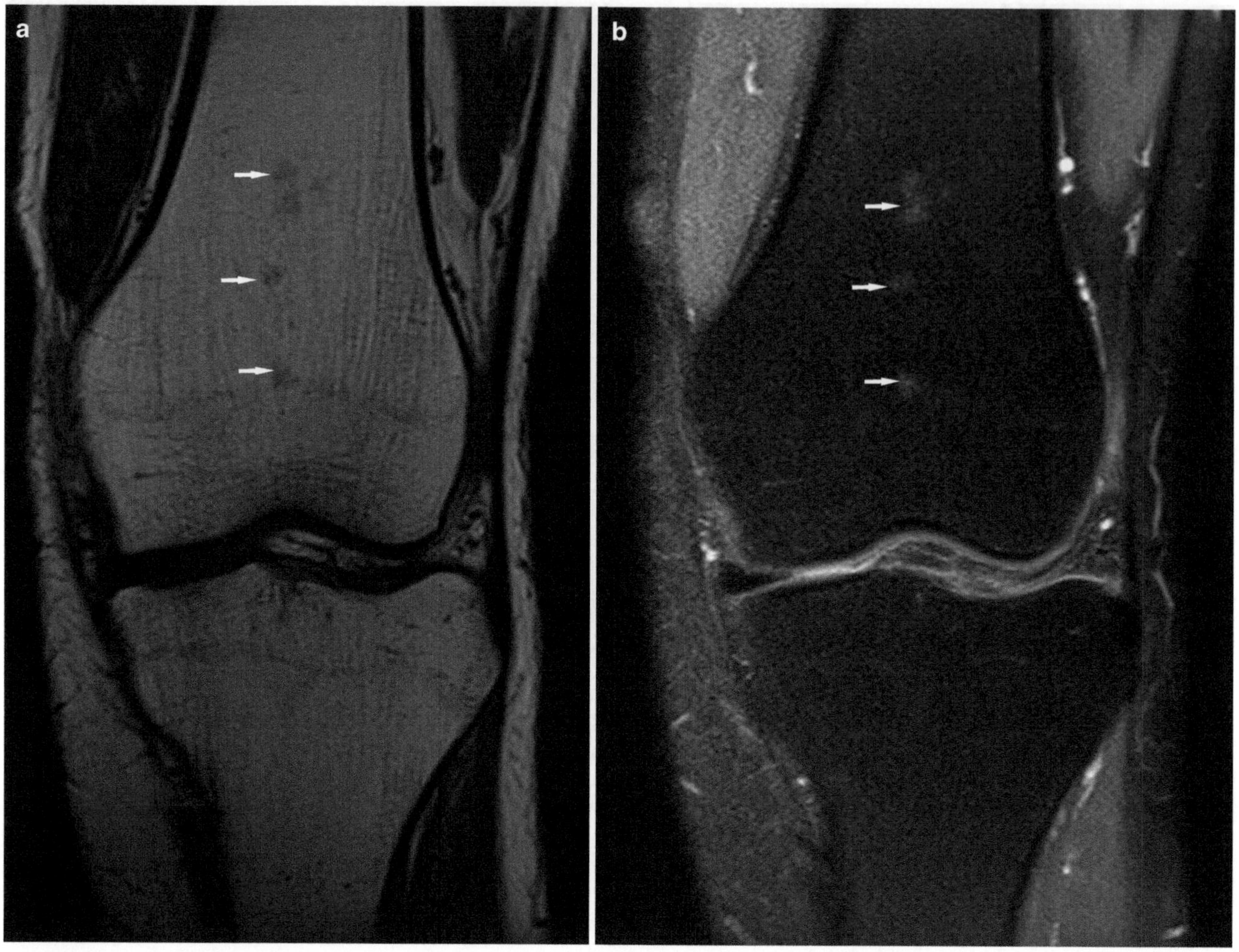

Fig. 1.34 A 37-year-old woman. Coronal T1-weighted (**a**) and T2-weighted (**b**) images of the left knee demonstrate several round small foci of red marrow in the distal femur (*arrows*)

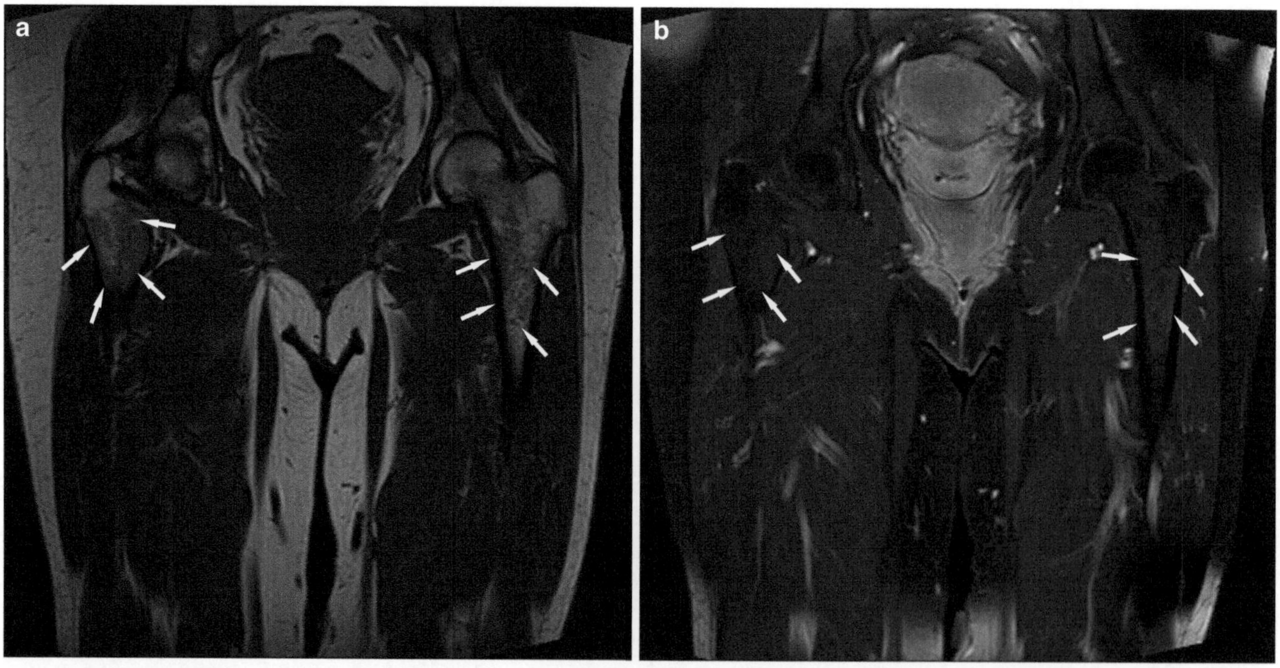

Fig. 1.35 A 33-year-old woman. Coronal T1-weighted (**a**) and T2-weighted (**b**) images show red marrow in proximal femora with areas of nodularity and patches (*arrows*)

Focal nodular hyperplasia of red marrow is the most extreme pattern of red marrow hypertrophy. It is characterized by one or more larger nodules of red marrow measuring up to several centimeters in diameter in the background of fatty marrow simulating a neoplastic disease process (Figs. 1.36, 1.37, and 1.38). The signal characteristics are similar to that of red marrow elsewhere. There may be none to moderate enhancement after gadolinium injection. It occurs relatively rarely in normal individuals but is frequent in patients with regenerating hematopoietic marrow after aplastic conditions or in response to the administration of hematopoietic stimulating drugs [24, 25].

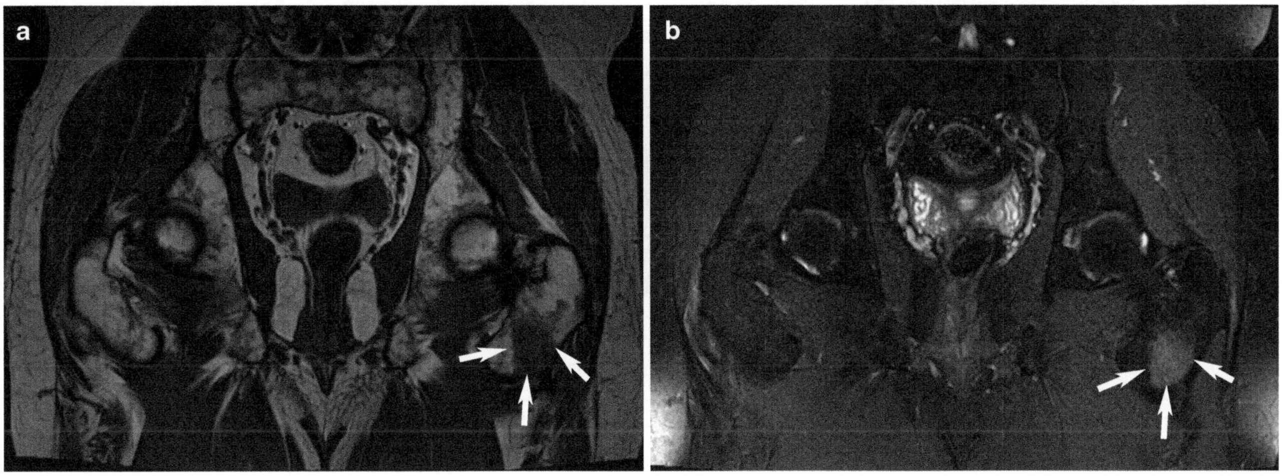

Fig. 1.36 A 58-year-old man. Coronal T1-weighted (**a**) and T2-weighted (**b**) images of the pelvis demonstrate a round mass-like area in the left intertrochanteric femur (*arrows*), with signal intensity similar to that of skeletal muscle on T1-weighted images. A mildly hyperintense signal is noted in this area on T2-weighted images. A CT-guided needle biopsy revealed hypercellular marrow without evidence of neoplasm

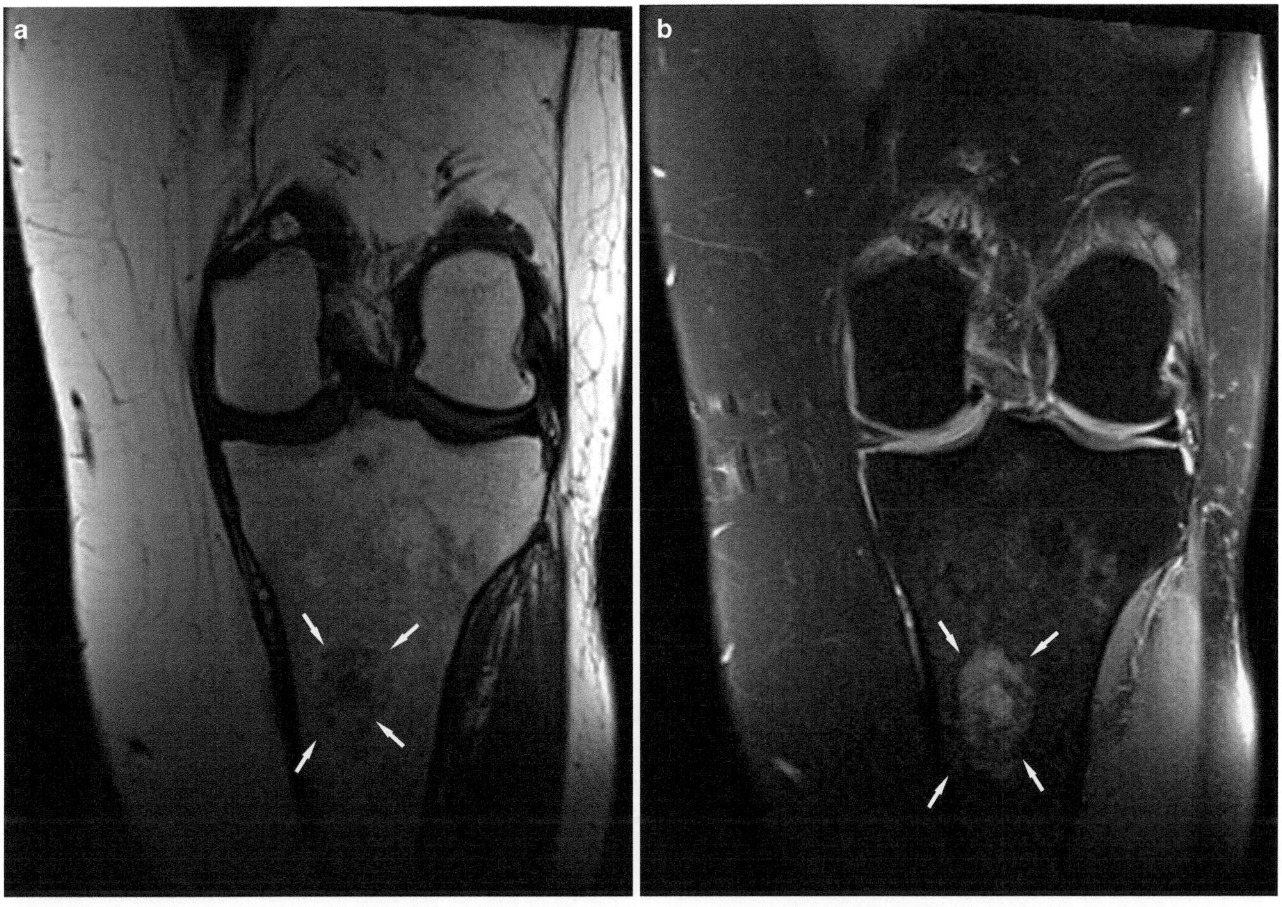

Fig. 1.37 A 60-year-old woman. Coronal T1-weighted (**a**) and T2-weighted (**b**) images show a large nodular area of red marrow in the proximal tibial diaphysis with intermixed fatty marrow signal (*arrows*)

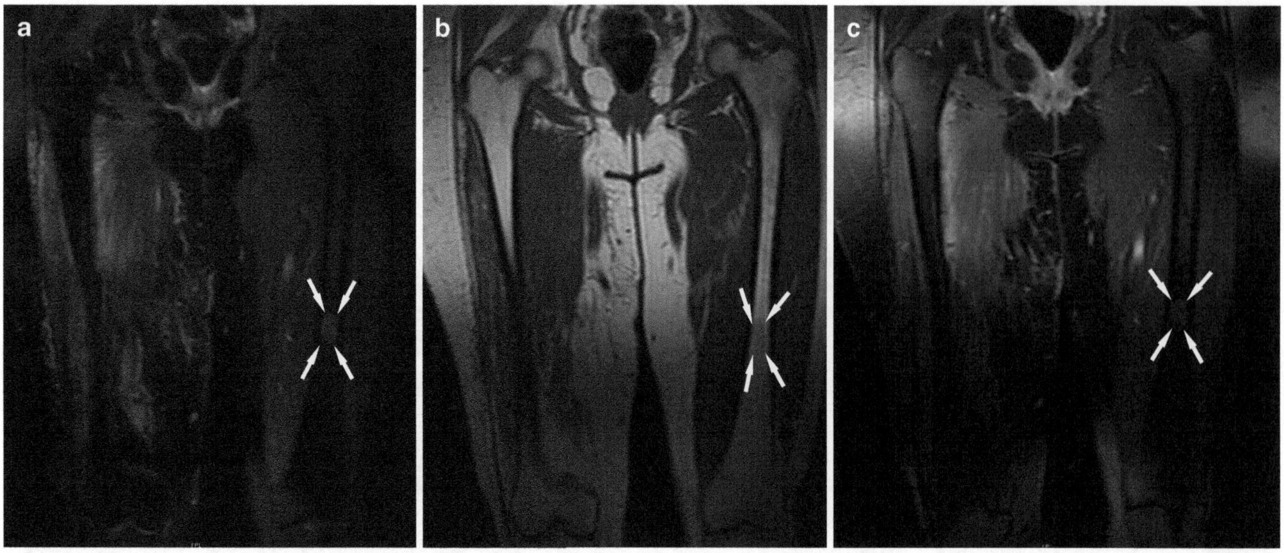

Fig. 1.38 A 57-year-old woman with a history of right proximal thigh myxoid liposarcoma resection, after radiation treatment. Follow-up MRI shows a large nodular area of red marrow in the opposite femoral shaft that appears prominent on coronal STIR sequence (**a**) and subtle hyperintensity on coronal T1-weighted images (*arrows*) (**b**). Mild enhancement is noted on a T1-weighted postcontrast fat-suppressed coronal image (**c**). Findings are consistent with nodular marrow hyperplasia, which likely developed as a compensatory phenomenon secondary to radiation of the right femur

Nutrient vessels are visualized on MR images of long bones within the marrow space as they enter through the cortex (Fig. 1.1A). In some instances, dilated vessels or so-called intraosseous varices could erroneously raise suspicion for a marrow-occupying neoplasm. Careful review of sequential images will show that continuity with proximal and distal vessels should preclude diagnostic equivocation (Figs. 1.39 and 1.40). Diffuse dilatation of intraosseous vessels are occasionally seen which are likely mild forms of vascular malformations (Fig. 1.41). When interval proliferation of intraosseous vasculature is noted on an MRI with a normal previous examination, an underlying pathology causing hyperemia or a diffuse marrow-infiltrating neoplasm such as multiple myeloma (Fig. 1.42) should be considered. Normal nutrient vessels should not be mistaken for longitudinal stress fractures, as there typically will not be surrounding bone marrow edema (Fig. 1.43). Red marrow, often present in the periphery of long bones and on T1-weighted sequences, may be identified on axial images as a subcortical low-signal structure distinct from marrow fat. On T2-weighted fat-suppressed images, the signal intensity corresponds to red marrow, less than that of edema, and should not be mistaken for stress reaction (Fig. 1.44).

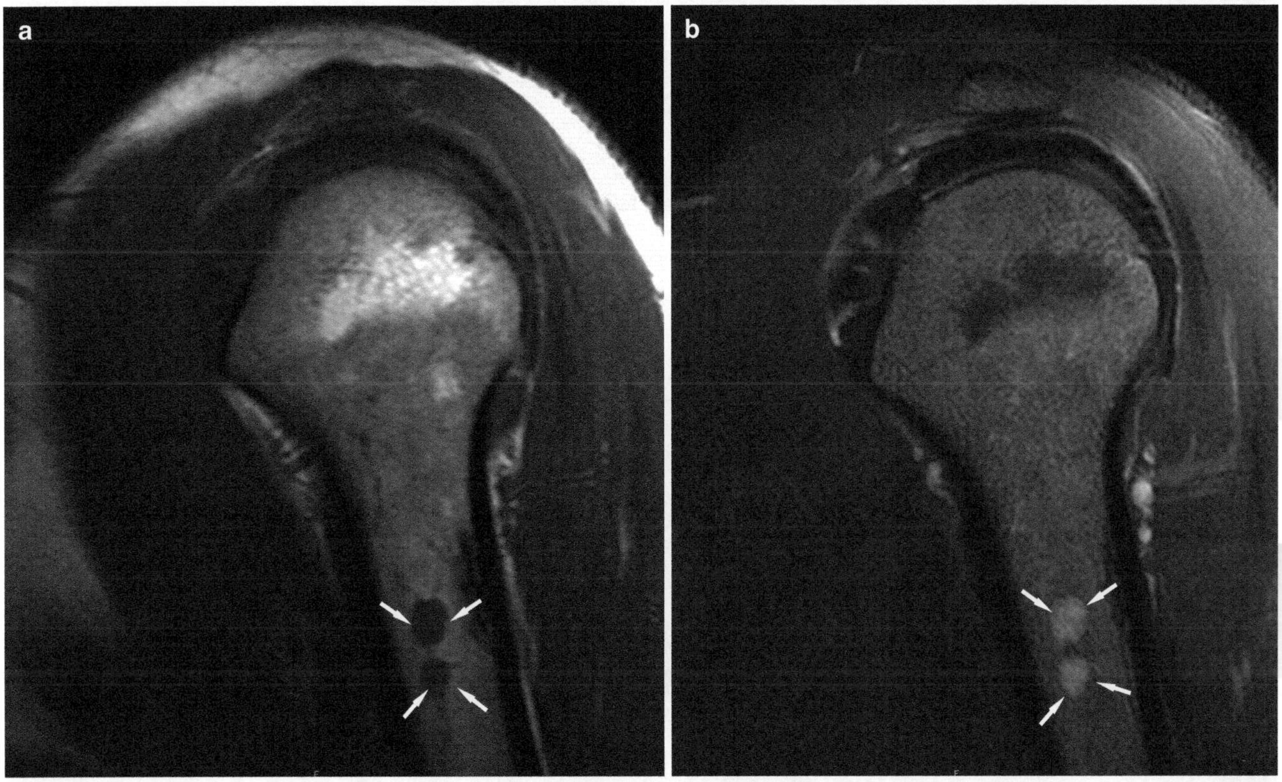

Fig. 1.39 A 44-year-old woman. Sagittal T1-weighted (**a**) and T2-weighted (**b**) images of the right shoulder demonstrate 2 focal areas of dilated intraosseous vessels (*arrows*) consistent with intraosseous varices

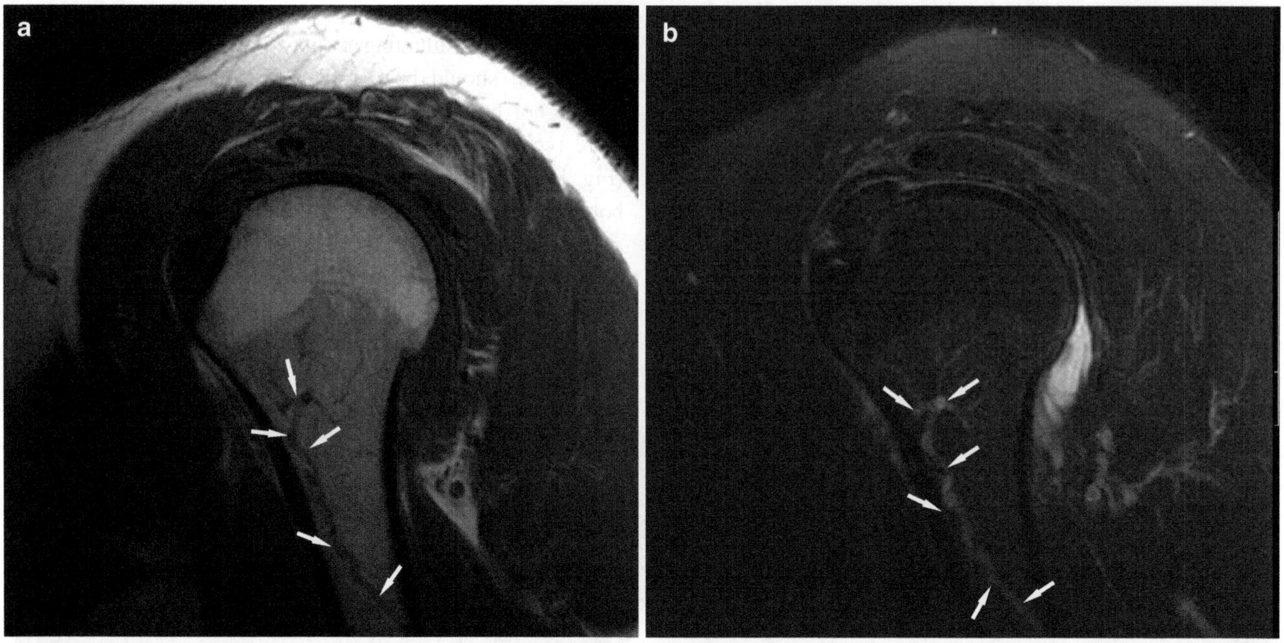

Fig. 1.40 A 32-year-old man. Sagittal T1-weighted (**a**) and T2-weighted (**b**) images demonstrate diffuse dilatation of the intraosseous vasculature of the proximal humerus (*arrows*)

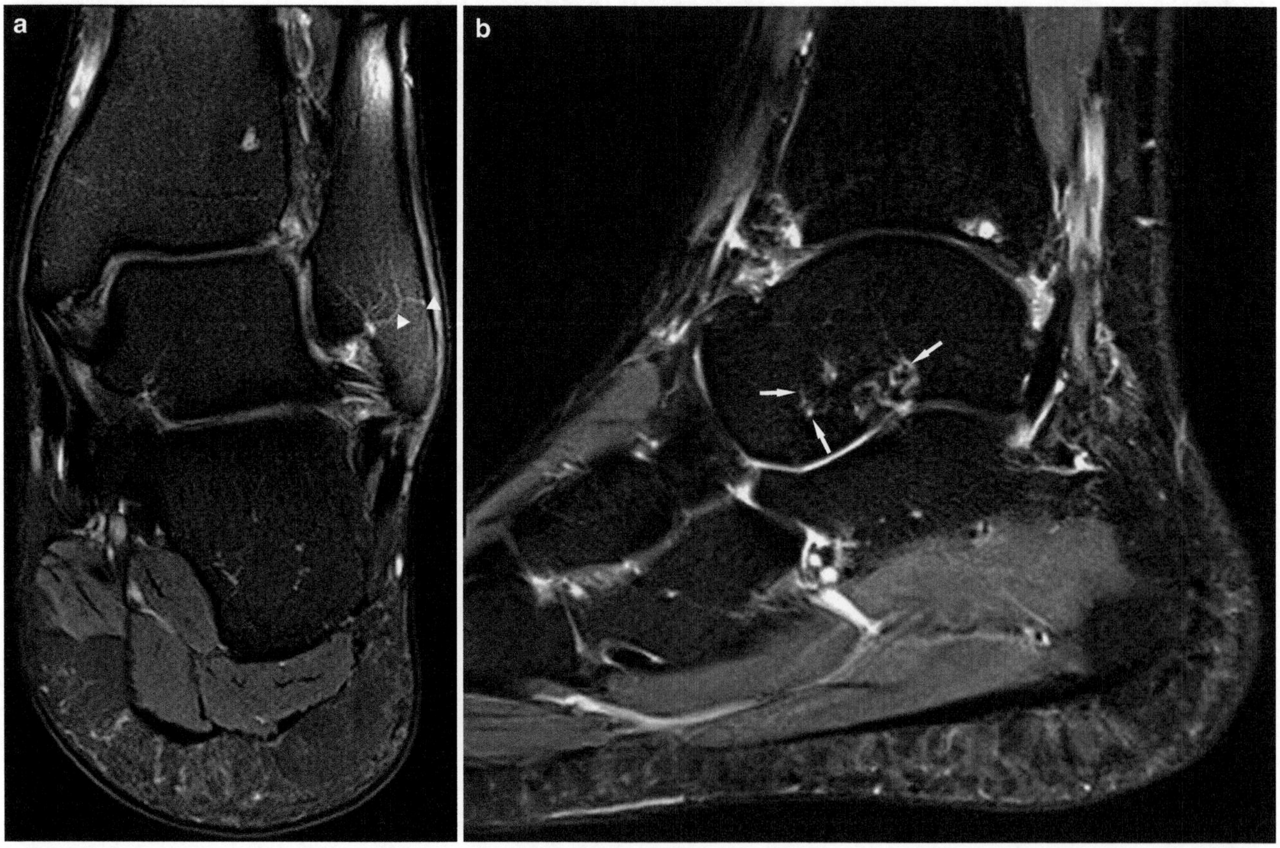

Fig. 1.41 A 39-year-old man. Sagittal (**a**) and coronal (**b**) T2-weighted images show prominent intraosseous vascularity and distal fibula (*arrowheads*) and talus (*arrows*)

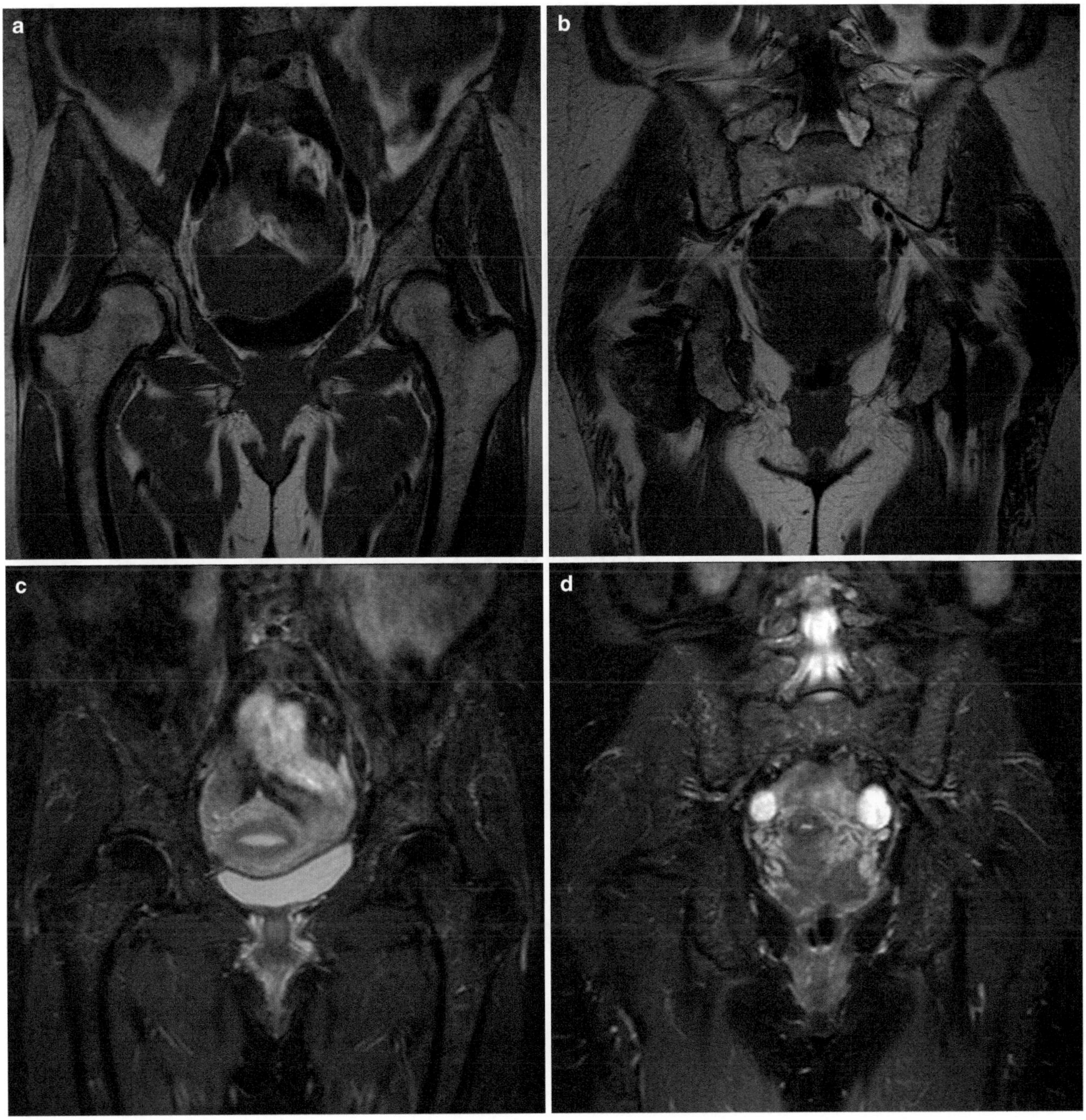

Fig. 1.42 A 69-year-old woman with recently diagnosed multiple myeloma. Coronal T1-weighted (**a**, **b**) and T2-weighted (**c**, **d**) images demonstrate diffuse proliferation of intraosseous vessels without discrete lesions. Findings are typical of bone marrow neovascularity in the setting of multiple myeloma

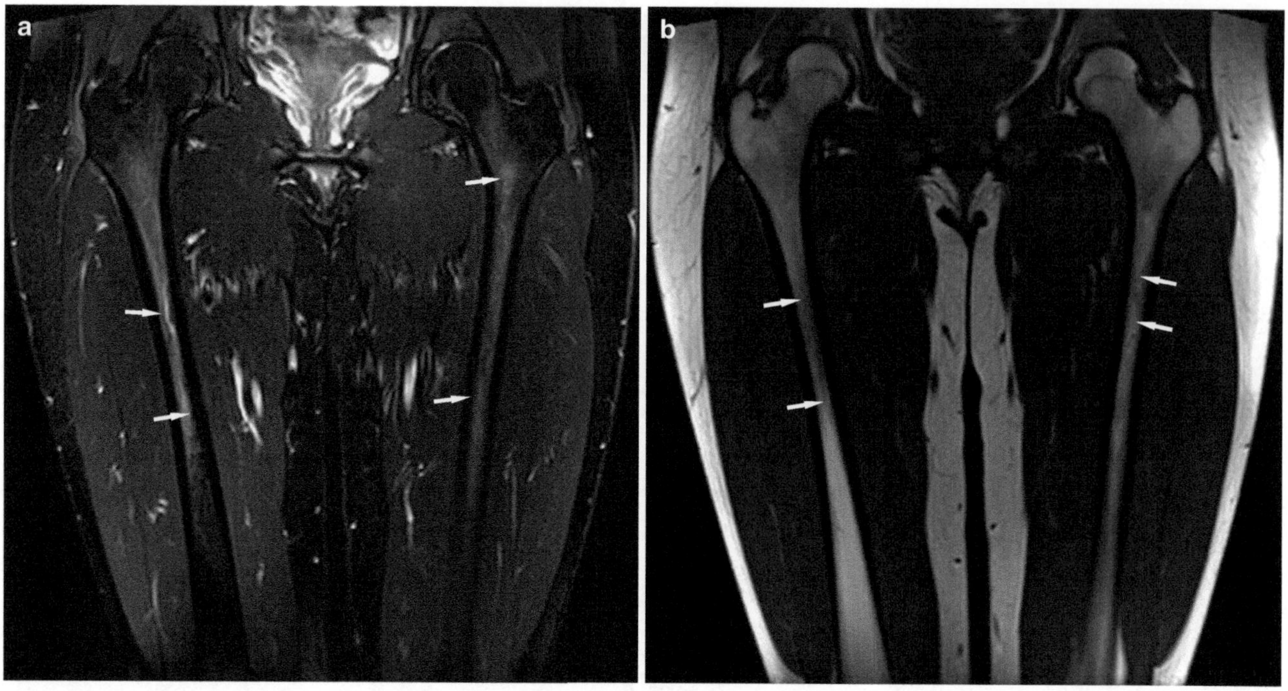

Fig. 1.43 A 19-year-old man. Coronal T2-weighted fat-suppressed (**a**) and T1-weighted (**b**) images demonstrate a linear T2 hyperintense structure (*arrows*) in the right femoral diaphysis consistent with intraosseous vessels (*arrows*). Note that the red marrow signal surrounding the vascularity is less hyperintense than bone marrow edema on T2-weighted images

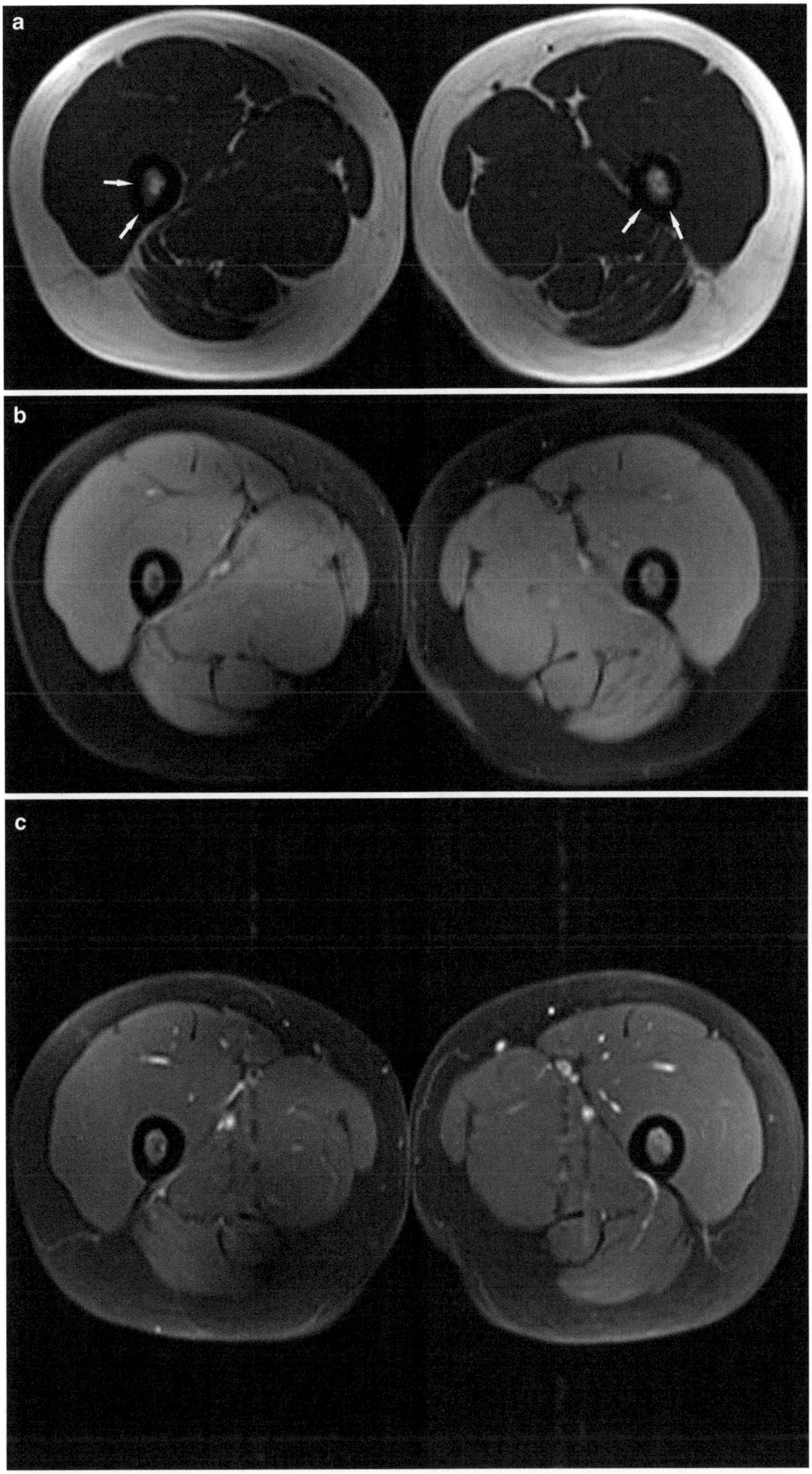

Fig. 1.44 A 17-year-old boy. Axial T1-weighted (**a**), T2-weighted fat-saturated (**b**), and postcontrast T1-weighted fat-saturated (**c**) images of bilateral thighs demonstrate peripheral red marrow signal (*arrows*) with central fatty marrow

1.5 MRI of Normal Axial Skeleton

In the skull, a thin layer of marrow is visualized between the inner and outer tables (Fig. 1.45). In the neonatal period, there is diffuse hematopoietic marrow in the calvarium and facial bones (Fig. 1.46). Low-signal serpentine areas are typically noted on all pulse sequences corresponding to sutures (Fig. 1.45). Conversion of marrow in the calvarium and facial bones typically progresses from front to rear. This occurs in an orderly fashion from midmandible and maxilla to the frontal bone and back over the calvarium [26]. The mandibular fatty marrow conversion starts in the midline and extends laterally [27] (Fig. 1.47). Fatty replacement of facial bone marrow precedes pneumatization of the sinuses. The timing and variability of sinus pneumatization is well established [28, 29]. Frontal sinuses appear around age 8. Sphenoid sinuses appear earlier, around age 4–5. Both frontal and sphenoid sinuses reach near adult size at age 12 [30]. In chronic anemic states, such as thalassemia, the frontal, sphenoid, and maxillary sinuses may not develop [30] to their normal capacity (Fig. 1.48). This raises the question of whether fatty replacement of marrow is a prerequisite for paranasal sinus development. In a normal adult, patches of hematopoietic marrow are most often seen in the parietal bone (Fig. 1.49), with fatty marrow signal in the rest of the skull and facial bones. It is not unusual to see patchy hematopoietic marrow in the skull and facial bones of adults (Fig. 1.50).

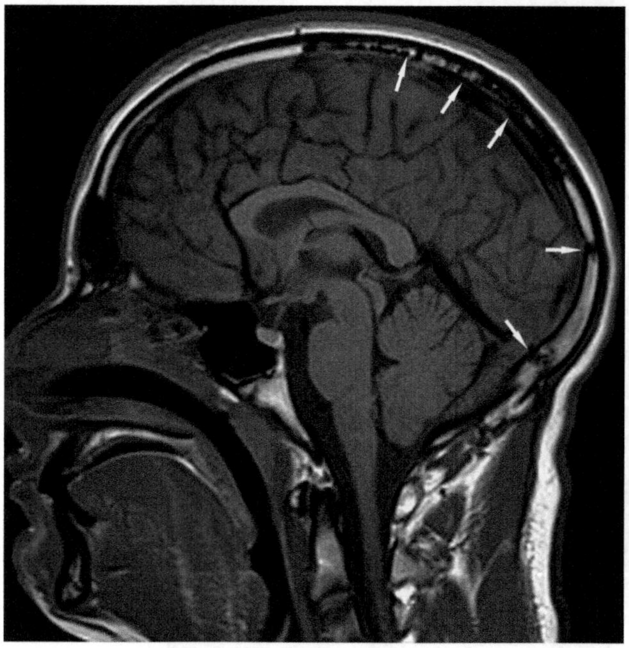

Fig. 1.45 Sagittal T1-weighted midline image of the skull demonstrates a thin layer of predominantly fatty bone marrow between the inner and outer tables. Please note hypointense signal in the region of sutures (*arrows*) in a 33-year-old man

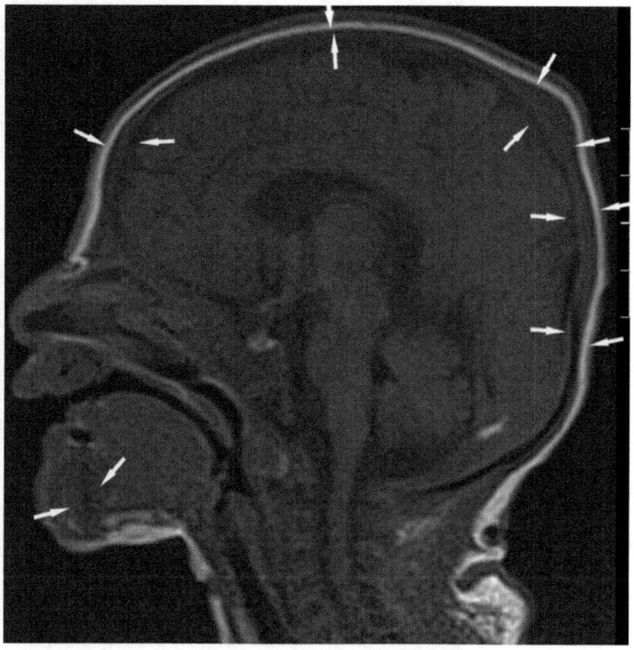

Fig. 1.46 A 19-day-old girl. Diffuse red marrow signal involving the skull (*arrows*) and facial bones is visualized on T1-weighted sagittal image

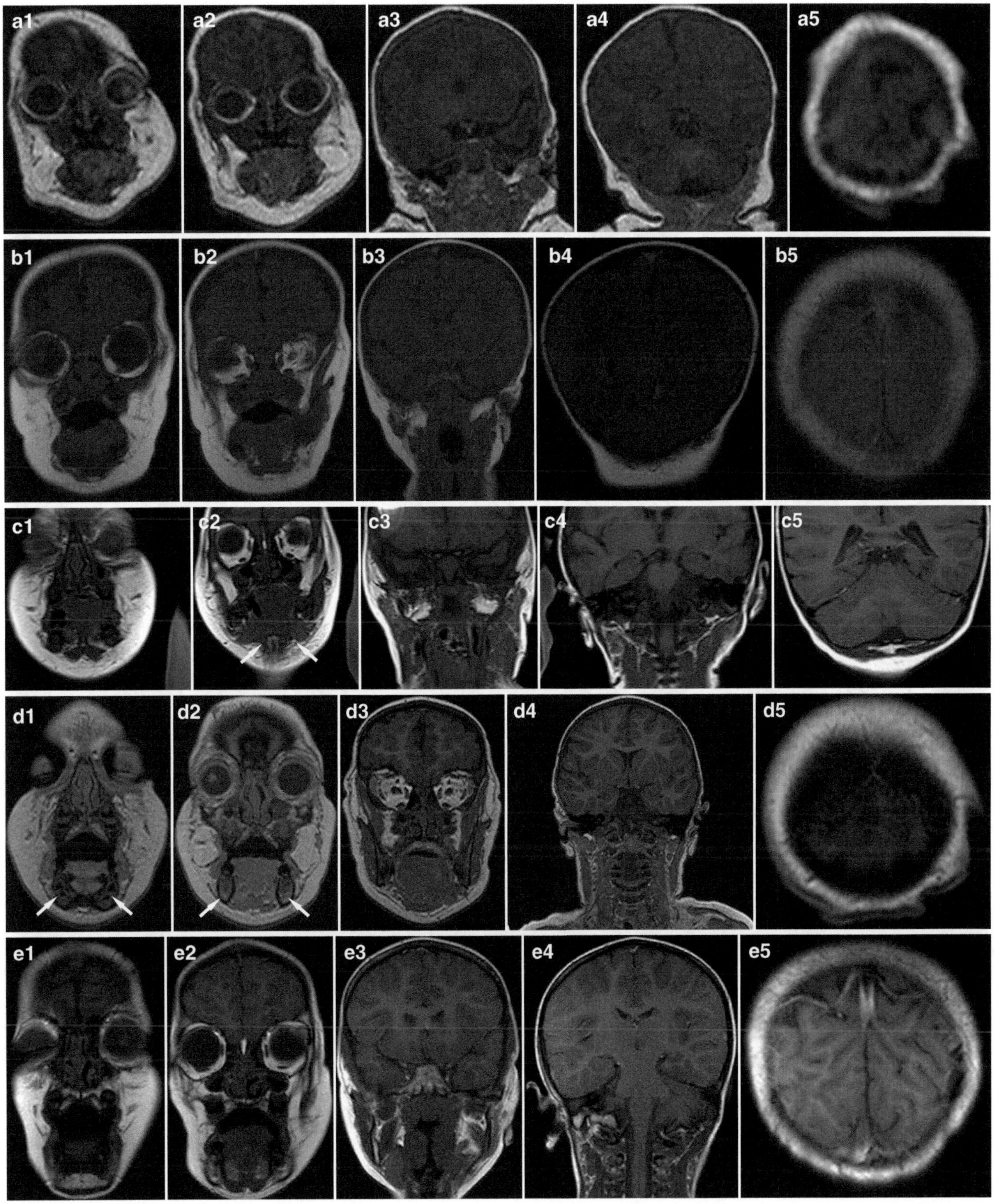

Fig. 1.47 Bone marrow signal about the skull and facial groups in various age groups on T1-weighted coronal images. Diffuse red marrow signal is noted throughout the facial bones and skulls of 1-day-old (**a**) and 2-month-old (**b**) infants. Early changes of fatty reconversion are noted in the mandible (*arrows*) of a 3-year-old girl (**c**). Partial fatty reconversion in the mandible is noted in a 5-year-old girl (**d**). Predominantly fatty marrow of the skull and facial bones is noted in a 10-year-old boy (**e**), a 16-year-old girl (**f**) and 19-year-old man (**g**)

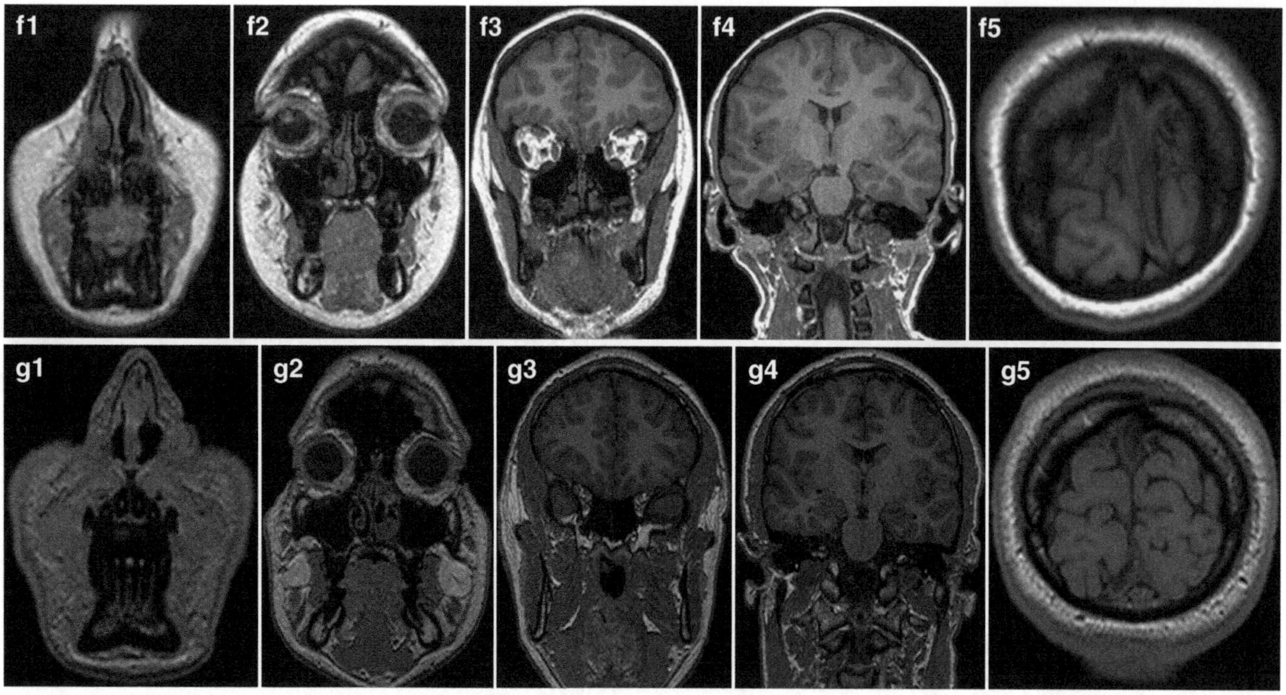

Fig. 1.47 (continued)

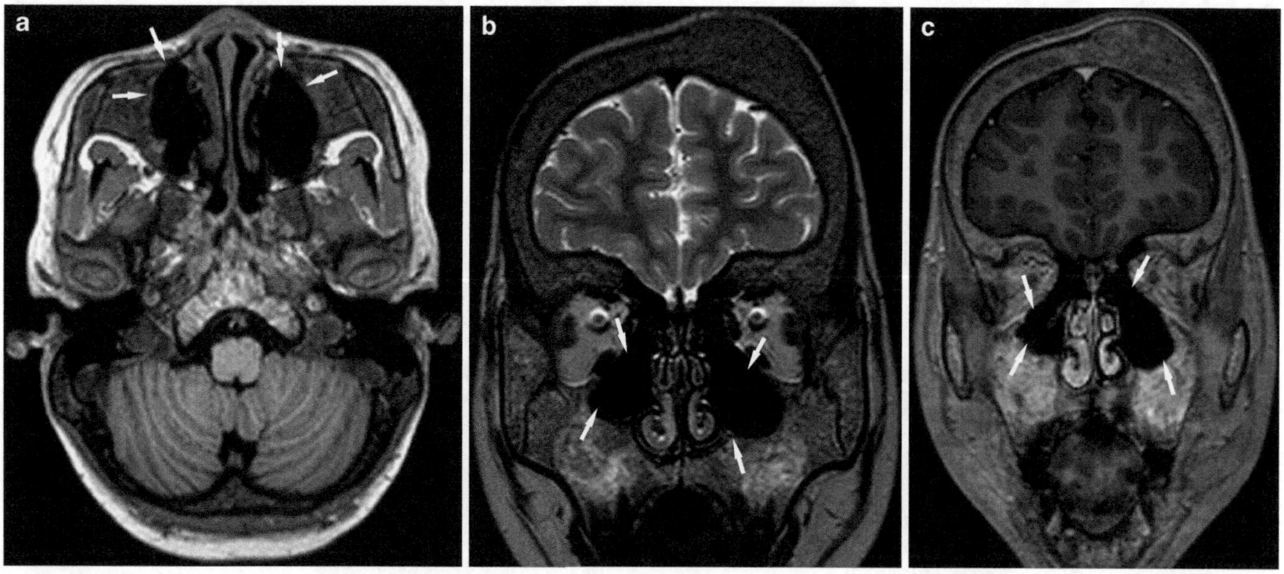

Fig. 1.48 A 9-year-old boy with history of thalassemia. Axial FLAIR (**a**), coronal T2-weighted (**b**) and coronal T1-weighted (**c**) images of skull demonstrate absent frontal and hypoplastic maxillary (*arrows*) paranasal sinuses

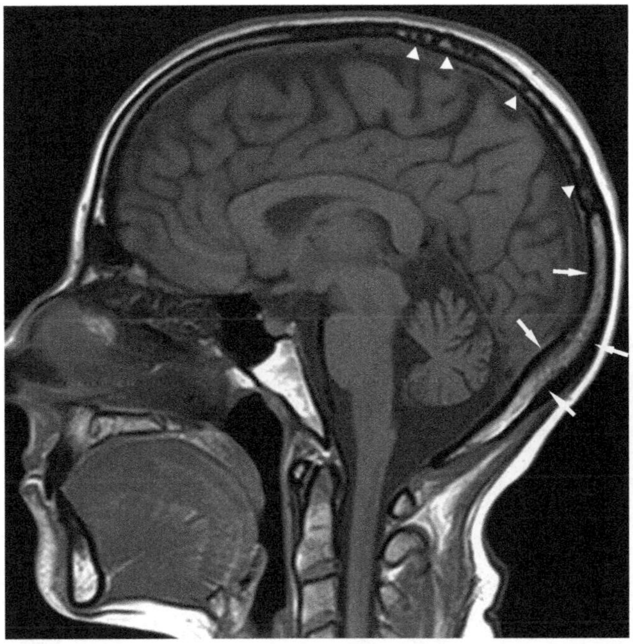

Fig. 1.49 A 40-year-old woman. Sagittal T1-weighted image of the skull demonstrates red marrow in the parieto-occipital region (*arrows*), with fatty marrow in the remainder of the skull. Note the markedly hypointense signal in the region of sutures (*arrowheads*)

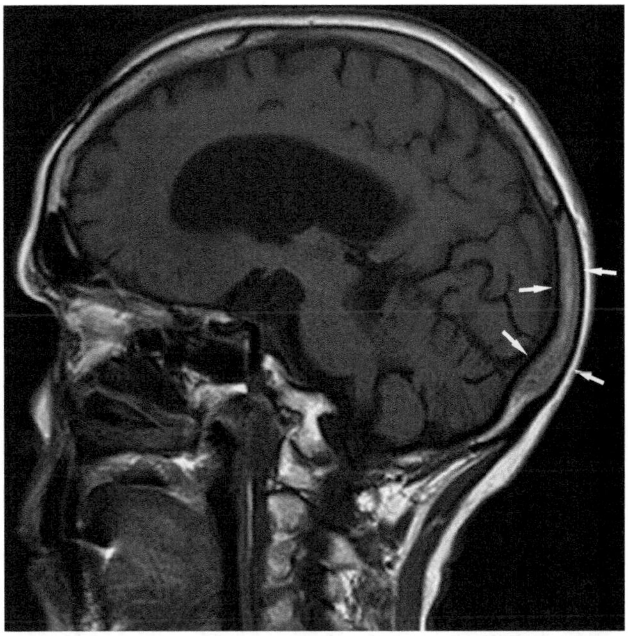

Fig. 1.50 A 79-year-old man. Sagittal T1-weighted image of the skull demonstrates patchy red marrow throughout the skull, especially about the parieto-occipital region (*arrows*)

The vertebra has predominantly hematopoietic marrow in the first decade except for the area around the basivertebral vein (Fig. 1.51). With few exceptions, the vertebra never fully converts to fatty marrow, but with age the amount of red marrow decreases, and fatty marrow increases resulting in increased T1 signal intensity compared to the adjacent intervertebral disc. The early MRI literature suggested that marrow conversion of vertebral bodies occurred after the first year of life and the T1 marrow signal relative to the intervertebral disc would be hypointense before 1 year of age (Fig. 1.52), isointense between 1 and 5 years, and hyperintense after 5 years [31]. The recent literature [3] and our own experience suggest an earlier time frame for this conversion (Fig. 1.53).

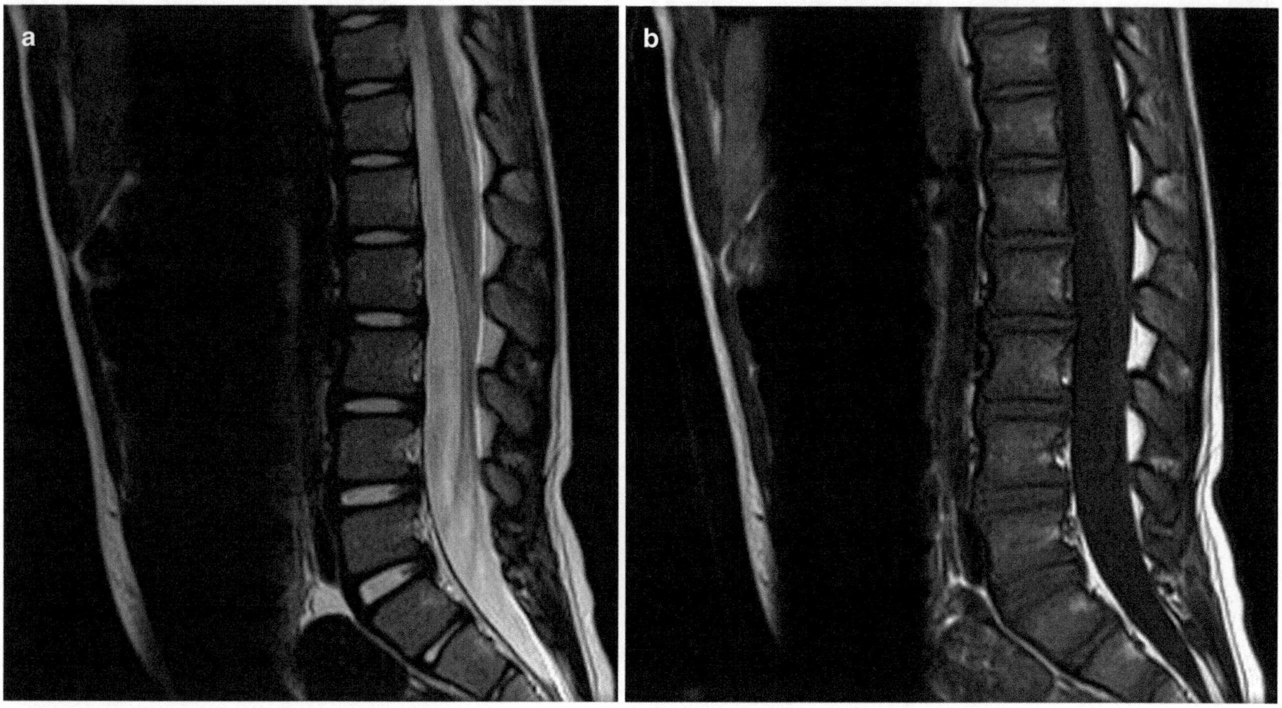

Fig. 1.51 A 14-year-old girl. Sagittal T2-weighted (**a**) and T1-weighted (**b**) images of the lumbar spine demonstrate predominantly red marrow in the vertebral body with fatty signal along the basivertebral vein

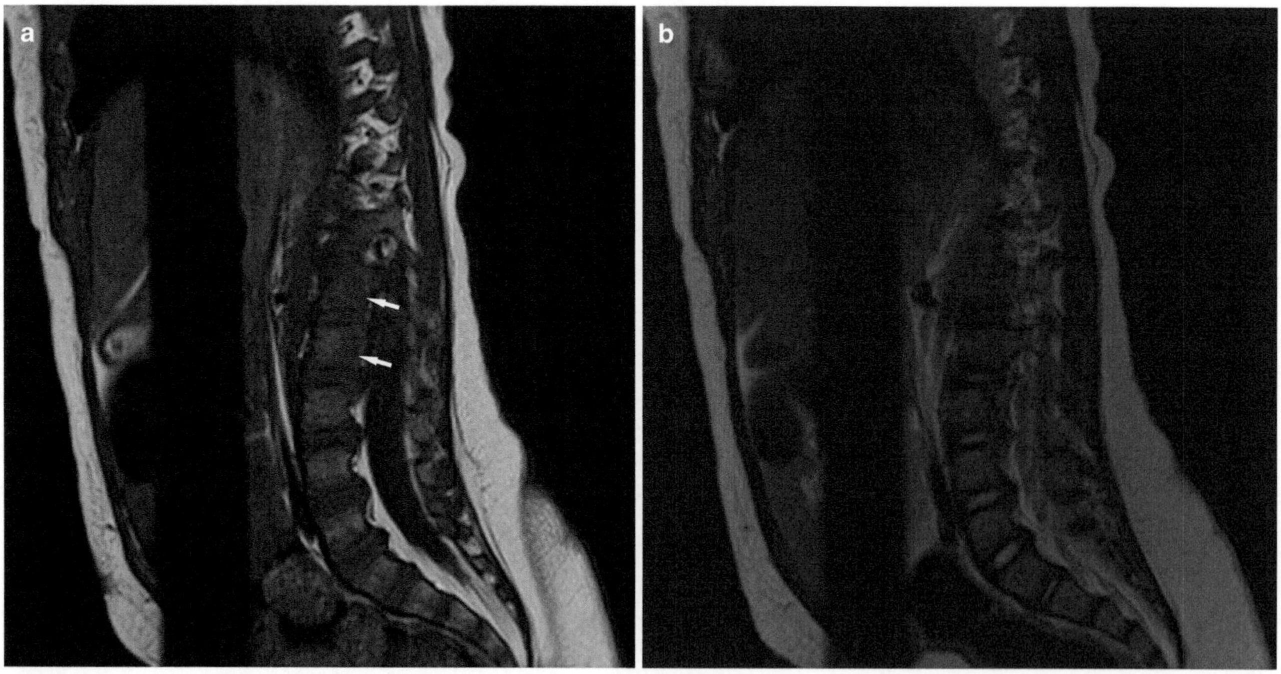

Fig. 1.52 An 8-month-old boy. Sagittal T1-weighted (**a**) and T2-weighted (**b**) images of the lumbar spine demonstrate foci of red marrow more hypointense than disc material on T1-weighted images (*arrows*)

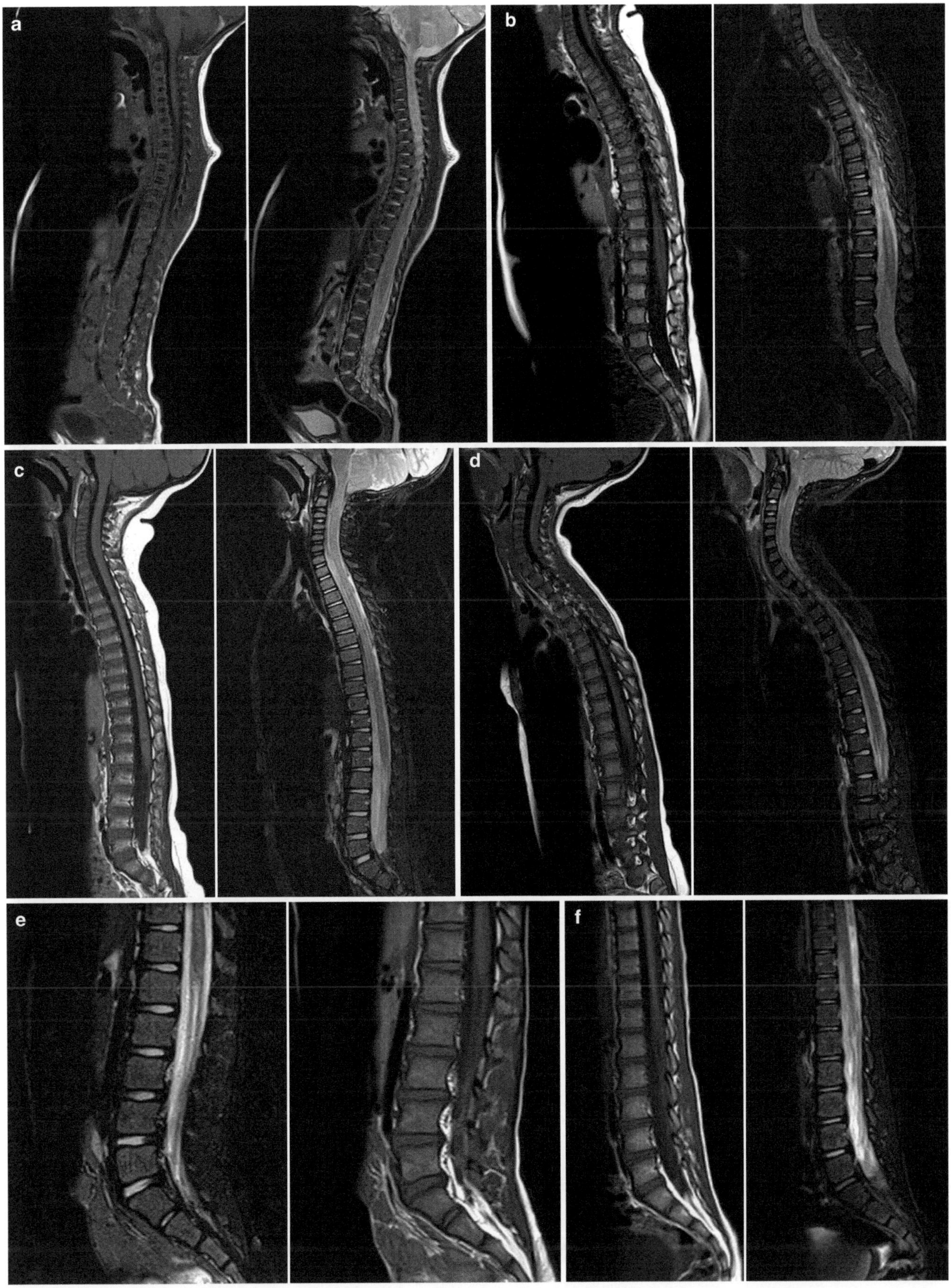

Fig. 1.53 The evolution of spinal bone marrow signal changes in the first 5 years of life. T1- and T2-weighted sagittal images of the entire spine in a 16-day-old newborn (**a**) show markedly hypointense T1 signal corresponding to red marrow. Early fatty marrow conversion changes are noted in a 12-month-old girl (**b**). There is progressive increase in fatty marrow conversion in a 24-month-old boy (**c**), a 3-year-old (**d**), and a 4-year-old boy (**e**). Slightly more fatty marrow signal is noted in a 5-year-old girl (**f**)

MR imaging of the vertebral column is routinely performed for the assessment of adult patients with spine-related symptoms, whereas pelvic bones are imaged in hip joint-related symptoms. On shoulder imaging, the glenoid and part of the scapular body are usually visualized. Similar to the appendicular skeleton, red marrow at these sites shows mild to moderate decrease in signal intensity on T1-weighted images, intermediate to low signal intensity on T2-weighted images, and moderate increase in signal intensity on fat-saturated intermediate or T2-weighted images (Fig. 1.54).

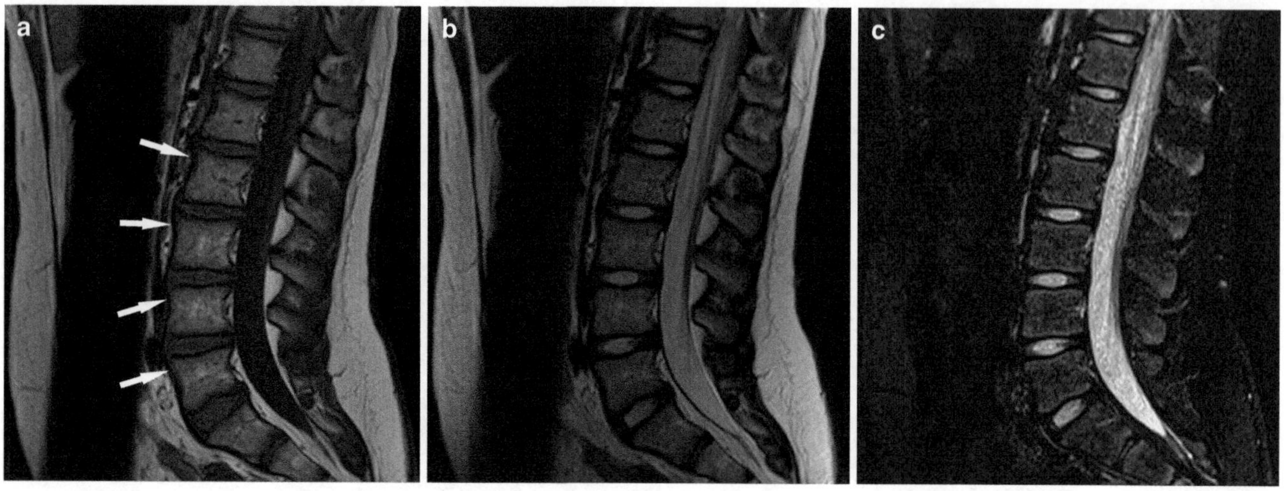

Fig. 1.54 A 16-year-old boy. Sagittal T1-weighted (**a**), T2-weighted (**b**), and T2-weighted fat-suppressed (**c**) images of the lumbar spine demonstrate patchy red marrow signal that is slightly hyperintense to intervertebral discs on T1-weighted image especially near endplates. There is mild to moderate hyperintensity on T2-weighted fat-suppressed images

Vertebral marrow of young adults typically shows intermediate signal intensity on T1-weighted images although diffuse fatty signal with minimal red marrow could also be seen. Conversely, older individuals can have relatively diffuse red marrow, instead of the expected age-related high signal intensity fatty marrow on T1-weighted images. Although technical parameters may partially account for variability among different individuals, variations in red marrow cellularity may play a role, regardless of the cause [25]. There is limited variation in marrow appearance among vertebral bodies of the same person, as opposed to marked variability in different people of similar age and demographics. Several patterns of vertebral marrow appearance can be recognized. These patterns are typically observed in all vertebral bodies of the same person [32, 33]. Red marrow is generally distributed in a homogeneous pattern within the vertebral body (Fig. 1.55). Sometimes, red marrow is more concentrated near the vertebral end plate (Fig. 1.56), which is a metaphyseal equivalent, an area where the bone is more vascular [13], particularly in children and young adults. Red marrow may also be more prominent in the anterior aspects of the vertebral bodies (Fig. 1.57). Red marrow could be diffuse with linear fatty signal around the basivertebral vein (Fig. 1.58), or in the middle between fatty marrow about the superior and inferior end plates (Fig. 1.59) [13]. Red marrow could also appear as small nodules (Fig. 1.60) or patchy areas (Fig. 1.61) in the background of fatty marrow. In general, these variations in vertebral marrow MR imaging appearance should involve virtually all vertebral bodies of an individual in a uniform manner, in the absence of prior trauma, surgery, or radiation. The exception to this rule is the sacrococcygeal region where partial or diffuse fatty infiltration is commonly seen (Fig. 1.62).

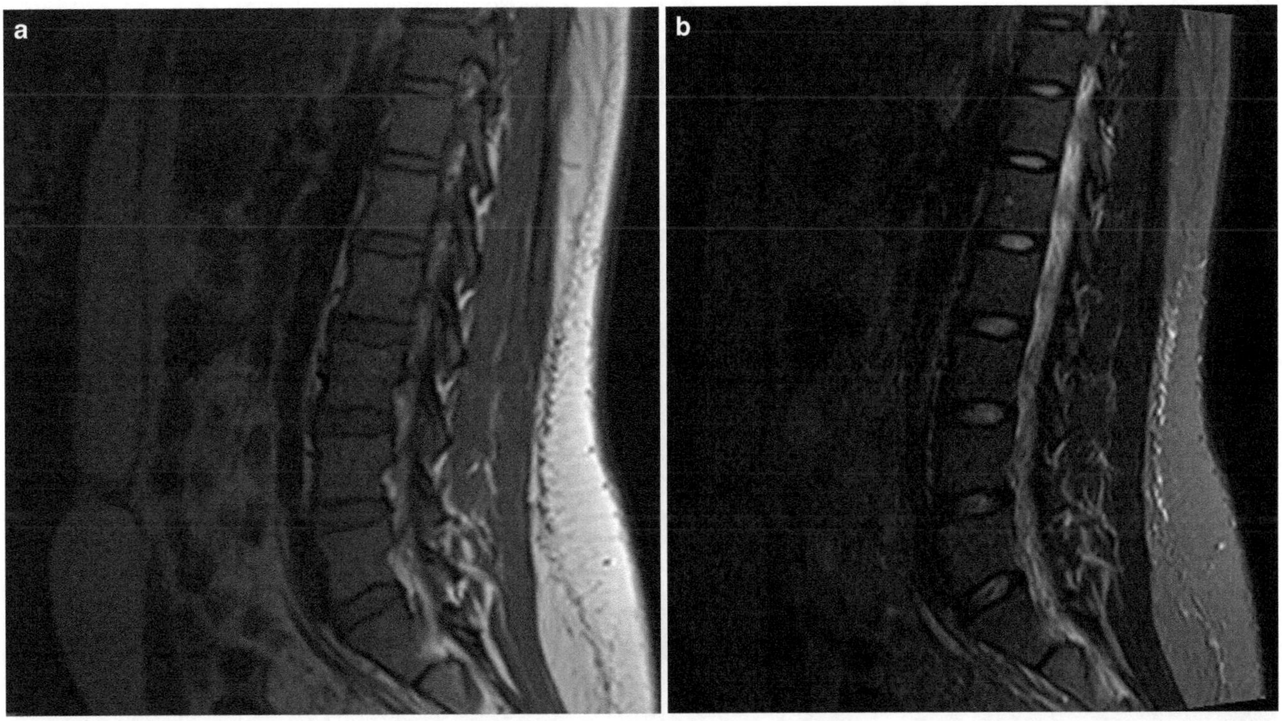

Fig. 1.55 A 27-year-old woman. T1-weighted (**a**) and T2-weighted (**b**) sagittal images of the lumbar spine demonstrate mild diffuse red marrow signal throughout the visualized thoracolumbar and sacral spine

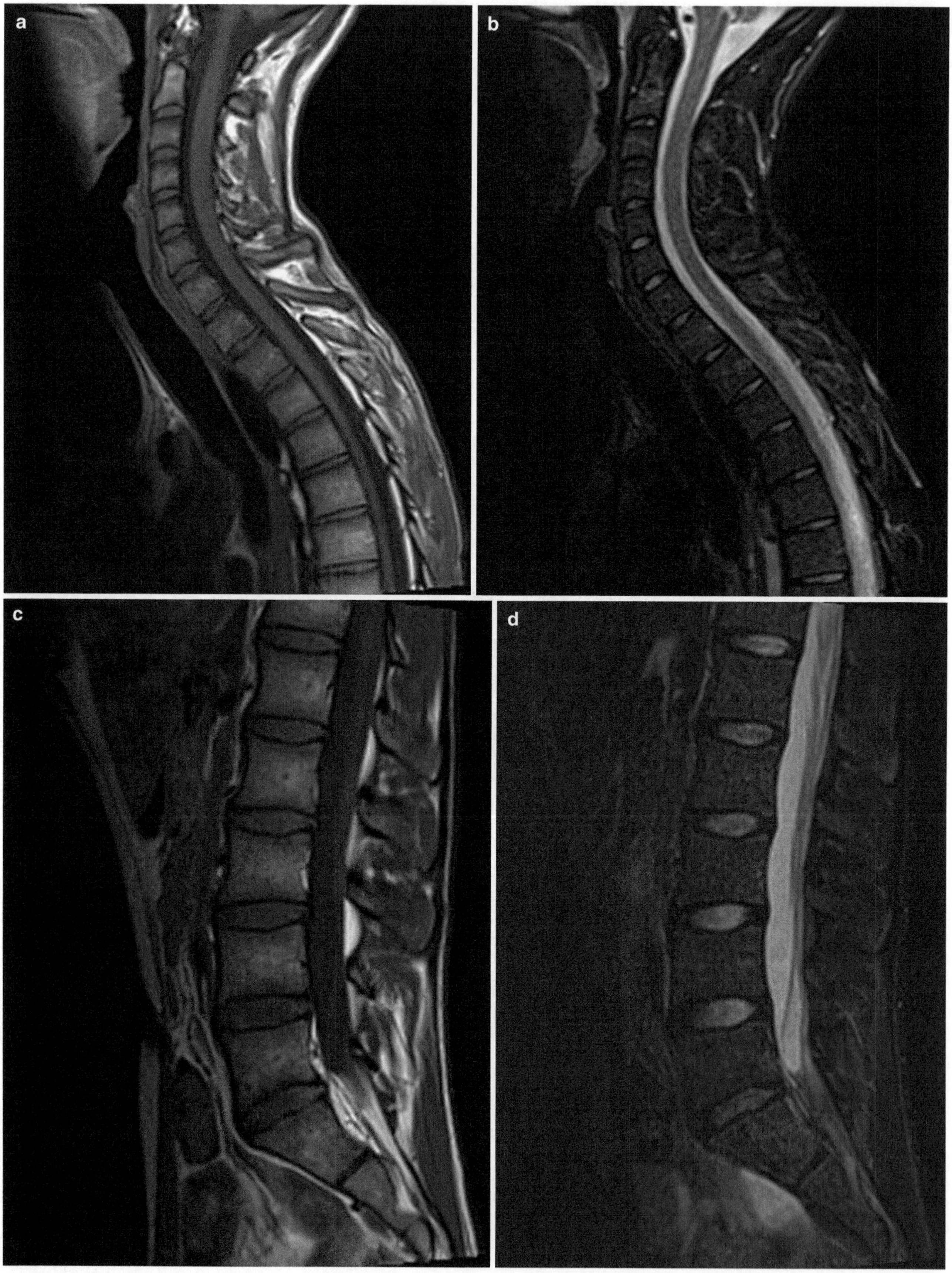

Fig. 1.56 A 19-year-old man. Sagittal T1-weighted (**a**, **c**) and T2-weighted fat-suppressed (**b**, **d**) images of the thoracolumbar spine showing red marrow signal more prominent about the end plates

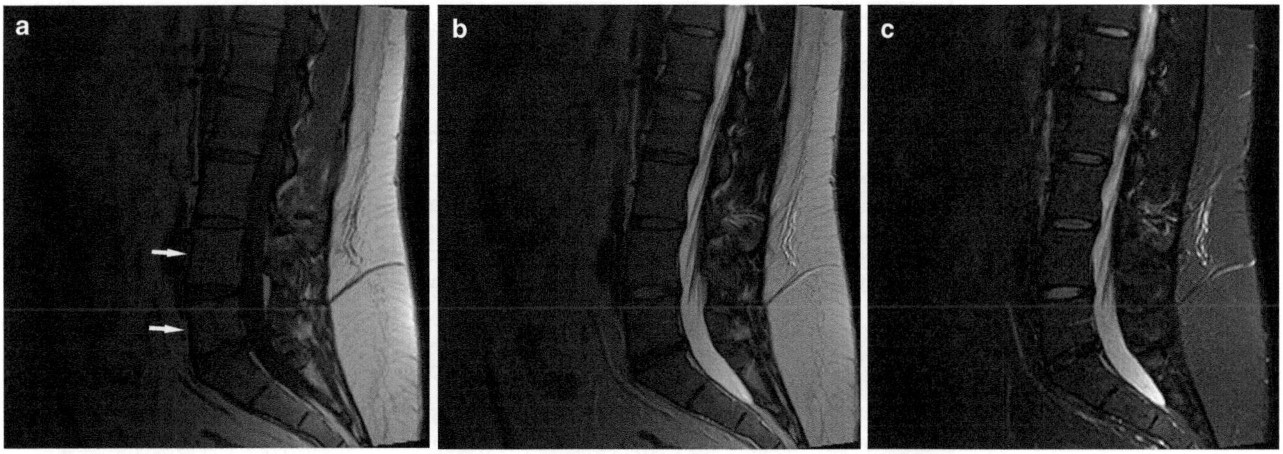

Fig. 1.57 A 23-year-old woman. T1-weighted (**a**), T2-weighted (**b**), and T2-weighted fat-suppressed (**c**) sagittal images of the lumbar spine demonstrate mild red marrow signal that is slightly more prominent in the anterior vertebral bodies (*arrows*)

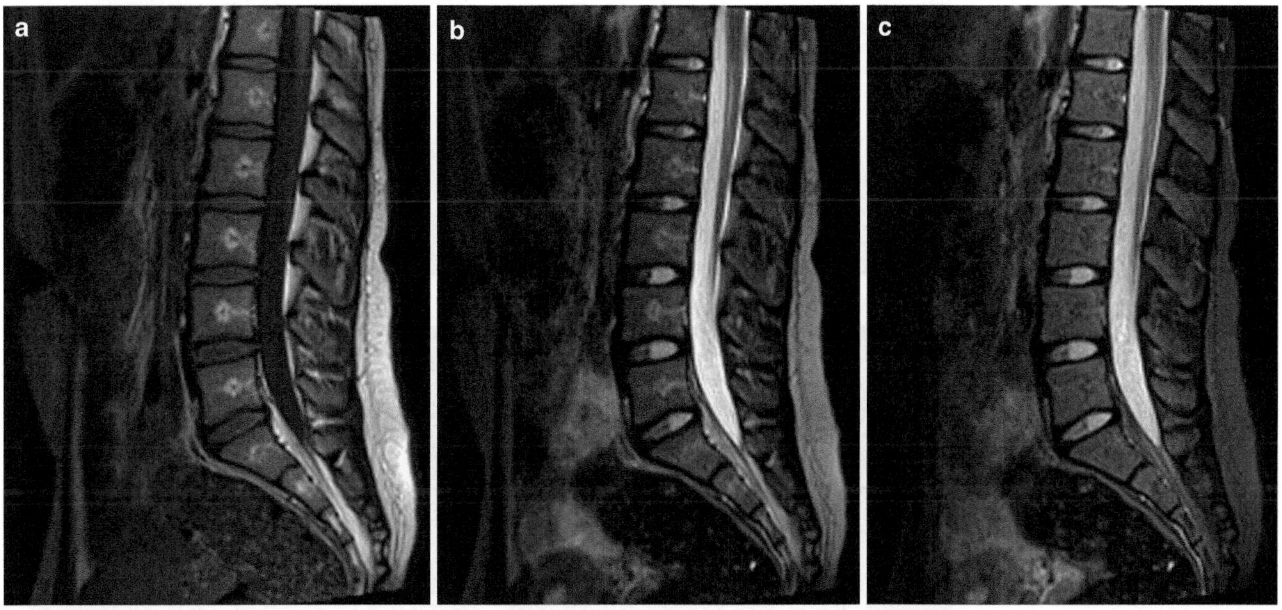

Fig. 1.58 A 16-year-old boy. T1-weighted (**a**), T2-weighted (**b**), and T2-weighted fat-suppressed (**c**) sagittal images of the lumbar spine demonstrate diffuse red marrow in the vertebral body with sparing of "key-shaped" fatty signal along the basivertebral veins

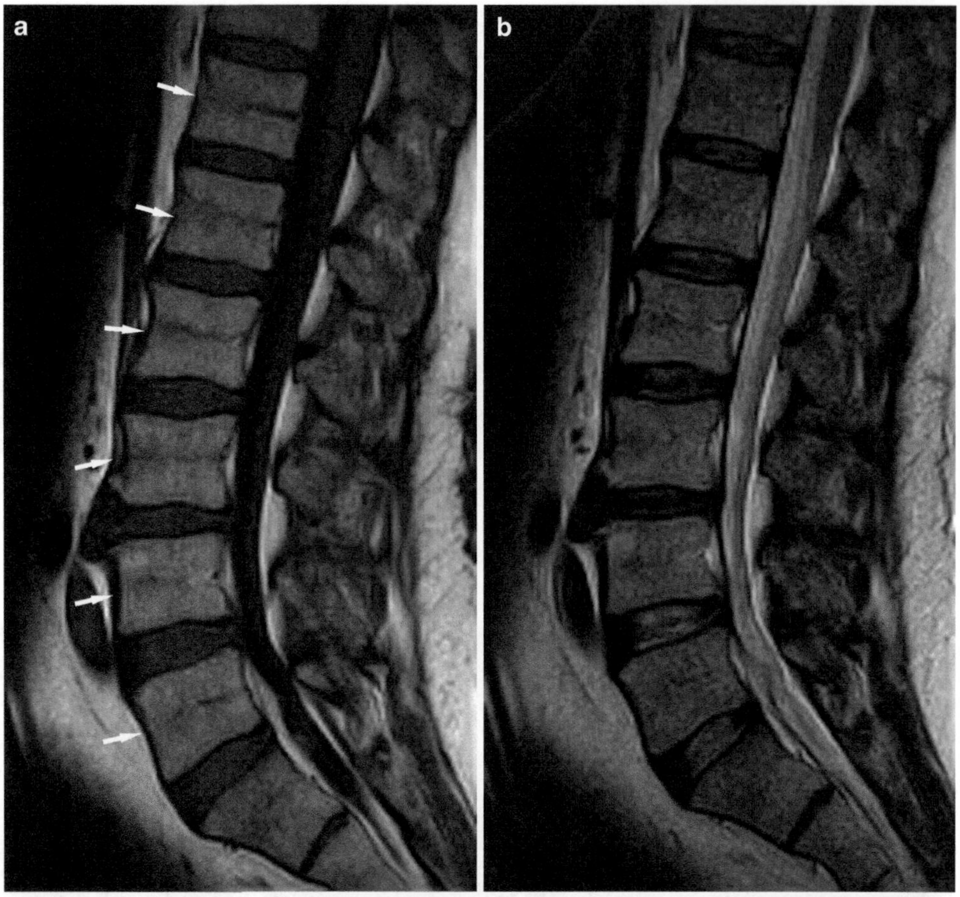

Fig. 1.59 A 33-year-old woman. T1-weighted (**a**) and T2-weighted (**b**) sagittal images of the lumbar spine demonstrate mild red marrow signal in the center of the vertebral bodies (*arrows*) accentuated by more fatty marrow signal in the end plates

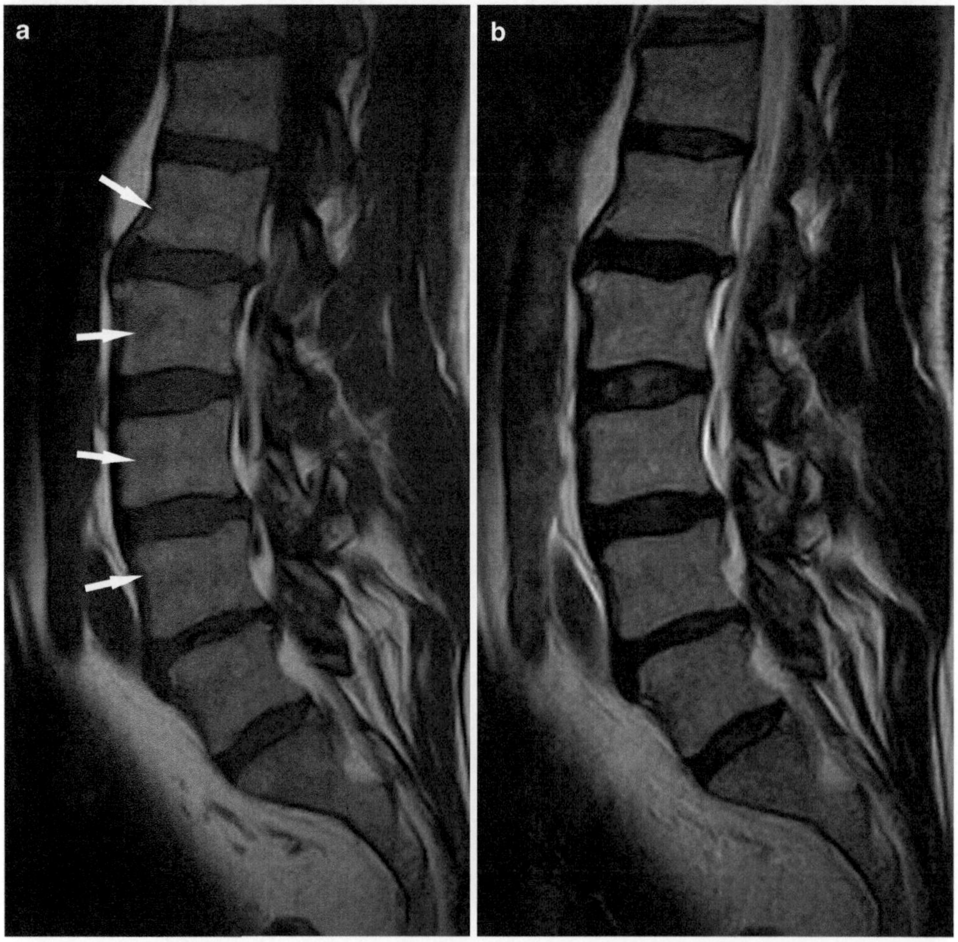

Fig. 1.60 A 39-year-old man. T1-weighted (**a**) and T2-weighted (**b**) sagittal images of the lumbar spine demonstrate slightly heterogeneous red marrow with areas of nodularity (*arrows*) in the background of fatty marrow

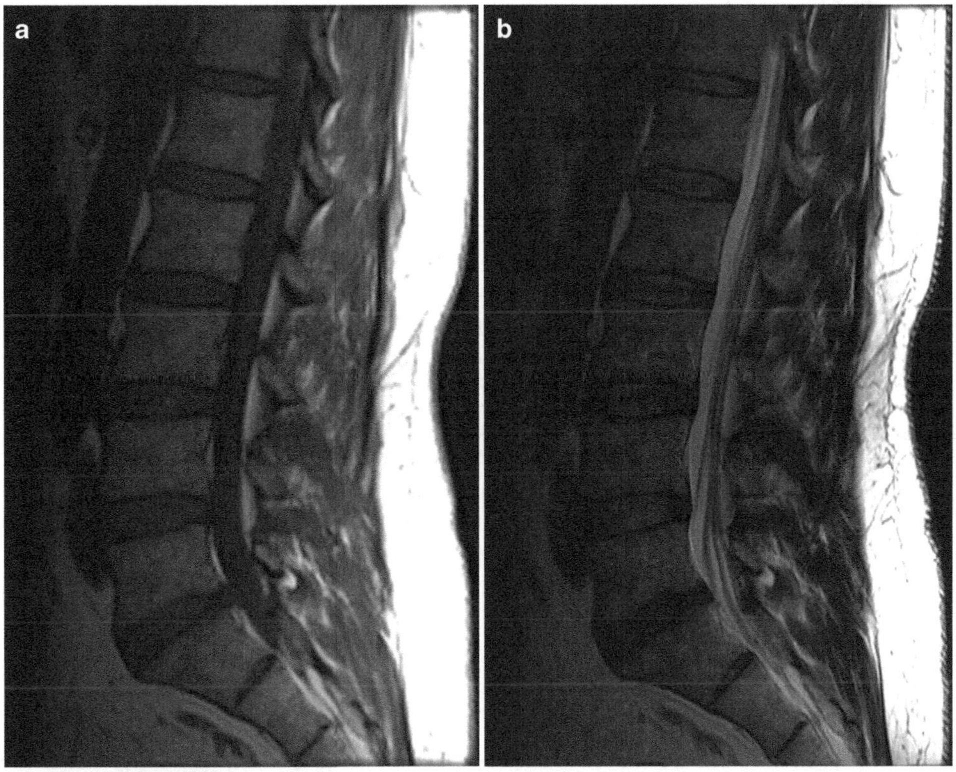

Fig. 1.61 A 48-year-old man. T1-weighted (**a**) and T2-weighted (**b**) sagittal images of the lumbar spine demonstrate slightly heterogeneous marrow with patchy areas of red marrow signal

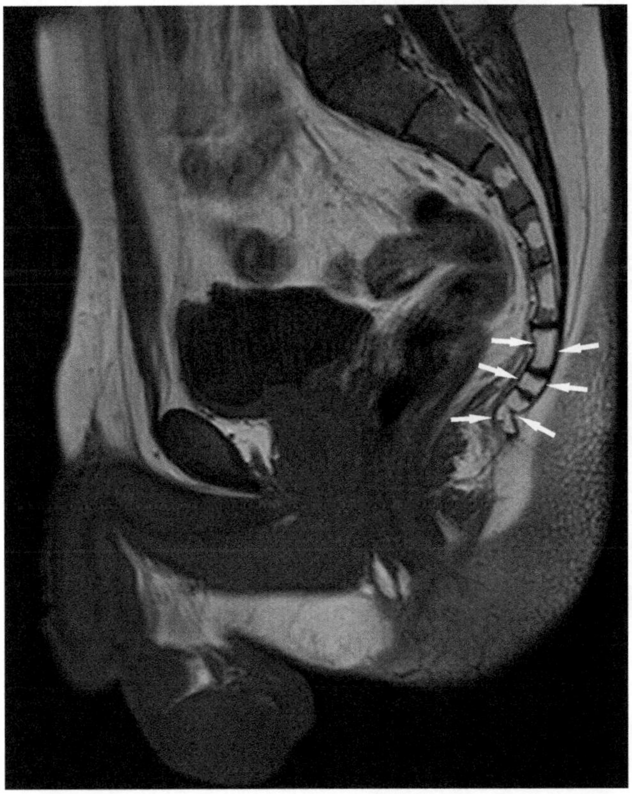

Fig. 1.62 A 40-year-old man. Sagittal T1-weighted image of the sacrococcygeal spine demonstrates fatty marrow signal in the center of the sacral segments with entirely fatty marrow signal within the coccygeal segments (*arrows*)

In the vertebral column, the signal intensity of the intervertebral disc is used as the internal standard on T1-weighted images. The majority of normal lumbar disc visualized is the central "nucleus pulposus" which consists of chondrocyte-like cells, collagen fibrils, and proteoglycan aggrecans that aggregate through hyaluronic chains which likely contributes the hypointense T1-weighted and hyperintense T2-weighted signal. The smaller annulus consists of both type I and type II collagen—the concentration of type I collagen increasing toward the periphery of the annulus showing hyperintense signal on both T1-weighted and hyperintense T2-weighted sequences. Red marrow signal is typically more hyperintense than intervertebral disc on T1-weighted images although it may appear more hypointense than annulus fibrosis at the end plates (Fig. 1.63). Improved signal to noise in higher magnetic strength allows differentiation of nucleus pulposus and annulus fibrosus on MRI. If possible, nucleus pulposus in the center of the disc should be used as the reference to compare with red marrow. In the thoracic and cervical spine, red marrow signal intensity can be lower than that of disc (Fig. 1.64) because the disc often shows higher signal intensity than in the lumbar spine. Throughout the spine, the collagen content of the nucleus pulposus has been shown to be the highest in cervical discs and lowest in lumbar discs [23] which may explain differences of signal intensities on MRI. With respect to age-related changes, the collagen content of the annulus fibrosus is higher in adults than in younger children [23]. Red marrow appears hyperintense on fat-suppressed intermediate, T2-weighted, and inversion recovery sequences with increased conspicuity in the background of fatty marrow (Fig. 1.65). On nonfat-suppressed T2-weighted images, the appearance of red marrow is visually less striking (Fig. 1.66). As in the appendicular skeleton, it is unreliable to assess bone marrow status solely on the basis of inversion recovery and T2-weighted images due to lack of an internal standard with which marrow signal intensity can be compared.

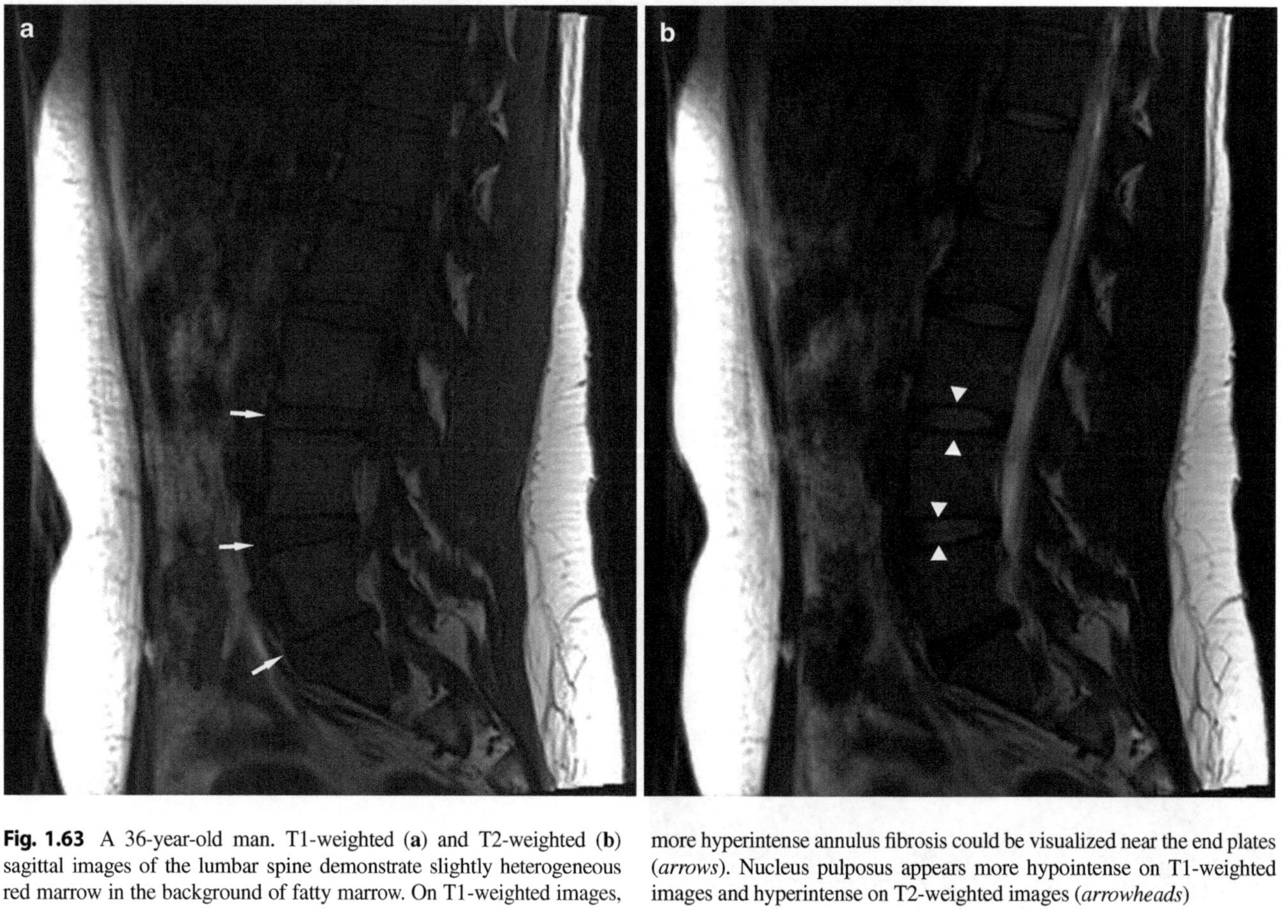

Fig. 1.63 A 36-year-old man. T1-weighted (**a**) and T2-weighted (**b**) sagittal images of the lumbar spine demonstrate slightly heterogeneous red marrow in the background of fatty marrow. On T1-weighted images, more hyperintense annulus fibrosis could be visualized near the end plates (*arrows*). Nucleus pulposus appears more hypointense on T1-weighted images and hyperintense on T2-weighted images (*arrowheads*)

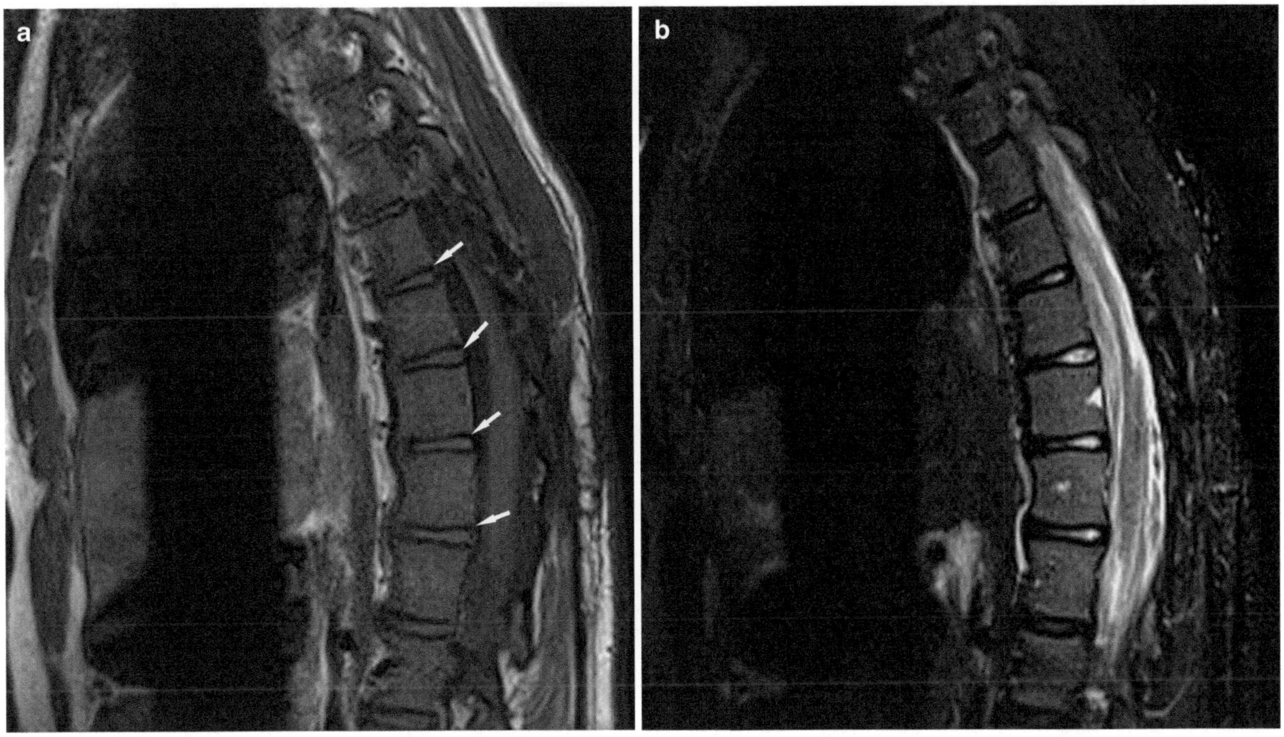

Fig. 1.64 A 9-year-old boy. Sagittal T1-weighted (**a**) and T2-weighted fat-suppressed (**b**) images of the thoracolumbar spine show diffuse red marrow that is slightly hyperintense on T2-weighted images. Note the hyperintense T1 signal of intervertebral discs (*arrows*) compared to vertebral body red marrow, which is a typical finding in the thoracic spine

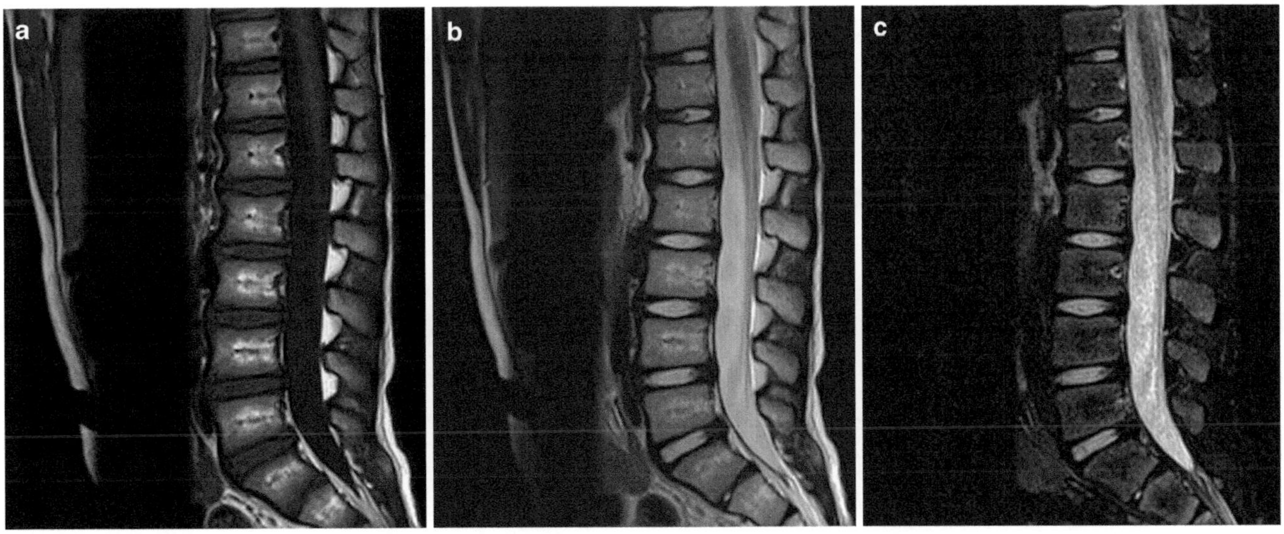

Fig. 1.65 A 11-year-old girl. T1-weighted (**a**), T2-weighted (**b**), and T2-weighted fat-suppressed (**c**) sagittal images of the lumbar spine demonstrate mild red marrow in the vertebral bodies with fatty signal along the basivertebral vein. Red marrow signal is more difficult to appreciate on a T2-weighted image without fat suppression (**b**)

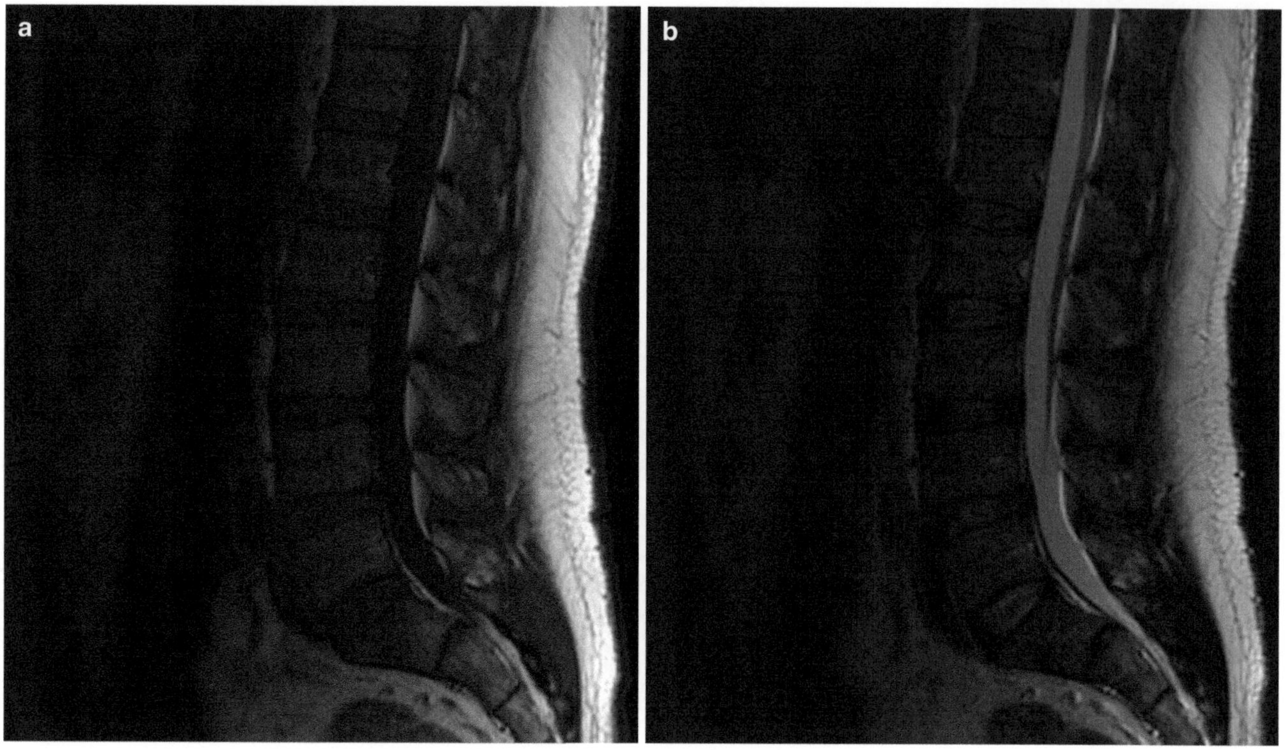

Fig. 1.66 A 38-year-old man. T1-weighted (**a**) and T2-weighted (**b**) sagittal images of the lumbar spine demonstrate patchy red marrow in the vertebral bodies. Red marrow signal is more difficult to appreciate on a T2-weighted image without fat suppression (**b**)

Unlike the appendicular skeleton, pelvic marrow is predominantly hematopoietic in the first two decades of life with marrow conversion typically beginning in the acetabulum superiorly and medially. The metaphyseal equivalents of flat bones have similar marrow signal intensity to those of metaphysis of a long bone, whereas epiphyseal equivalents demonstrate cartilage in young children and fatty signal after fusion. These are abundant in the pelvis and include areas surrounding triradiate cartilage (Fig. 1.67), ischiopubic synchondrosis (Fig. 1.68), and sacroiliac joints [3] (Fig. 1.69).

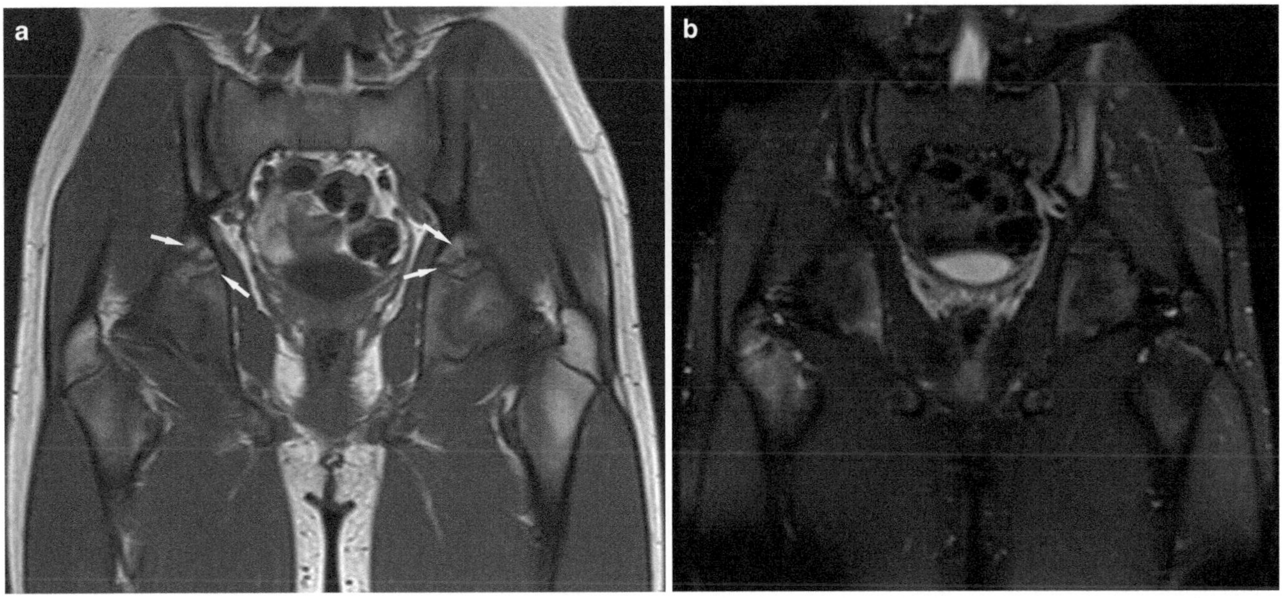

Fig. 1.67 A 9-year-old boy. Coronal T1-weighted (**a**) and T2-weighted (**b**) images of the pelvis demonstrate fatty signal surrounding the triradiate cartilage (*arrows*), which is an epiphyseal equivalent

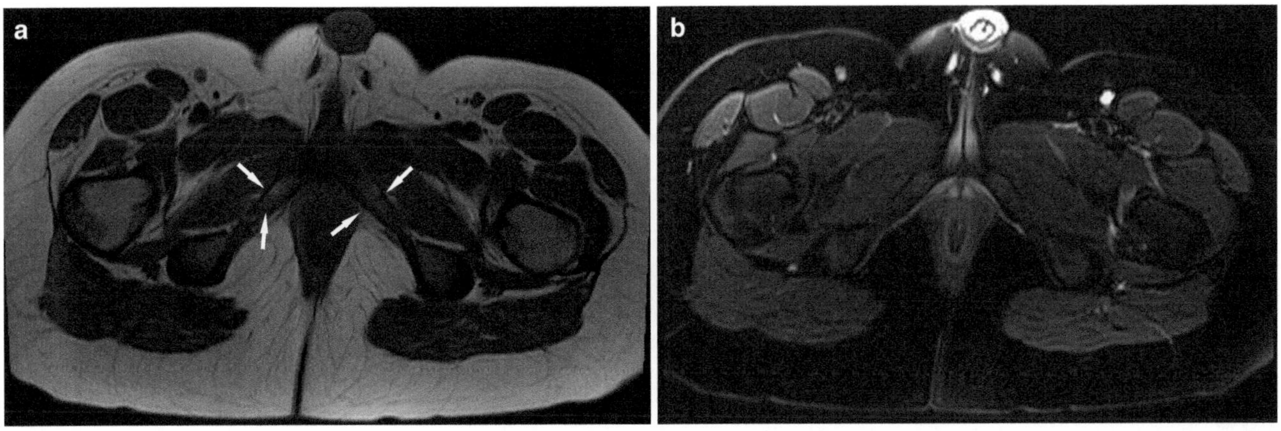

Fig. 1.68 A 11-year-old boy. Sagittal T1-weighted (**a**) and T2-weighted fat-suppressed (**b**) images of the pelvis show fatty bone marrow signal surrounding the ilioischial synchondrosis (*arrows*)

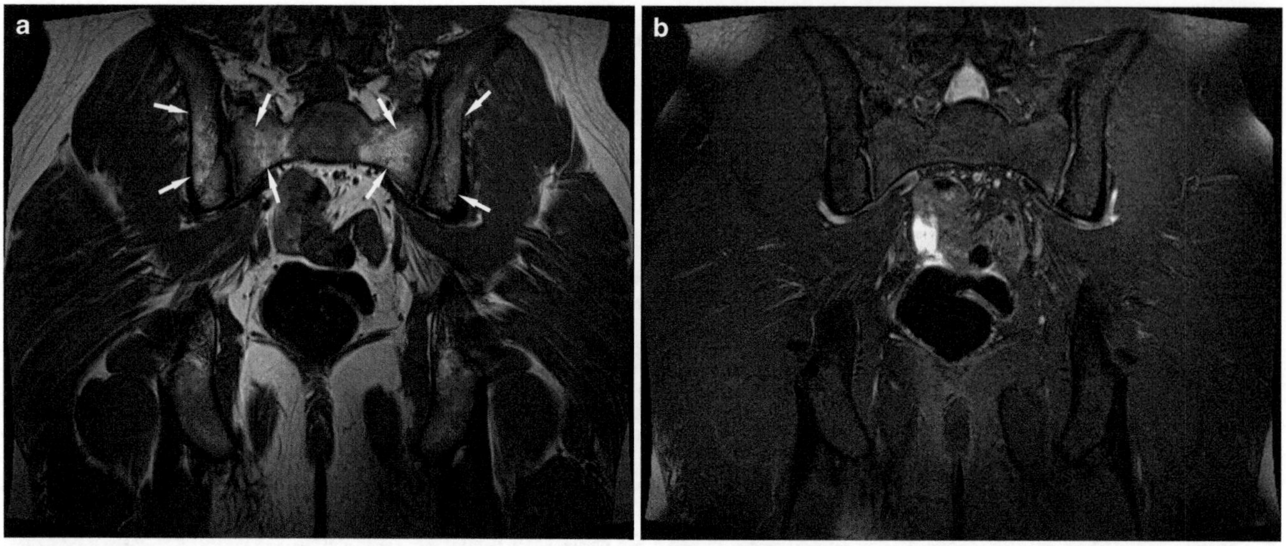

Fig. 1.69 A 37-year-old woman. Coronal T1-weighted (**a**) and T2-weighted fat-suppressed (**b**) images of the pelvis demonstrate fatty marrow signal adjacent to the sacroiliac joints (*arrows*) with more central red marrow signal

In the pelvis, a relatively large proportion of bone marrow remains cellular through the adult years. Small patches of red marrow could be scattered about the acetabula, sacrum, and ileum. The distribution is usually symmetric although slight asymmetry is not uncommon. Diffuse fatty (Fig. 1.70) or diffuse red marrow patterns (Fig. 1.71) may also be encountered. A heterogeneous appearance of pelvic marrow is not uncommon due to admixed red and yellow marrow (Fig. 1.72).

Sternum and scapula typically show areas of red marrow throughout life. Familiarity with the MRI appearance of sternum in different age groups could be helpful in the recognition of normal patterns (Fig. 1.73).

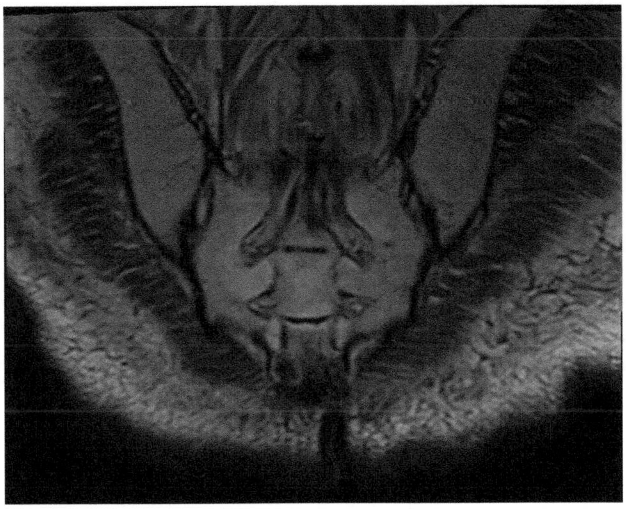

Fig. 1.70 A 62-year-old woman. Coronal T1-weighted image of the pelvis shows diffuse fatty marrow signal without appreciable red marrow

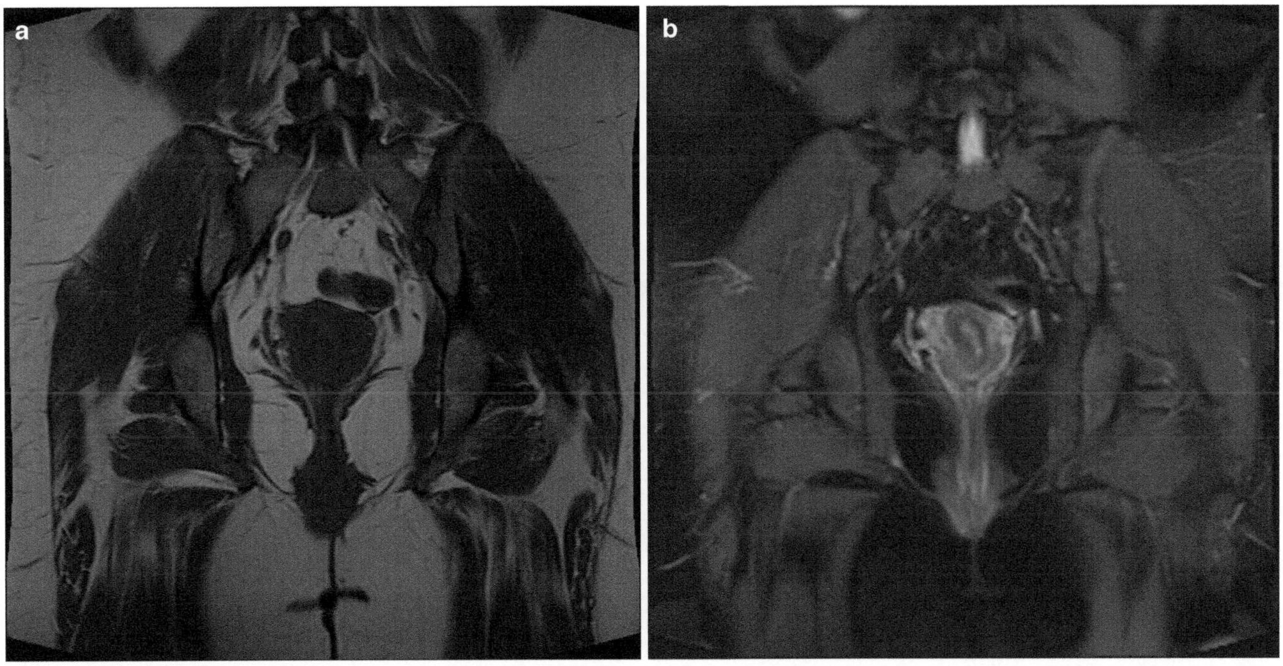

Fig. 1.71 A 39-year-old woman. T1-weighted (**a**) and T2-weighted fat-suppressed (**b**) images of the pelvis demonstrate diffuse red marrow with minimal intermixed marrow fat

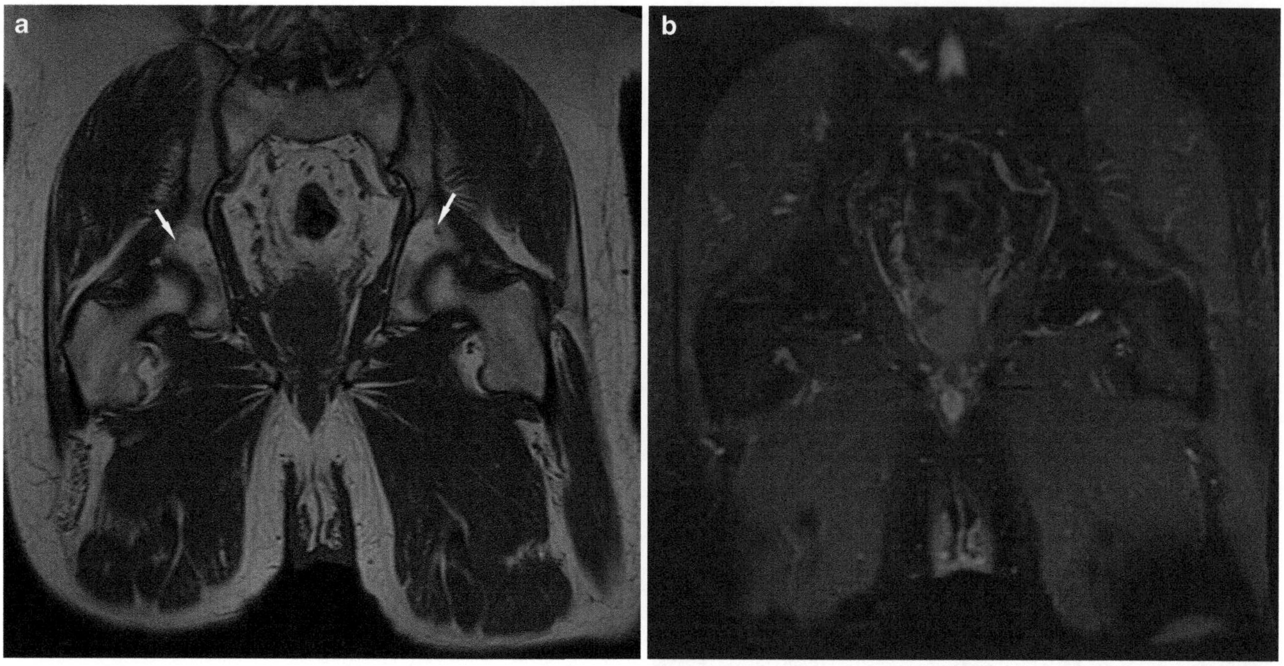

Fig. 1.72 A 38-year-old man. T1-weighted (**a**) and T2-weighted fat-suppressed (**b**) images of the pelvis show heterogeneous red marrow with intermixed marrow fat. Note the fatty marrow signal in the region of the epiphyseal equivalents about the triradiate cartilage bilaterally (*arrows*)

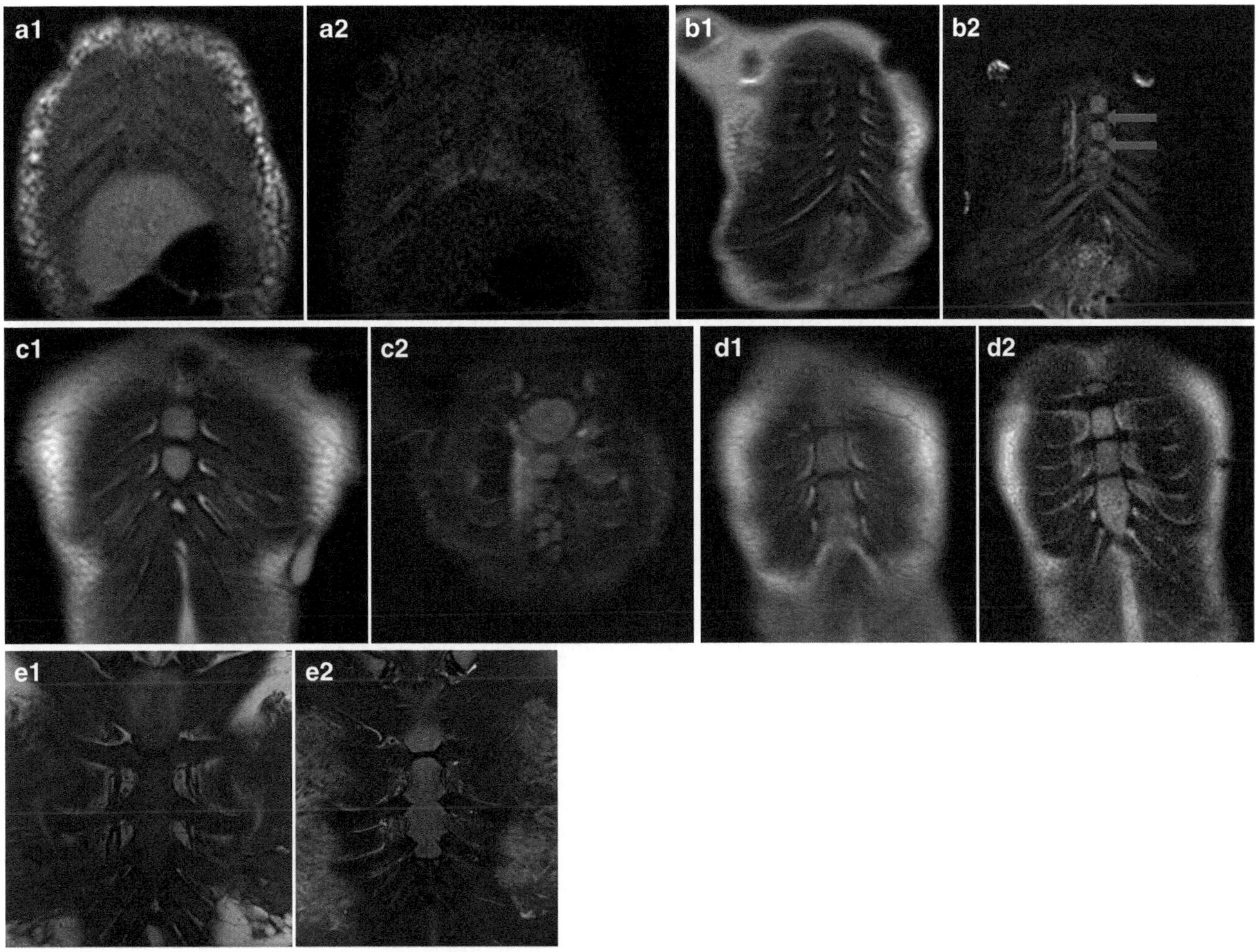

Fig. 1.73 Evolution of the bone marrow signal changes of the sternum on coronal MRI examinations. (**a**) A 7-day-old newborn girl. T1-weighted (**a1**) and T2-weighted fat-suppressed (**a2**) images show a diffuse red marrow signal. Hypointense signal is noted in the costal cartilages. (**b**) A 6-month-old infant boy. T1-weighted (**b1**) and T2-weighted fat-suppressed (**b2**) images show a diffuse red marrow signal. A cartilaginous signal separating the sternal segments is particularly evident on T2-weighted images (*arrows*). (**c**) A 4-year-old boy. T1-weighted (**c1**) and T2-weighted fat-suppressed (**c2**) images show predominantly fatty marrow signal with minimal scattered red marrow. Hypointense signal is again noted in the costal cartilages and between sternal segments. (**d**) A 9-year-old boy. T1-weighted (**d1**) and T2-weighted (**d2**) images show fatty marrow signal with mild scattered red marrow. Less pronounced separation of the sternal segments is noted. (**e**) A 16-year-old boy. T1-weighted (**e1**) and T2-weighted (**e2**) images show mixed fatty and red marrow signal. Overall morphology of the sternum is similar to that of an adult at this age

Focal nodular hyperplasia of red marrow, although rare, frequently creates a diagnostic dilemma in the spine and pelvis, especially in patients with a history of malignancy [33, 34]. In patients with history of malignancy, hyperplasia of the hematopoietic marrow can be attributed to the administration of granulocyte colony-stimulating factors, used as an adjunct to radiation or chemotherapy to decrease the myelosuppression effects of these treatments [35, 36]. They appear as diffuse or nodular red marrow simulating neoplastic marrow infiltration (Fig. 1.74). Focal nodular red marrow hyperplasia may show increased uptake on FDG-PET and therefore may be confused with other causes of increased uptake including neoplasm or infection [36]. Focal nodular hyperplasia of red marrow should have characteristic T1-weighted appearance, same as red marrow elsewhere with ill-defined margins (Fig. 1.75). There is an overlap between certain multiple myeloma lesions and focal nodular red marrow hyperplasia on T1-weighted signal although myeloma lesions tend to have well-defined margins and are likely to be numerous. A follow-up MRI and laboratory testing could help in ruling out neoplastic etiology although some cases may require biopsy confirmation.

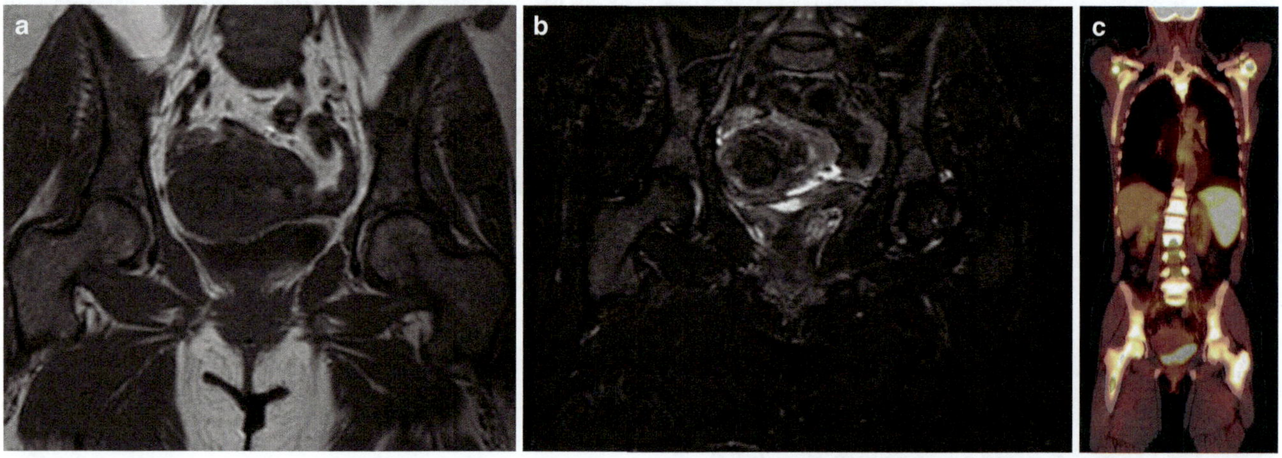

Fig. 1.74 A 43-year-old woman who was recently treated with chemotherapy and Neulasta (recombinant human granulocyte colony-stimulating factor analog). Coronal T1-weighted (**a**) and STIR (**b**) images of the pelvis demonstrate diffuse red marrow throughout the visualized skeleton with scattered tiny foci of fatty signal. Moderately increased metabolic activity is noted about the red marrow on the fused PET/CT image (**c**)

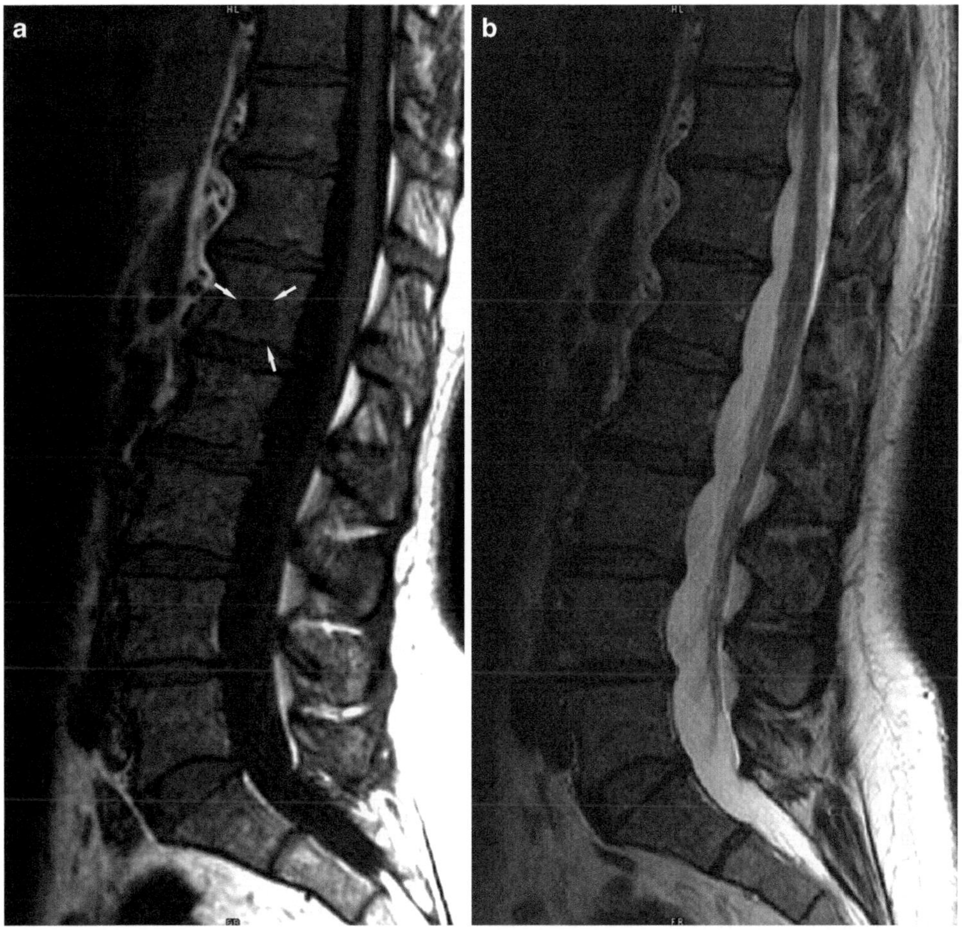

Fig. 1.75 Sagittal T1-weighted (**a**) and T2-weighted (**b**) images of the lumbar spine demonstrate round focus of prominent red marrow in L1 vertebral body (*arrows*) simulating a lesion. Note that this area is difficult to visualize on T2-weighted images

References

1. Steiner RM, Mitchell DG, Rao VM, Schweitzer ME. Magnetic resonance imaging of diffuse bone marrow disease. Radiol Clin North Am. 1993;31:383–409.
2. Burdiles A, Babyn PS. Pediatric bone marrow MR imaging. Magn Reson Imaging Clin N Am. 2009;17(3):391–409, v.
3. Laor T, Jaramillo D. MR imaging insights into skeletal maturation: what is normal? Radiology. 2009;250(1):28–38.
4. Vogler 3rd JB, Murphy WA. Bone marrow imaging. Radiology. 1988;168(3):679–93.
5. Moore SG, Dawson KL. Red and yellow marrow in the femur: age-related changes in appearance at MR imaging. Radiology. 1990; 175:219–23.
6. Kuntz A, Richins CA. Innervation of the bone marrow. J Comp Neurol. 1945;83:213–22.
7. DePace DM, Webber RH. Electrostimulation and morphologic study of the nerves of the bone marrow of the albino rat. Acta Anat. 1975;93:1–18.
8. Trubowitz S, Davis S. The bone marrow matrix. In: The human bone marrow: anatomy, physiology and pathophysiology. Boca Raton: CRC; 1982. p. 43–75.
9. Siegel MJ. MRI of bone marrow. In: Ho VB, Kransdorf MJ, Reinhold C, editors. Body MRI. Reston: American Roentgen Ray Society; 2006. p. 169–78.
10. Darge K, Jaramillo D, Siegel MJ. Whole-body MRI in children: current status and future applications. Eur J Radiol. 2008;68(2): 289–98.
11. Foster K, Chapman S, Johnson K. MRI of the marrow in the paediatric skeleton. Clin Radiol. 2004;59:651–73.
12. Jaramillo D, Laor T, Hoffer FA, et al. Epiphyseal marrow in infancy: MR imaging. Radiology. 1991;180:809–12. 2002;224:669–74.
13. Ricci C, Cova M, Kang YS, et al. Normal age-related patterns of cellular and fatty bone marrow distribution in the axial skeleton: MR imaging study. Radiology. 1990;177:83–8.
14. Zawin JK, Jaramillo D. Conversion of bone marrow in the humerus, sternum, and clavicle: changes with age on MR images. Radiology. 1993;188:159–64.
15. Taccone A, Oddone M, Dell'Acqua A, Occhi M, Ciccone MA. MRI "road-map" of normal age-related bone marrow. Pediatr Radiol. 1995;25:596–606.
16. Emery JL, Follett GF. Regression of bone marrow haemopoiesis from the terminal digits in the foetus and infant. Br J Haematol. 1964;10:485–9.
17. Haines RW. The histology of epiphyseal union in mammals. J Anat. 1975;120:1–25.
18. Ogden J. Anatomy and physiology of skeletal development: skeletal injury in the child. New York: Springer; 2000. p. 17–8.
19. Harcke HT, Snyder M, Caro PA, Bowen JR. Growth plate of the normal knee: evaluation with MR imaging. Radiology. 1992;183: 119–23.
20. Sasaki T, Ishibashi I, Okamura Y, Toh S, Sasaki K. MRI evaluation of growth plate closure rate and pattern in the normal knee joint. J Knee Surg. 2002;15:72–6.
21. Zbojniewicz AM, Laor T. Focal Periphyseal Edema (FOPE) zone on MRI of the adolescent knee: a potentially painful manifestation of physiologic physeal fusion? AJR Am J Roentgenol. 2011;197(4):998–1004.
22. Shabshin N, Schweitzer ME, Morrison WB, Carrino JA, Keller MS, Grissom LE. High-signal T2 changes of the bone marrow of the foot and ankle in children: red marrow or traumatic changes? Pediatr Radiol. 2006;36:670–6.
23. Scott JE, Bosworth TR, Cribb AM, Taylor JR. The chemical morphology of age-related changes in human intervertebral disc glycosaminoglycans from cervical, thoracic and lumbar nucleus pulposus and annulus fibrosus. J Anat. 1994;184(Pt 1):73–82.
24. Mirowitz SA. Hematopoietic bone marrow within the proximal humeral epiphysis in normal adults: investigation with MR imaging. Radiology. 1993;188(3):689–93.
25. Vande Berg BC, Lecouvet FE, Galant C, Maldague BE, Malghem J. Normal variants and frequent marrow alterations that simulate bone marrow lesions at MR imaging. Radiol Clin North Am. 2005;43(4):761–70, ix.
26. Okada Y, Aoki S, Barkovich AJ, Nishimura K, Norman D, Kjos BO, Brasch RC. Cranial bone marrow in children: assessment of normal development with MR imaging. Radiology. 1989;171(1): 161–4.
27. Yamada M, Matsuzaka T, Uetani M, Hayashi K, Tsuji Y, Nakamura T. Normal age-related conversion of bone marrow in the mandible: MR imaging findings. AJR Am J Roentgenol. 1995;165(5): 1223–8.
28. Dolan KD. Paranasal sinus radiology, part IA: introduction and the frontal sinuses. Head Neck Surg. 1982;4(4):301–11.
29. Dolan KD. Paranasal sinus radiology, Part 3A: sphenoidal sinus. Head Neck Surg. 1982;5(2):164–76.
30. Simonson TM, Kao SC. Normal childhood developmental patterns in skull bone marrow by MR imaging. Pediatr Radiol. 1992;22(8):556–9.
31. Sebag GH, Dubois J, Tabet M, Bonato A, Lallemand D. Pediatric spinal bone marrow: assessment of normal age-related changes in the MRI appearance. Pediatr Radiol. 1993;23:515–8.
32. De Bruyn PPH, Breen PC, Thomas TB. The microcirculation of the bone marrow. Anat Rec. 1970;168:55–68.
33. Weiss L. The structure of bone marrow functional interrelationships of vascular and hematopoietic compartments in experimental hemolytic anemia: an electron microscopic study. J Morphol. 1965;117:467–538.
34. Yao WJ, Hoh CK, Hawkins RA, et al. Quantitative PET imaging of bone marrow glucose metabolic response to hematopoietic cytokines. J Nucl Med. 1995;36:794–9.
35. Hollinger EF, Alibazoglu H, Ali A, Green A, La-Monica G. Hematopoietic cytokine-mediated FDG uptake simulates the appearance of diffuse metastatic disease on whole-body PET imaging. Clin Nucl Med. 1998;23:93–8.
36. Bordalo-Rodrigues M, Galant C, Lonneux M, Clause D, Vande Berg BC. Focal nodular hyperplasia of the hematopoietic marrow simulating vertebral metastasis on FDG positron emission tomography. AJR Am J Roentgenol. 2003;180(3):669–71.

Posttreatment-Related Marrow Changes

2

Kathleen Ruchalski, Kambiz Motamedi,
and Leanne L. Seeger

2.1 Radiation Therapy

Radiation therapy induces dynamic changes in bone marrow in both a time- and dose-dependent fashion. During the first week of treatment, localized doses of 20 Gy have been shown to reduce hematopoietic cellularity with corresponding histologic findings of edema, hemorrhage, and microvascular damage. Within the following week, early fatty conversion of marrow and cellular migration from surrounding unirradiated tissue has been described. These postradiation inflammatory changes and edema may be seen on magnetic resonance imaging (MRI) as early as 7 days after the initiation of radiation therapy. Early postradiation changes are characterized by diffuse hyperintensity on fluid-sensitive sequences: fat-saturated T2-weighted or short tau inversion recovery (STIR) images without significant signal changes on T1-weighted images (Fig. 2.1) [1]. During this acute phase, focal areas of T1 hyperintensity with reciprocal T2/STIR hypointensity within the bone marrow may represent hemorrhage [2]. Signal changes are more pronounced in the marrow closest to radiation port (Figs. 2.2 and 2.3). Although not necessary for the evaluation of bone marrow, the use of dynamic MR may demonstrate transient contrast enhancement during the first 2 weeks and is thought to be related to capillary damage and vascular congestion [3].

With time, bone marrow edema subsides, and the consequences of microvascular damage and sinusoidal destruction are better delineated. In addition to early fatty conversion of marrow, histologic evaluation of bone marrow between 1 and 3 months postradiation demonstrates early endosteal fibrosis with a decrease in the number of sinusoids. Early fatty infiltration and fibrosis is characterized by heterogeneous T1 hyperintensity compared to muscle and may occasionally demonstrate centrally located areas of fat signal intensity (Fig. 2.4). While these changes may be detected as early as 1 week after radiation therapy initiation (Fig. 2.1), the majority of characteristics are visible after 3–6 weeks (Figs. 2.3 and 2.4). Eventually, the MRI signal changes evolve into homogeneous and diffusely hyperintense T1 with corresponding hypointense STIR signal, the intensity compatible with fatty conversion [1] (Figs. 2.5 and 2.6) within the boundaries of radiation port. These findings are diffuse when total body radiation is applied without identifiable radiation port (Fig. 2.7).

Fatty marrow conversion is not necessarily permanent, as hematopoietic and sinusoidal regeneration has been demonstrated 6 months after a single dose of 20 Gy. It is suggested that radiation doses over 40 Gy cause irreversible injury [3]. Comparable changes in bone marrow signal due to fatty conversion may be seen adjacent to the radiation field and are thought to be related to very low doses of radiation scatter [2].

H. Ilaslan, M. Sundaram, *Pediatric and Adult MRI Atlas of Bone Marrow: Normal Appearances, Variants and Diffuse Disease States*, DOI 10.1007/978-3-642-02740-6_2

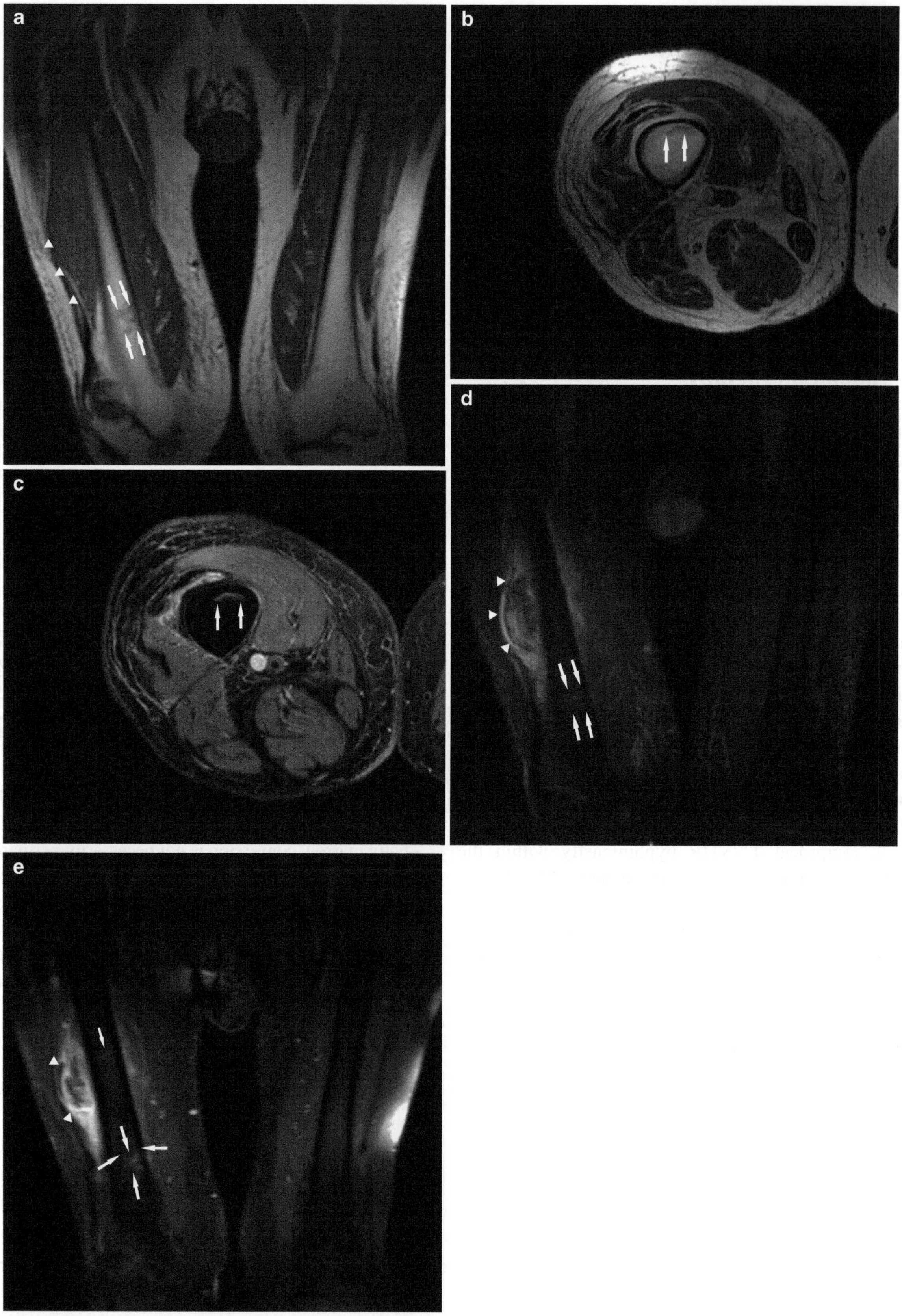

Fig. 2.1 MRI of the right femur obtained shortly after completion of radiation therapy for right thigh sarcoma (*arrowheads*). T1-weighted coronal (**a**) and axial (**b**), T2-weighted fat-suppressed axial, (**c**) STIR coronal (**d**), and fat-saturated T1-weighted postcontrast coronal (**e**) images demonstrate mild bone marrow edema (*short arrows*) and lobulated subcortical foci of abnormal marrow signal along the right proximal femoral shaft (*long arrows*) consistent with early radiation changes

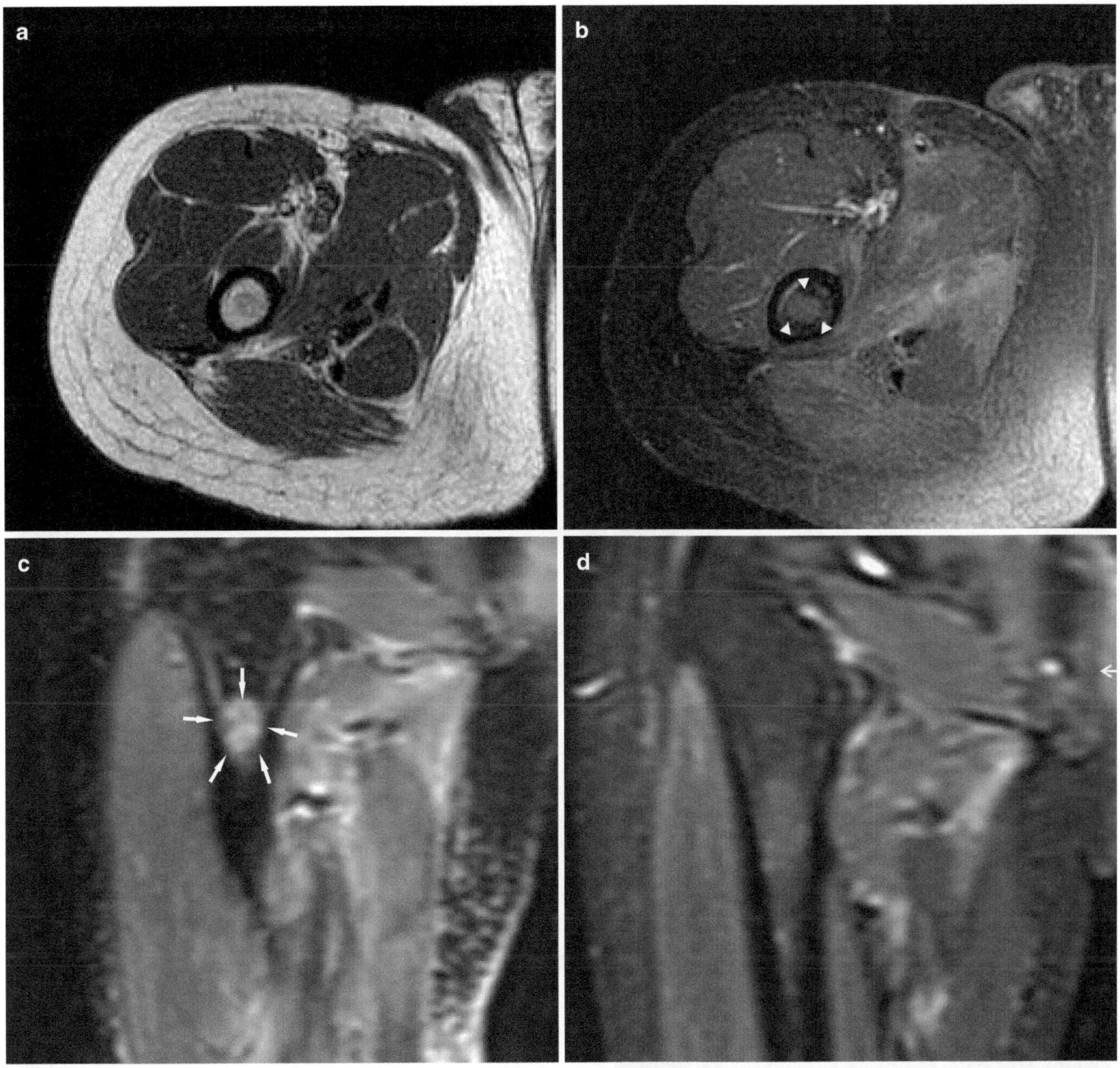

Fig. 2.2 Coronal T1-weighted (**a**) and fat-saturated T1-weighted postcontrast (**b**) images as well as coronal inversion recovery image (**c**) of the right femur obtained shortly after surgical resection and radiation therapy for right proximal thigh sarcoma. There is heterogeneous marrow signal along the right proximal femoral shaft. There is increased marrow signal on inversion recovery (*arrows*) and subtle enhancement on postcontrast images (*arrowheads*) of subtrochanteric region of the right femoral shaft which demonstrates consistency with early postradiation changes. Coronal inversion recovery image acquired several months later (**d**) illustrates improvement in signal changes in proximal femur marrow and overlying soft tissues

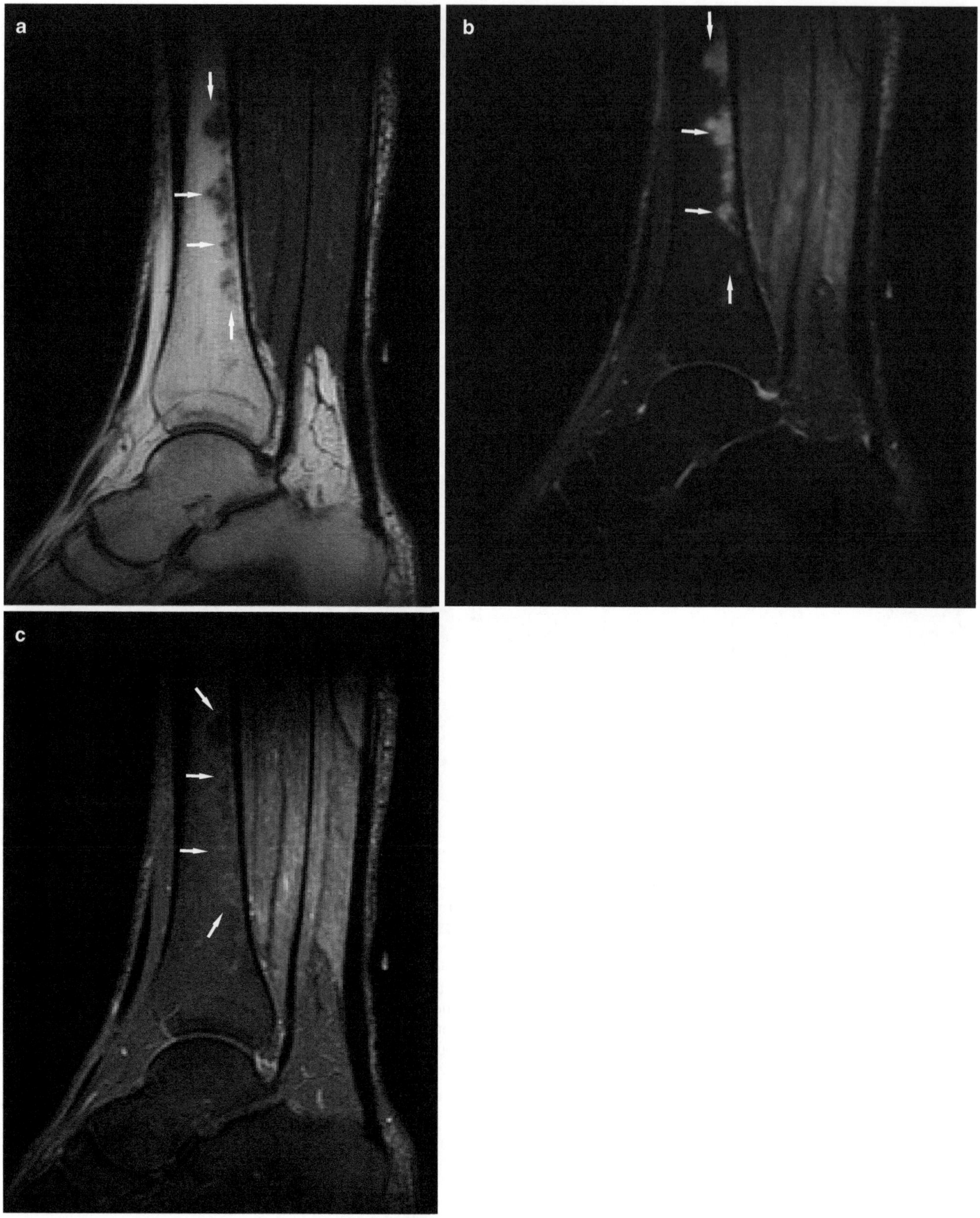

Fig. 2.3 Sagittal T1-weighted (**a**), STIR (**b**), and postcontrast fat-suppressed T1-weighted (**c**) images of the ankle in a patient with distal calf sarcoma resection and 11 months after completion of radiation therapy demonstrate foci of hypointense T1 and hyperintense STIR signal with minimal enhancement consistent with radiation changes. Please note the subcortical location of these changes closer to radiation port (*arrows*) and the overlying muscle edema

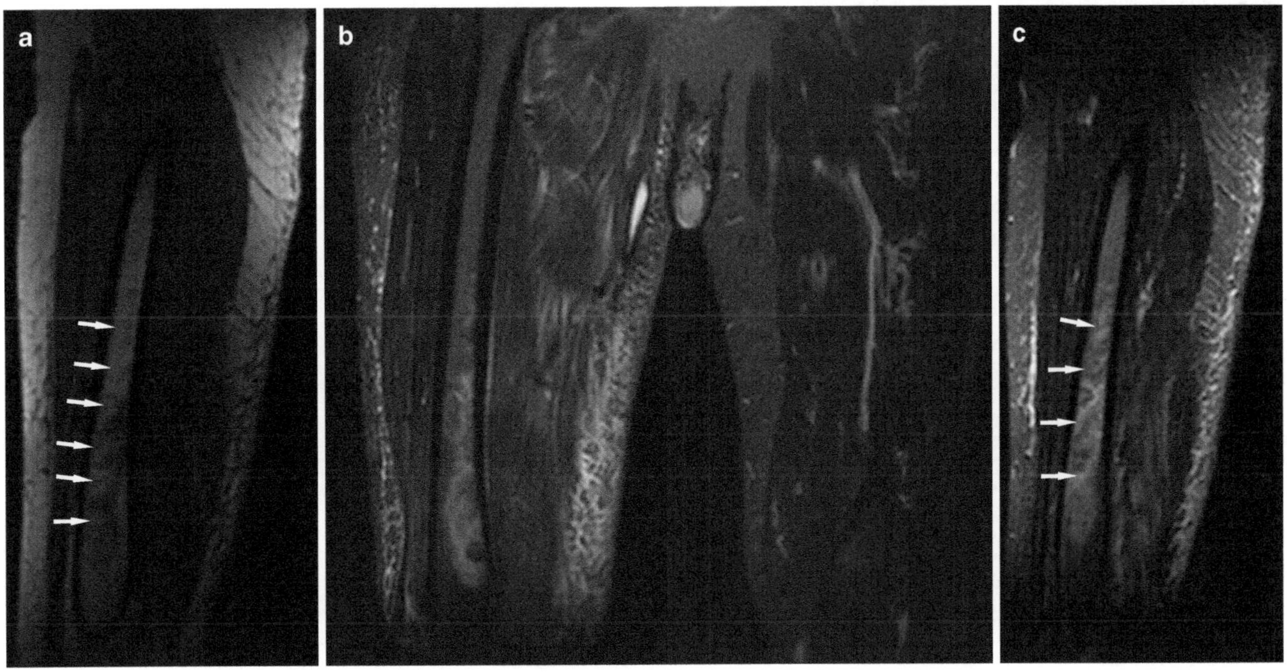

Fig. 2.4 Sagittal T1-weighted (**a**), sagittal T2-weighted (**b**), and coronal inversion recovery (**c**) images of the right femur approximately 1 year after completing radiation therapy illustrate a long segment heterogeneous foci of T2/STIR hyperintensity (*arrows*) with intermixed fatty signal

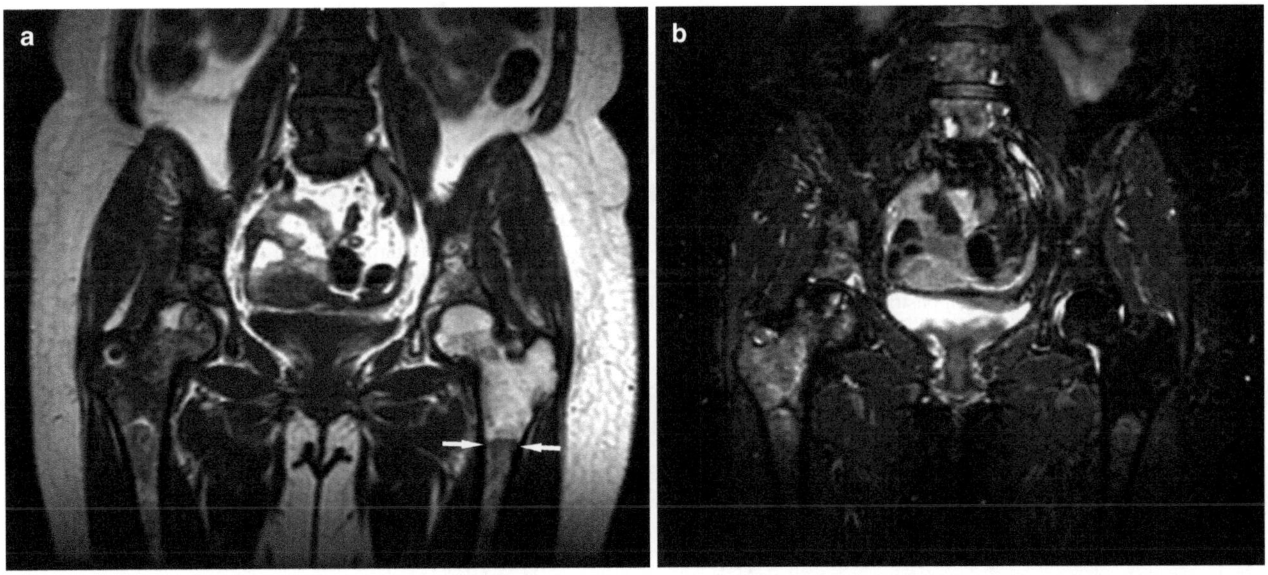

Fig. 2.5 MRI of the pelvis with coronal T1-weighted (**a**) and STIR (**b**) images. Within the proximal left femur, including the head, neck, and proximal shaft, there is heterogeneously increased T1 signal intensity with corresponding decreased STIR intensity, consistent with fatty marrow replacement. The sharp demarcation between this region of fatty signal and the more distal femoral shaft is consistent with a radiation port (*arrows*)

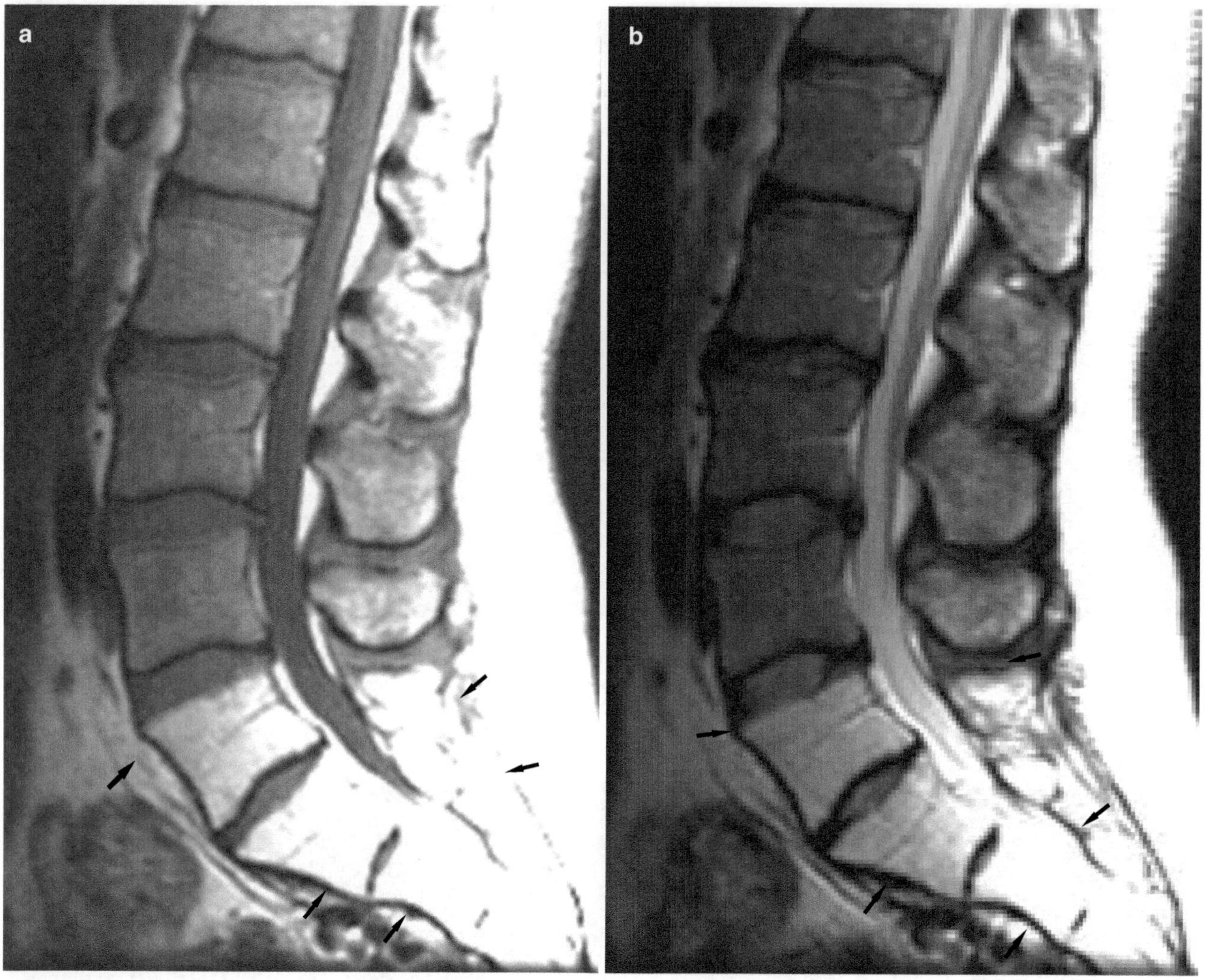

Fig. 2.6 MRI of the lumbar spine with T1-weighted (**a**) and fat-suppressed T2-weighted images (**b**) approximately 2 years after radiation therapy for colon cancer demonstrate increased T1-weighted marrow signal intensity throughout the sacrum and at the L5 vertebral body (*arrows*), consistent with postradiation changes

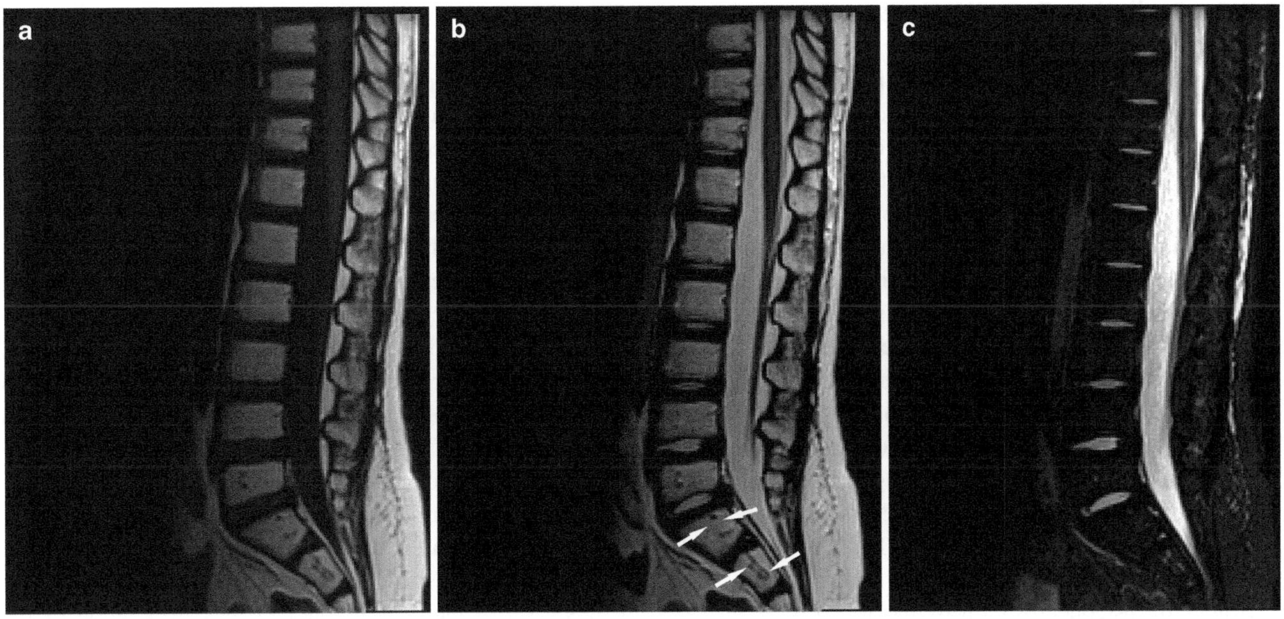

Fig. 2.7 A 4-year-old boy, status post total body radiation 4 months prior. T1-weighted (**a**), T2-weighted (**b**), and STIR (**c**) sagittal images of the thoracolumbar spine and sacrum demonstrate diffuse fatty marrow signal consistent with postradiation changes. Please note small foci of marrow infarctions in the S1 and S2 segments (*arrows*)

2.1.1 Radiation Complications

Osseous complications related to radiation therapy depend on multiple factors, including radiation dose, fractionation and duration, as well as the patient's age and the particular bones involved [4]. Exposure to radiation may lead to acute complications in addition to latent consequences [5].

Radiation osteitis is caused by vascular damage as well as osteoblastic and osteoclastic injury without bone infarction. Radiographic findings are typically visible within the first 3 years after irradiation. Radiation osteitis is usually associated with lower doses of radiation exposure and is potentially reversible. Radiographic findings consist of a disorganized trabecular pattern and focal areas of osteopenia intermixed with dense sclerotic bone. On MR imaging, radiation osteitis may be considered in the differential diagnosis for heterogeneous T1 hypointensity with T2/STIR hyperintensity [3] (Fig. 2.8).

Radiation osteonecrosis (avascular necrosis) is an early complication of radiation therapy, particularly with higher dosages. This disease process is fundamentally similar to radiation osteitis as it involves radiation-induced arteritis and fibrosis, as well as vascular obstruction. Radiation osteonecrosis, however, also leads to bone infarction. MRI is the preferred and most sensitive method for evaluating osteonecrosis. Bone marrow edema is the earliest sign, with MRI findings of diffusely increased T2-weighted signal. The classic double-line sign eventually forms as a low signal intensity line on T1- or T2-weighted images circumscribing a region of high signal intensity (Fig. 2.9). The centrally located focus of high signal intensity represents hyperemic granulation tissue and is peripherally surrounded by sclerotic bone [3] (Fig. 2.10).

Insufficiency fractures may be a primary consequence of radiation therapy or occur secondarily from radiation osteitis and osteonecrosis (Figs. 2.11 and 2.12). These fractures are caused by normal stress on architecturally altered bone. The imaging characteristics of insufficiency fractures depend on the acuity of the injury. A fracture line may demonstrate hyperintensity on fluid-sensitive sequences with reciprocal T1 hypointensity, as well as enhancement on postcontrast T1-weighted images. With acute fractures, bone marrow edema often accompanies the fracture line and is visualized on T1-weighted and/or fluid-sensitive sequences. In the setting of malignancy, visualization of linear fracture line on T1-weighted images may aid in differentiating associated bone marrow edema from infiltrating tumor, as both will demonstrate hyperintense T2-weighted signal [3]. Radiographic correlation often helps in demonstrating the fracture line and showing signs of healing in follow-up.

Exposure to radiation doses as low as 1200 Gy in children has been associated with alterations in skeletal maturation. Children are particularly sensitive to radiation exposure during early childhood and adolescent growth spurts [5]. Radiation of the growth plate interferes with chondrogenesis and causes cartilage and bone calcium reabsorption, with abnormal mineral deposition. In addition to the marrow edema and fatty conversion also seen in adults, radiation of the growth plate causes metaphyseal sclerosis and fraying, as well as epiphyseal widening [6]. On MR imaging, these growth arrest lines are seen as metaphyseal hypointense bands on T1- and T2-weighted images. Irradiation of the spine may lead to decreased vertebral body height, scalloping of the end plates, as well as scoliosis. Radiation-induced scoliosis commonly presents during the adolescent growth spurt and is concave to the radiation field. Bowing of irradiated bone and limb length discrepancy has also been described. Radiation of the proximal femur predisposes children to an increased risk of slipped capital femoral epiphysis [3] (Fig. 2.13). Craniofacial bony deformities caused by therapeutic radiation-induced bone growth inhibition can occur in nearly all survivors of childhood head and neck cancers [7] with variable bone marrow signal changes (Fig. 2.14).

Delayed complications of radiation therapy include benign and malignant tumors. Benign entities include osteochondroma, fibrous dysplasia, and aneurysmal bone cysts [8]. Although rare, treatment-related sarcomas have been described to occur within previous radiation beds at least 3 years and usually after 10 years or more after treatment [9]. The criteria of radiation-induced sarcoma diagnosis proposed by Cahan et al. [10] and modified by Arlen et al. [11] are treatment with therapeutic irradiation at least 3 years prior to development of sarcoma, a sarcoma arising within the field of previous therapeutic irradiation, and histology that is different from the primary tumor that required radiotherapy. These sarcomas are typically high grade and large tumors.

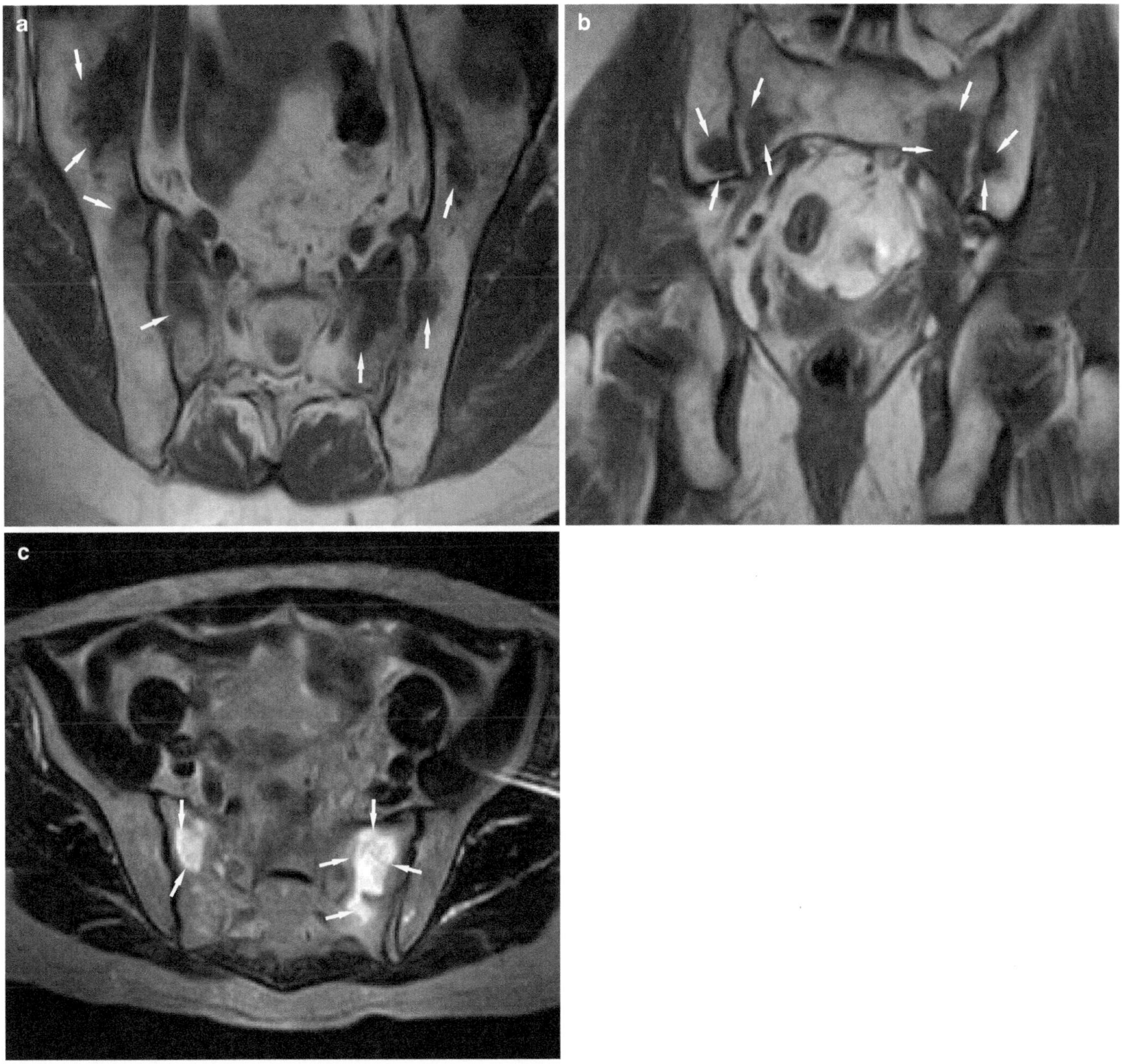

Fig. 2.8 A 54-year-old male, status post pelvic radiation. Axial (**a**) and coronal (**b**) T1-weighted images as well as axial (**c**) T2-weighted images of the pelvis. There are geographic areas of signal abnormality along the iliac sides of the sacroiliac joints bilaterally (*arrows*). These areas demonstrate primarily isointense T1 signal and hyperintense T2/STIR signal consistent with radiation-induced osteitis

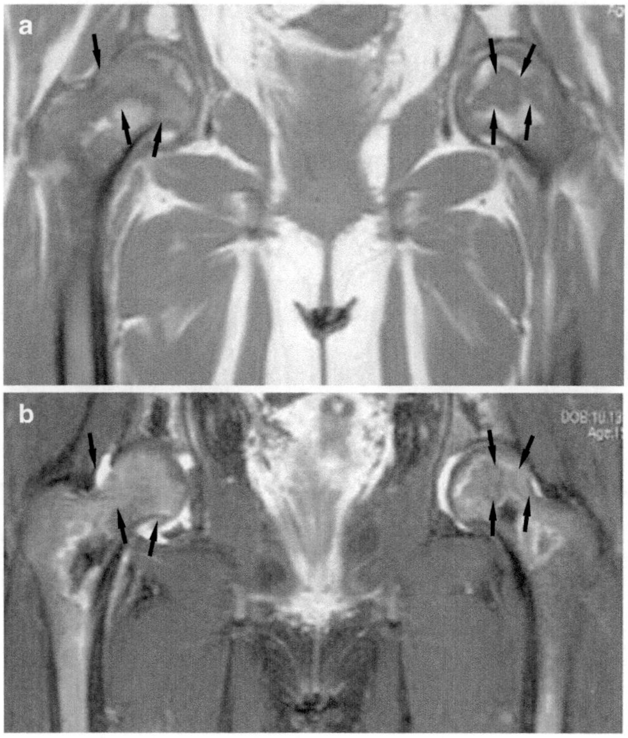

Fig. 2.9 A 78-year-old female, status post chemotherapy. Coronal T1-weighted (**a**) and inversion recovery images (**b**) of the pelvis demonstrate bone infarction of the femurs with a T1 hypointense and T2 hyperintense line (*arrows*) circumscribing the region of necrotic bone

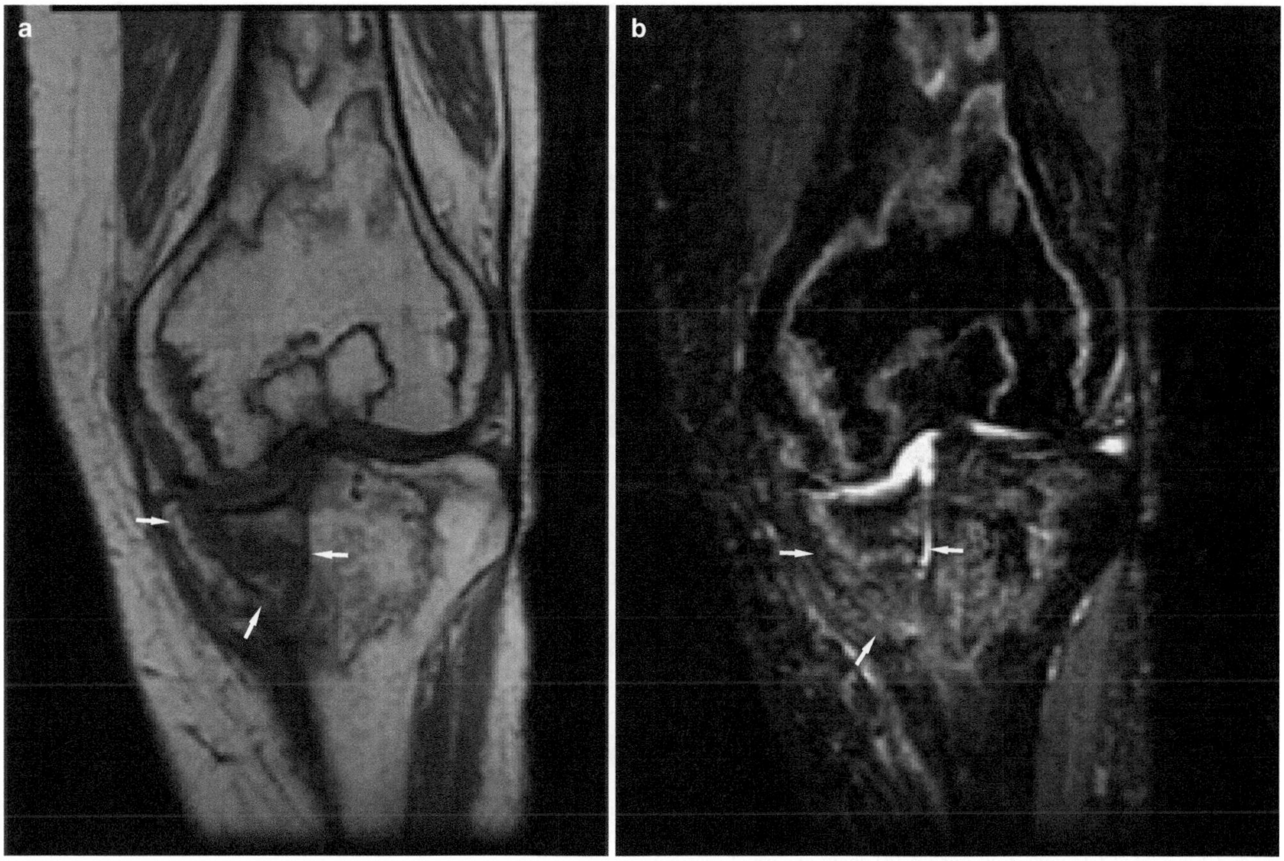

Fig. 2.10 Coronal T1-weighted (**a**) and inversion recovery images (**b**) of the knee demonstrate bone infarction of the distal femur, with a T1 hypointense and T2 hyperintense line circumscribing the region of necrotic bone. Also of note is a tibial plateau subchondral collapse with associated bone marrow edema (*arrows*)

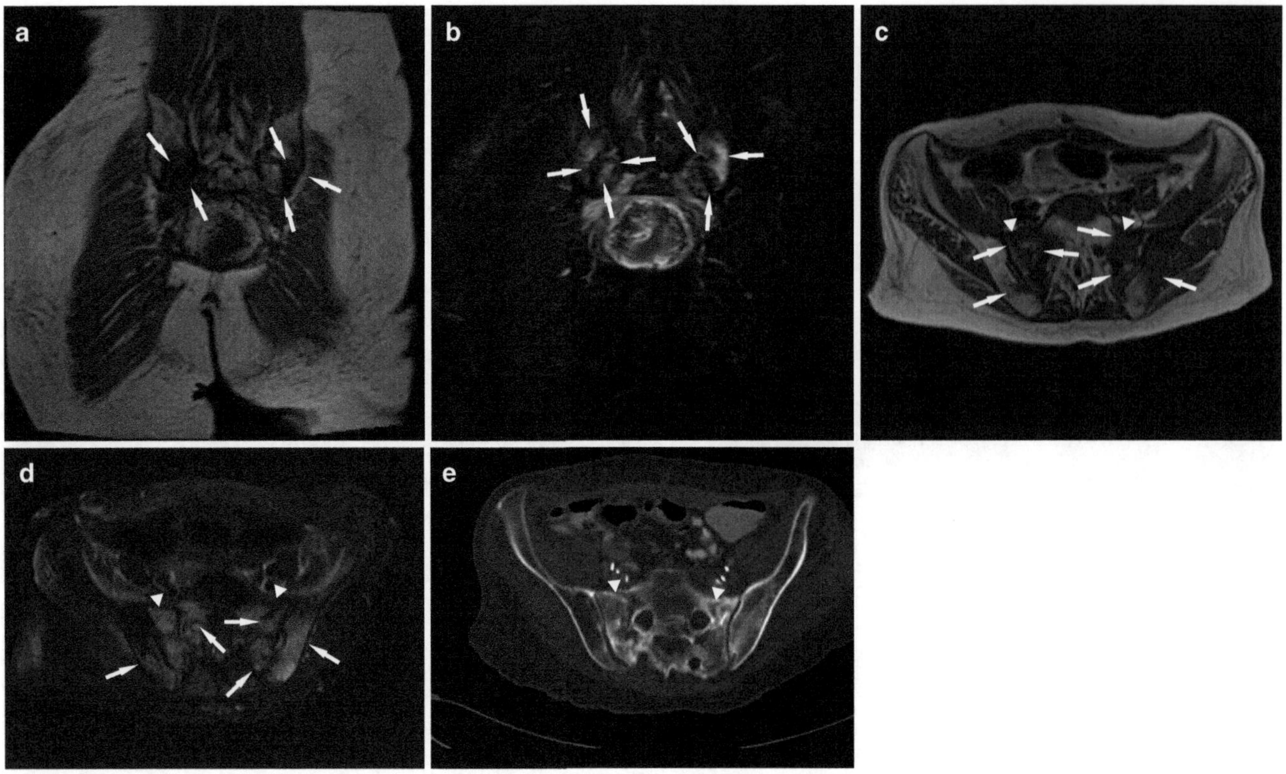

Fig. 2.11 A 67-year-old male after radiation treatment of the pelvis. Coronal T1-weighted (**a**), coronal STIR (**b**), axial T1-weighted (**c**), and axial T2-weighted fat-suppressed images (**d**) show abnormal marrow signal (*arrows*). Fracture lines (*arrowheads*) could be seen on MR images although they appear more discrete on CT image (**e**)

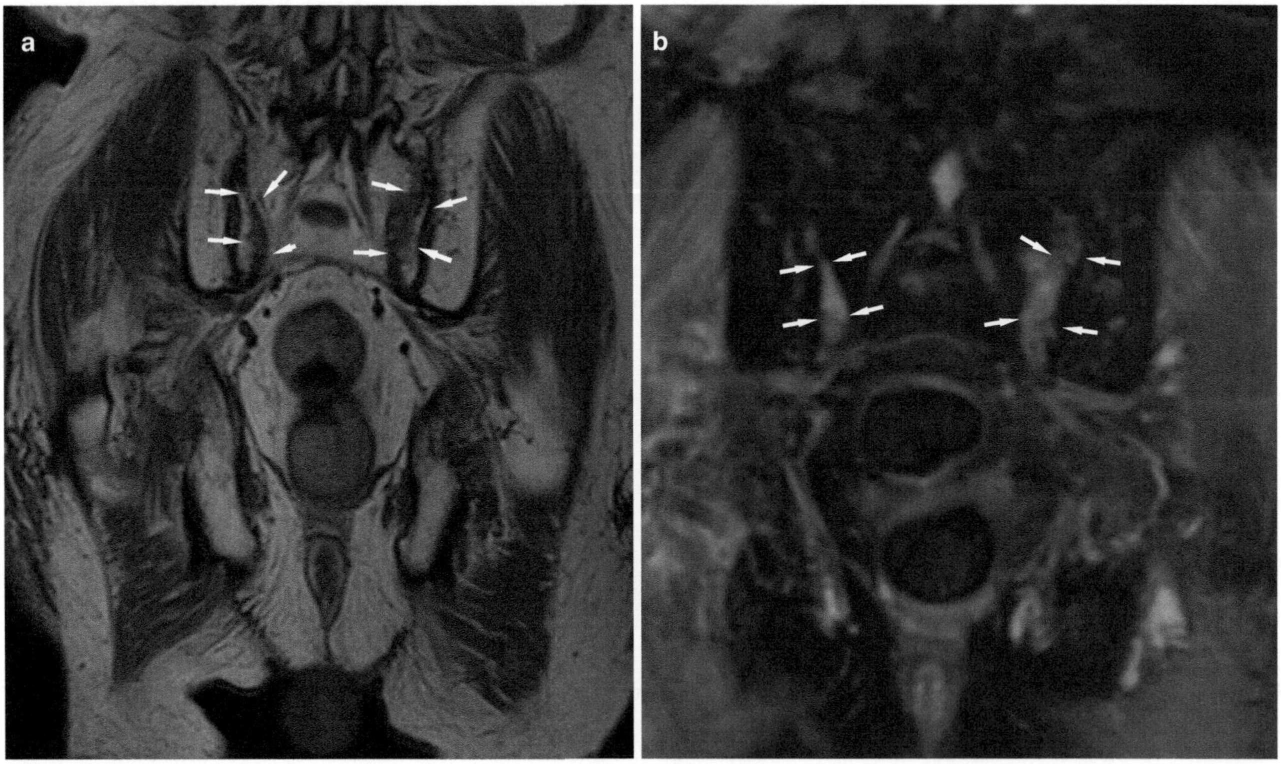

Fig. 2.12 A 72-year-old male 2 years after pelvic radiation. Coronal T1-weighted (**a**) and coronal STIR (**b**) images demonstrate linear insufficiency fracture lines of the sacral ala parallel to SI joints bilaterally (*arrows*) in the background of fatty marrow

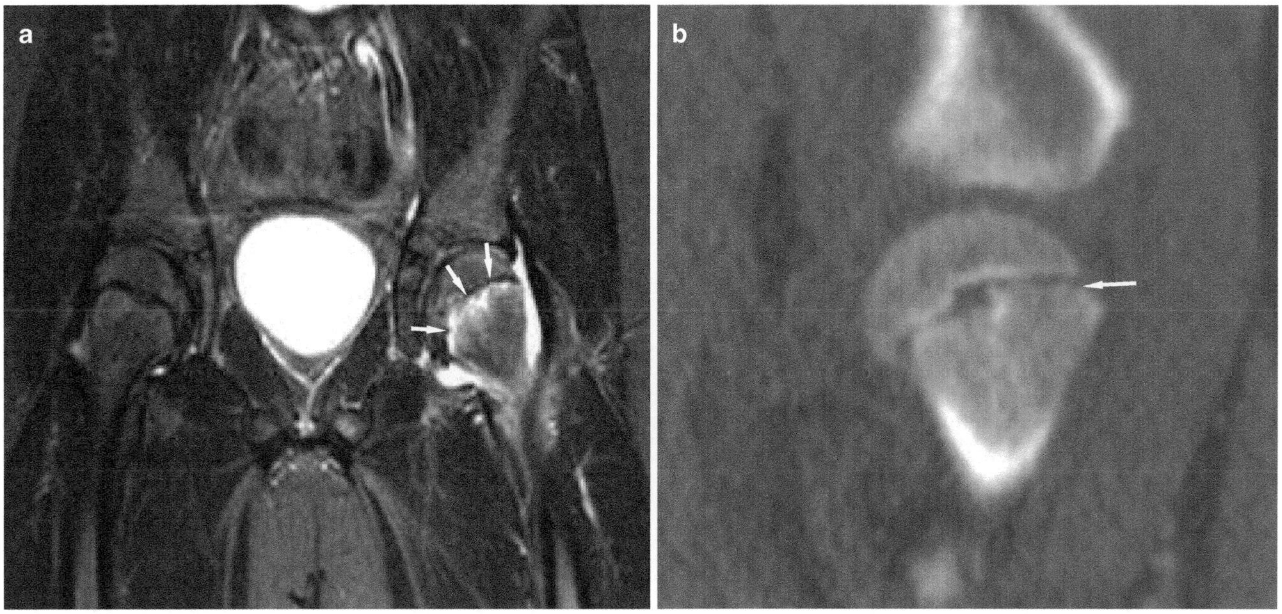

Fig. 2.13 Coronal STIR (**a**) image of the pelvis shows increased signal within the physis of the femoral head with medial and posterior displacement of the capital epiphysis (*arrows*) and surrounding bone marrow edema. A sagittal CT of the hip (**b**) better demonstrates displacement of the femoral head (*arrow*)

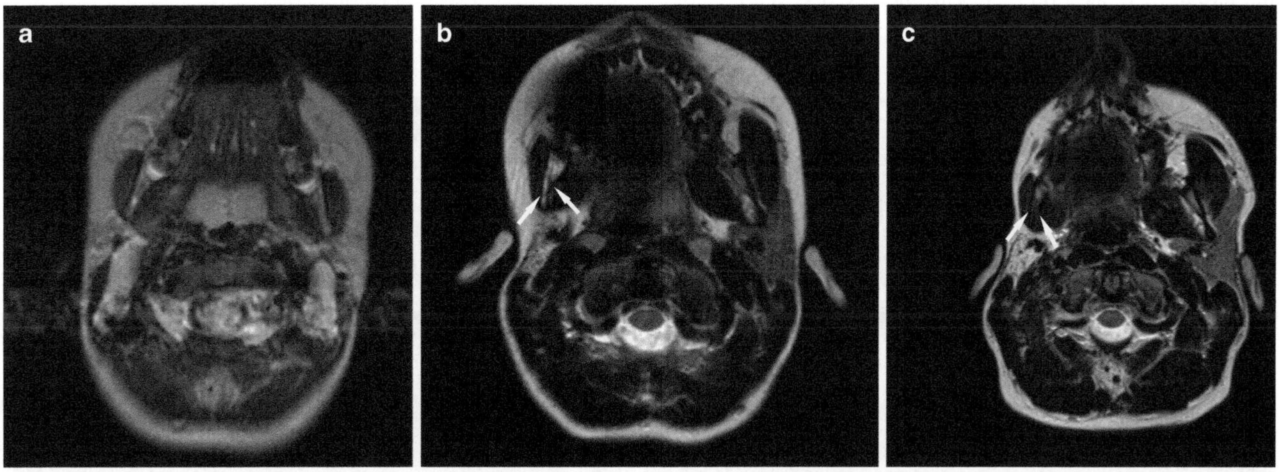

Fig. 2.14 Status post right masticator space rhabdomyosarcoma resection and radiation treatment at the age of 4. Serial T2-weighted axial MR images of the mandible demonstrate symmetric mandibular condyles bilaterally in the immediate postoperative and postradiation MRI of 2001 (**a**). Follow-up MRIs from 2006 (**b**) and 2013 (**c**) demonstrate smaller right mandibular condyle with radiation-related marrow signal changes (*arrows*). Overall findings are consistent with radiation-induced bone growth inhibition

2.2 Chemotherapy

Hematologic malignancies such as leukemia, lymphoma, and multiple myeloma infiltrate bone marrow, causing neoplastic replacement of the normal fat-containing marrow. Tumor infiltration produces distinct changes in MR signaling, including prolongation of T1 relaxation times. Hypercellularity and subsequent increased intracellular water content is visualized as an increased signal intensity on fluid-sensitive sequences when compared to normal bone marrow. These areas demonstrate reciprocal hypointense T1-weighted signaling compared to muscle. Detection and signal features vary based on tumor burden and distribution [3]. Although bone marrow aspiration and biopsy are the preferred methods for diagnosing, staging, and monitoring treatment response of bone marrow malignancies, imaging has provided an additional tool for the evaluation of disease activity [12].

There are three histologic stages of bone marrow remodeling after the initiation of chemotherapy. During the first week, increased permeability and dilatation of the bone marrow sinuses causes acute edema [13]. Evaluation with MR imaging during initiation of chemotherapy demonstrates increased T1 relaxation time with increased signal on fluid-sensitive sequences and a corresponding decrease in T1-weighted intensity (Fig. 2.15) [14].

The second stage of bone marrow remodeling occurs as early as the second week after chemotherapy initiation. Histologically, there is decreased marrow cellularity, as well as early fatty conversion to multilocular adipocytes [13]. On MR imaging, these pathologic changes cause an increased T1-weighted signal and decreased intensity on fluid-sensitive sequences, with a corresponding increase in T1 relaxation times [3] (Fig. 2.16).

Finally, with the completion of chemotherapy, multilocular adipocytes are replaced by unilocular fat cells. These unilocular adipocytes and stromal cells form multifocal aggregates and are thought to be necessary for regeneration of normal hematopoietic tissue [13]. Early reconversion on MR imaging is seen as diffuse hematopoietic foci of T1 hypointensity and modest hyperintensity on fluid-sensitive sequences (Fig. 2.17). In the setting of malignancy, regeneration of hematopoietic tissue may be differentiated from clinical relapse on T1-weighted postcontrast images. Given the hypervascular nature of malignant cells, avid contrast enhancement would suggest a neoplastic process. In addition to contrast enhancement, increase in size of known infiltrates and findings of new focal marrow lesions are compatible with clinical relapse [3].

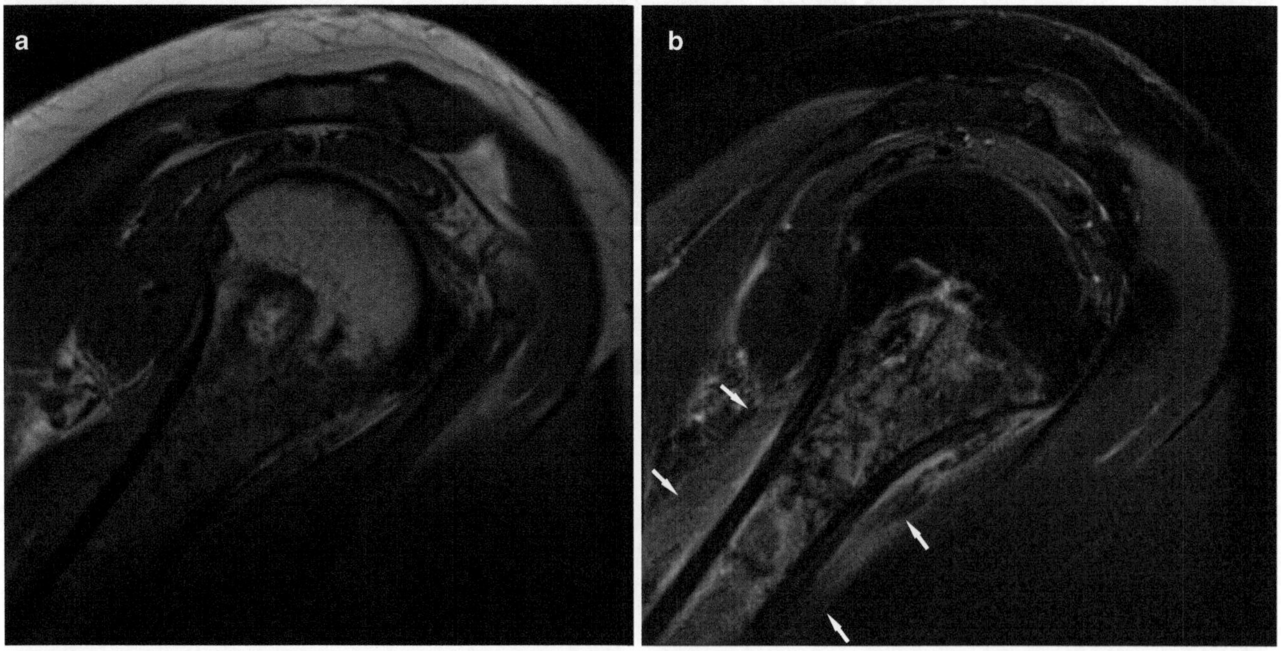

Fig. 2.15 A 38-year-old female with known lymphoma. An MRI of the right shoulder was obtained 6 days after the start of chemotherapy regimen. T1-weighted (**a**) sagittal image demonstrates heterogeneously hypointense marrow signal in proximal humerus with corresponding heterogeneously hyperintense signal on T2-weighted fat-suppressed sagittal image (**b**). Soft tissue edema and periostitis noted on T2-weighted images (*arrows*)

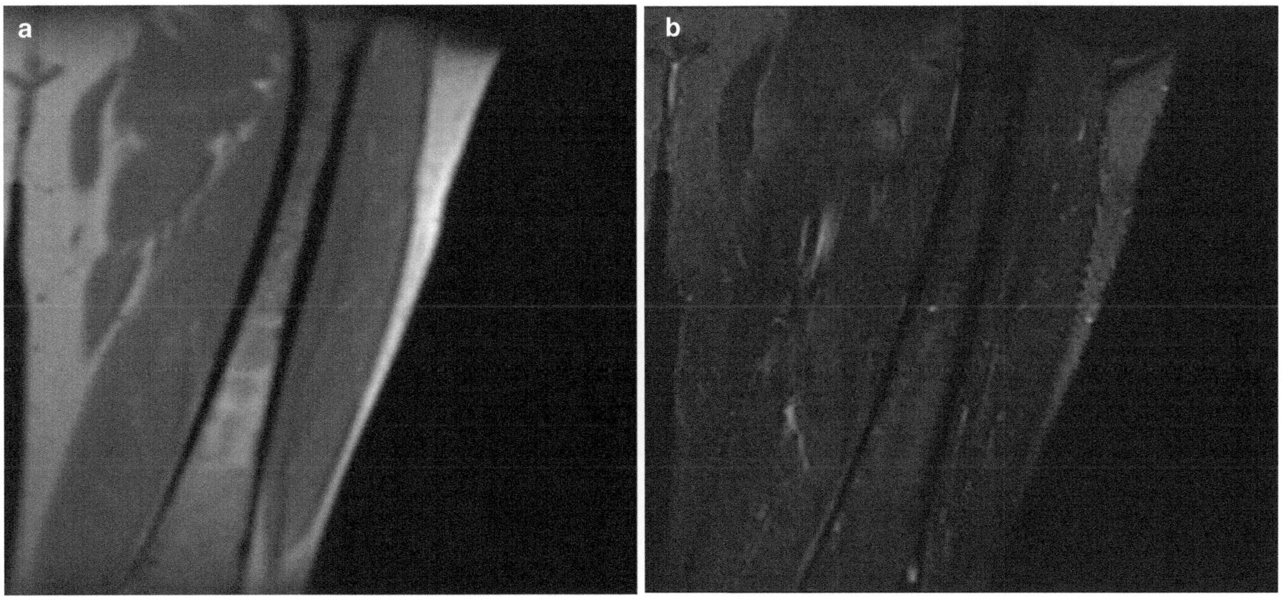

Fig. 2.16 Coronal T1-weighted image of the left femur (**a**) of a 38-year-old female 3 weeks into chemotherapy demonstrates diffuse hematopoietic marrow proliferation. No corresponding hyperintense bone marrow signal on T2-weighted fat-suppressed image (**b**)

Fig. 2.17 Sagittal T1- (**a**) and T2-weighted (**b**) images of the thoracic spine with scattered foci of increased T1-weighted intensity consistent with fatty infiltration (*arrows*) 1 year after chemotherapy

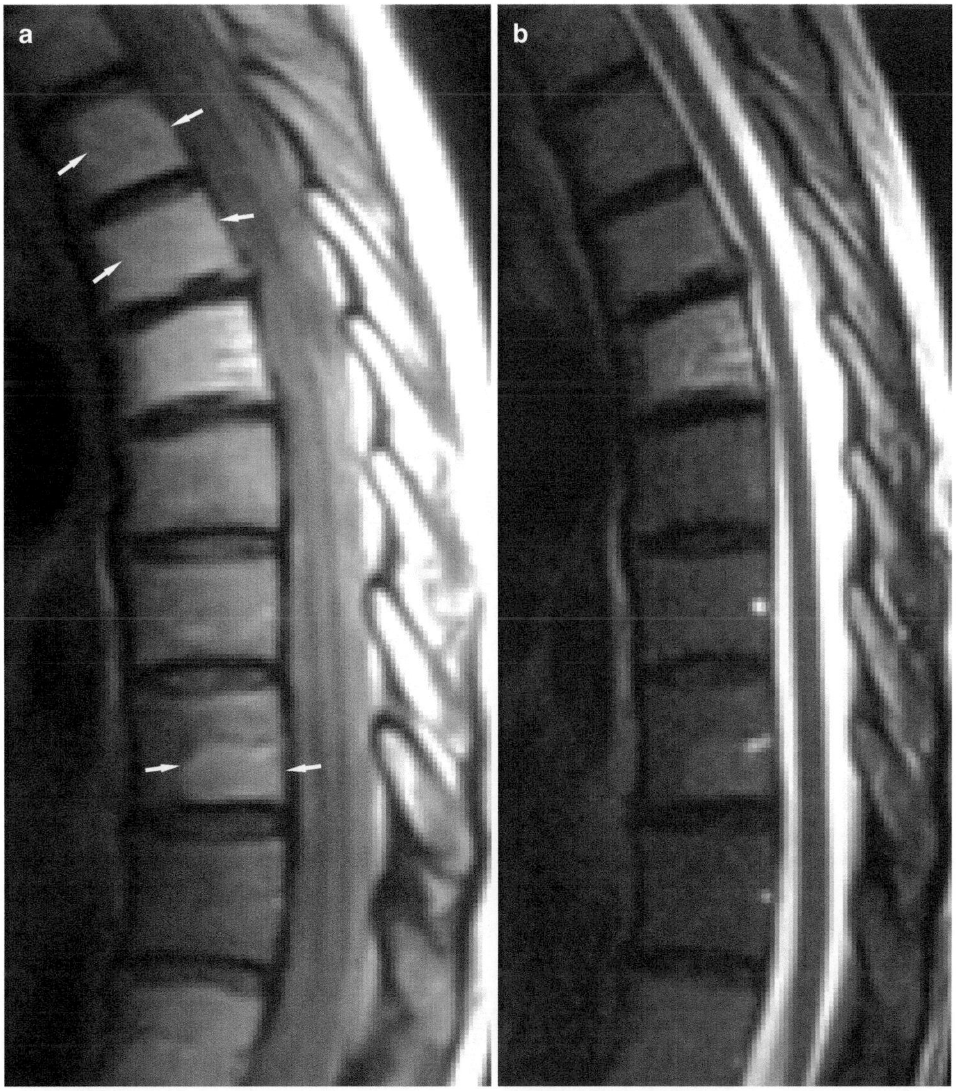

2.2.1 Lymphoma/Leukemia

Diagnosis, prognosis, and imaging characteristics of lymphoma depend on the cell lineage and degree of differentiation. Hodgkin's lymphoma represents approximately 25 % of lymphomas. Although bone marrow involvement is an uncommon presentation of Hodgkin's lymphoma, approximately 5–32 % may have bone marrow involvement with disseminated disease. Bone marrow infiltration usually presents as focal areas, with near-complete normalization of bone marrow signal after the initiation of chemotherapy (Fig. 2.18) [15]. Non-Hodgkin's lymphomas are more likely to involve bone marrow, and account for 20–40 % of patients [16].

Bone marrow changes after chemotherapy for lymphoma are usually similar to those of leukemia and myeloma, with eventual normalization of bone marrow signal with small foci of residual signal abnormalities. There is, however, a case series of patients with the nodular sclerosis subtype of Hodgkin's lymphoma where complete reversal of tumor signal, with diffuse hyperintense T1 and hypointense STIR signal within bone marrow after the completion of chemotherapy, was reported. The signal characteristics are similar to those described after radiation therapy and are also thought to be related to complete fatty conversion of marrow [17].

Osteonecrosis (avascular necrosis) may also be seen in this patient subset following chemotherapy and should not be confused with residual/recurrent tumor (Fig. 2.19) given the typical imaging of preserved fatty signal surrounded by serpentine areas of abnormal signal.

Treated focal lymphoma lesions may show imaging features reminiscent of osteonecrosis (Fig. 2.20). In the lower extremities, fractures could develop due to weakening of bone simulating tumor recurrence clinically which, if present, could be diagnosed on imaging, unequivocally (Fig. 2.21).

Chemotherapy produces similar marrow responses in patients with leukemia (Fig. 2.22). Although not used clinically, sequential quantitative MRI has been shown to be useful for monitoring treatment response in acute lymphoid leukemia (ALL) more so than for acute myeloid leukemia (AML). During the second week of chemotherapy, an increase in T1 values may be seen with AML, whereas T1 values decrease in ALL. It is presumed that the increased T1 value seen in AML is related to a larger amount of edema and necrosis associated with the highly toxic chemotherapeutic agents [3] (Fig. 2.23).

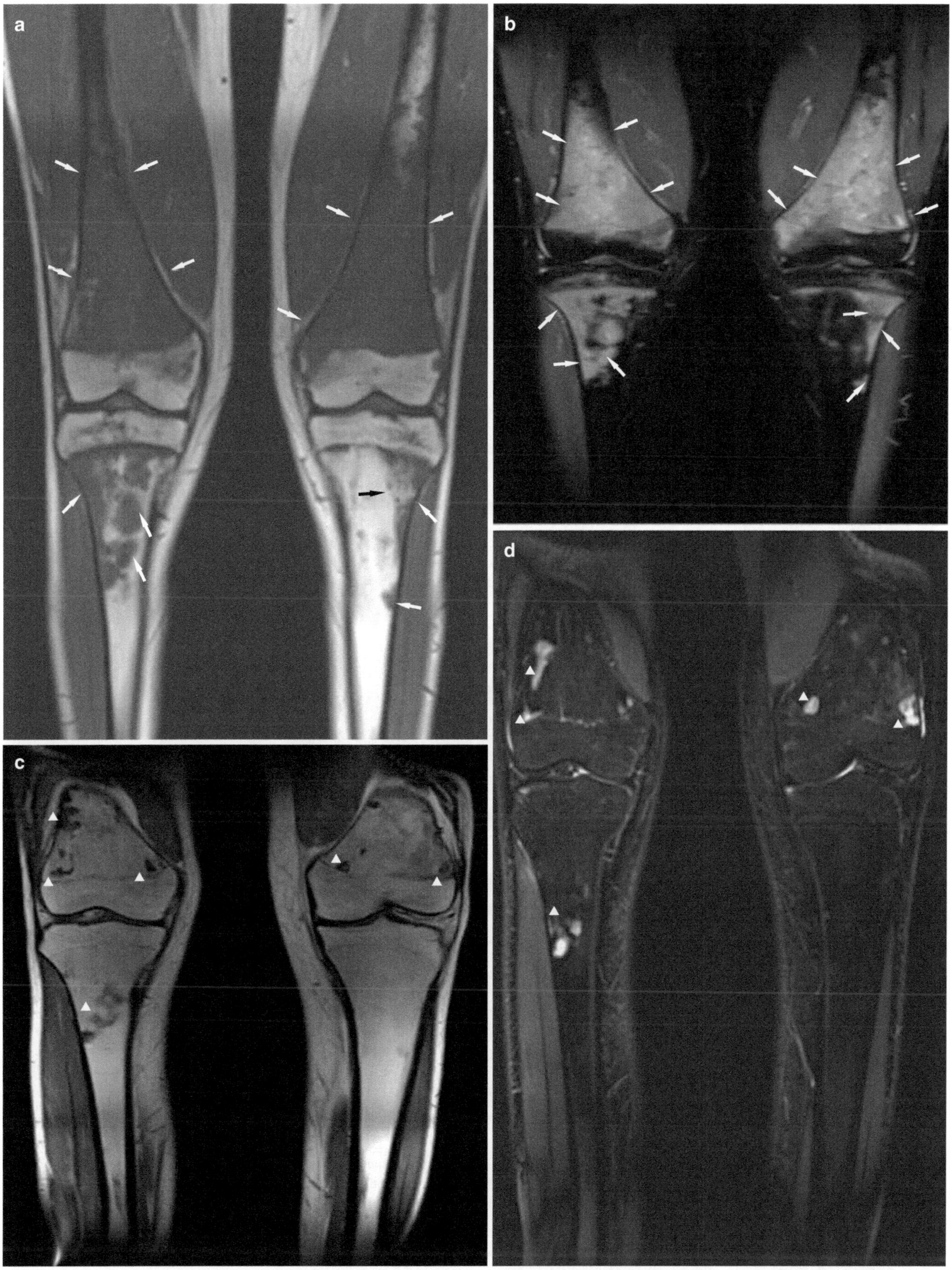

Fig. 2.18 A 17-year-old patient with diffuse large B cell lymphoma. Coronal T1-weighted (**a**) and T2-weighted fat-suppressed (**b**) images of the lower extremities at the time of initial diagnosis show large areas of bone marrow infiltration most marked about the distal femurs bilaterally (*arrows*). Three-month follow-up MRI after completion of chemotherapy demonstrates near normal bone marrow signal with small foci of hypointense T1 (**c**) and hyperintense T2 signal (**d**) likely representing infarcts (*arrowheads*)

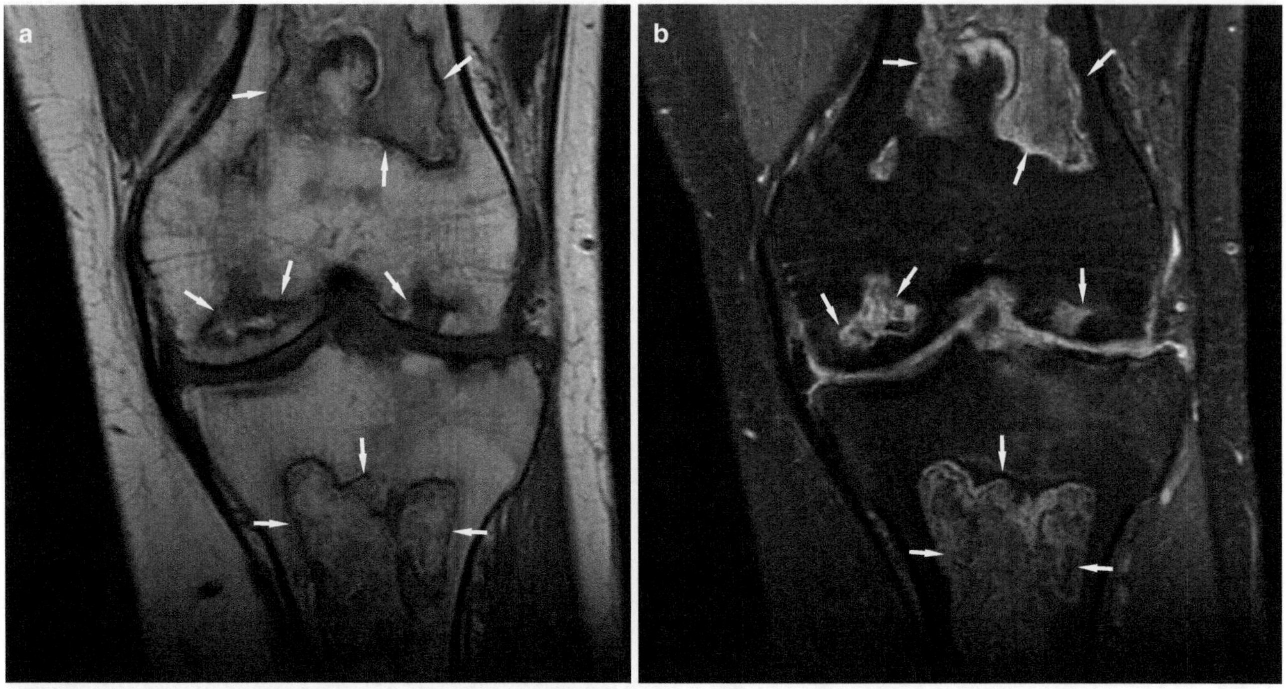

Fig. 2.19 A 58-year-old male, status post chemotherapy for systemic lymphoma. Coronal T1-weighted image (**a**) and T2-weighted fat-suppressed image (**b**) demonstrate large areas of serpentine signal abnormalities (*arrows*) with preservation of fatty signal centrally consistent with bone infarcts

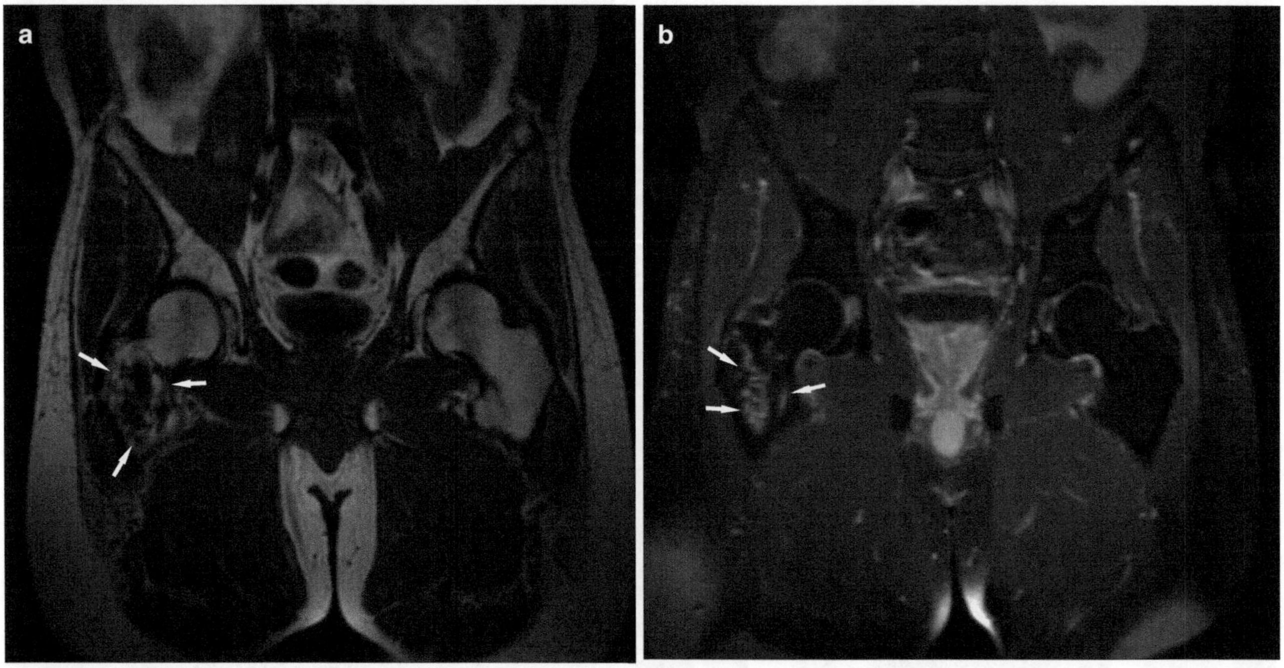

Fig. 2.20 Coronal T1-weighted precontrast (**a**) and T1-weighted fat-suppressed postcontrast (**b**) images demonstrate serpentine areas of hypointense signal with intermixed fatty marrow (*arrows*) and linear areas of enhancement. Findings correspond to a treated lymphoma lesion in a patient with clinical remission

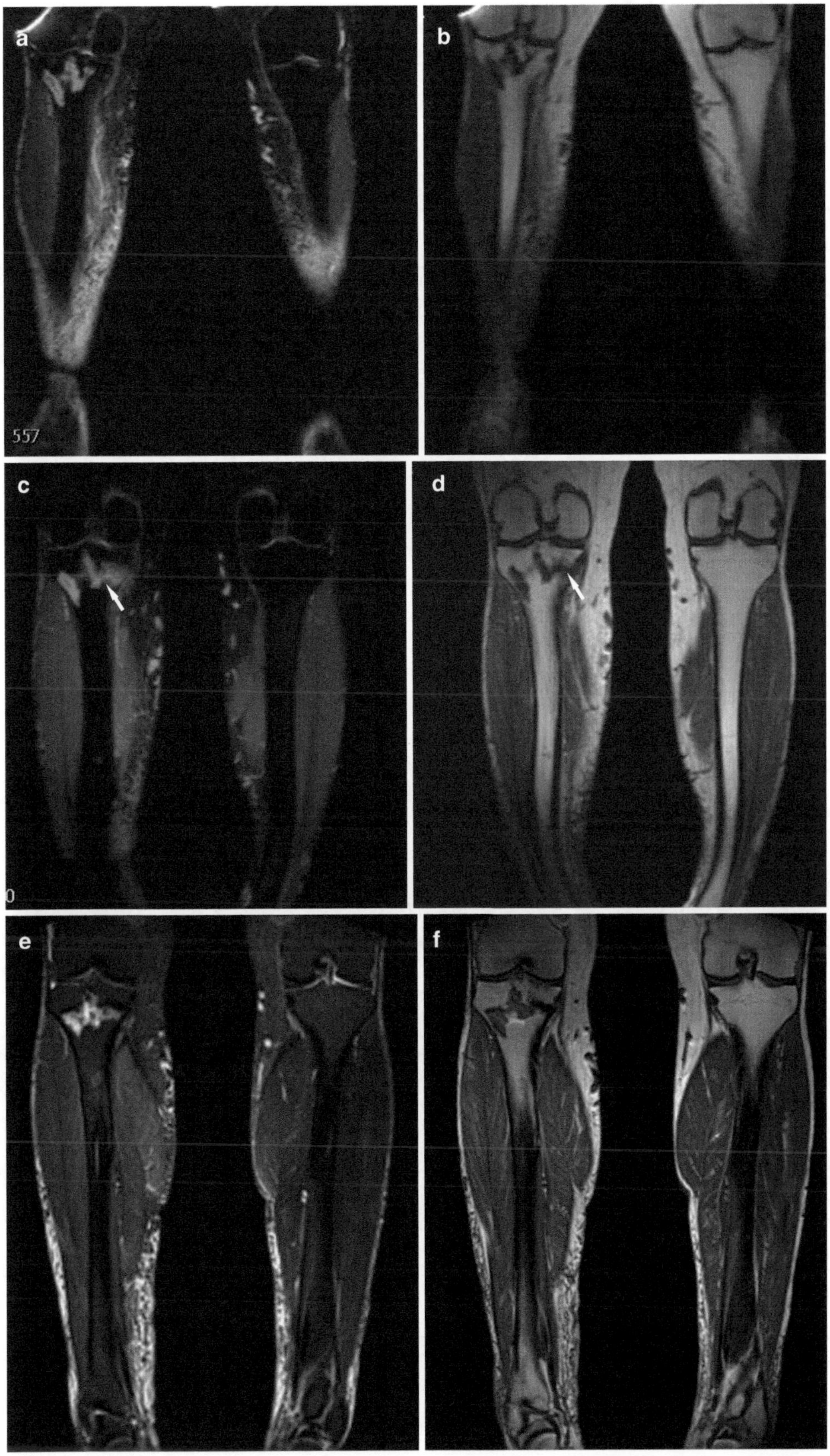

Fig. 2.21 A 43-year-old male, status post chemotherapy for lymphoma. T1-weighted (**a**) and hyperintense STIR image (**b**) six months after completion of chemotherapy shows a treated lesion in right proximal tibia with serpentine areas of hypointense signal. Patient came back with right knee pain 1 year after; MRI shows a fracture line (*arrow*) on T1-weighted image (**c**) with surrounding bone marrow edema extending to medial cortex on STIR image (**d**). Eleven months after conservative treatment, there is widening of fracture line consistent with nonunion on T1-weighted (**e**) and STIR (**f**) images

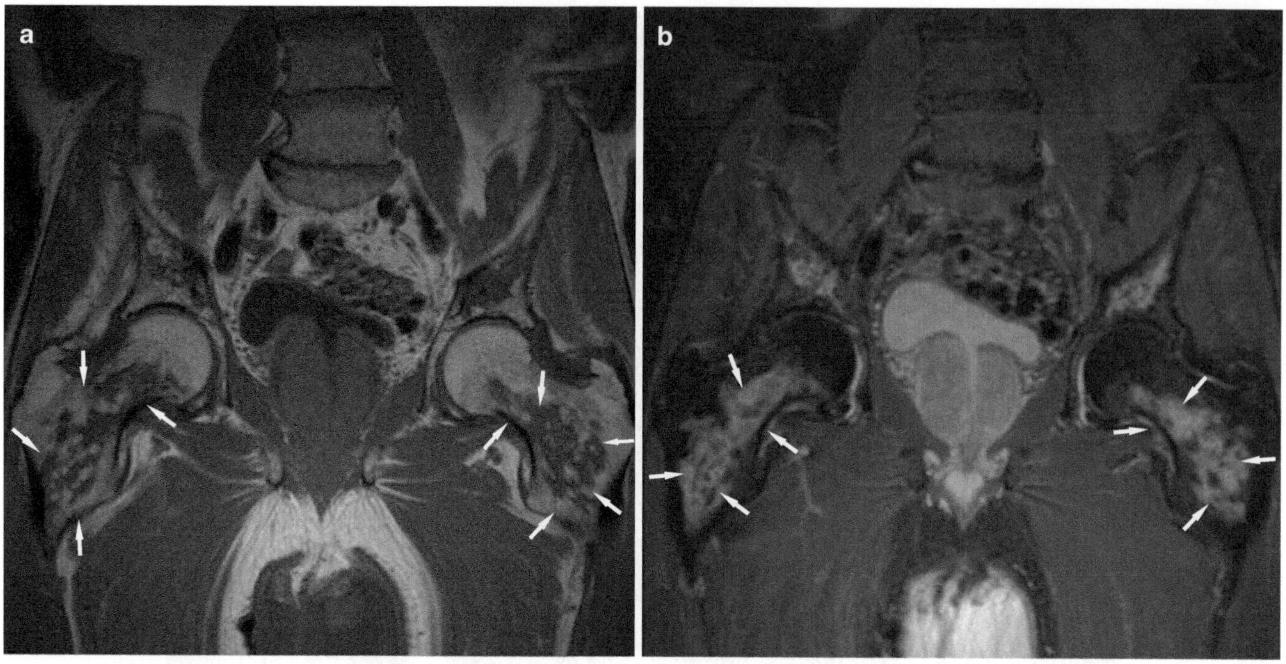

Fig. 2.22 A 67-year-old male patient who completed chemotherapy for acute myelogenous leukemia 6 months earlier. Coronal T1-weighted (**a**) and T2-weighted fat-suppressed (**b**) images of the pelvis demonstrate patchy areas of abnormal signal with intermixed fatty marrow about the proximal femurs and acetabula bilaterally (*arrows*) consistent with treated leukemia lesions

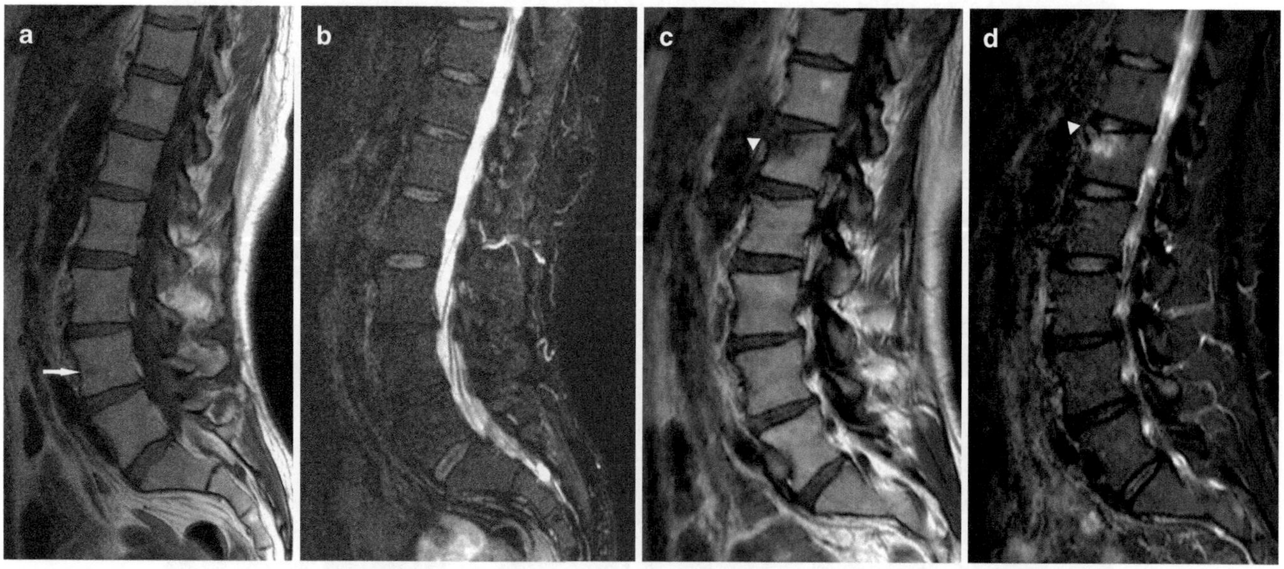

Fig. 2.23 A 51-year-old female with known multiple myeloma. Sagittal T1-weighted (**a**) image of lumbar spine shows diffuse red marrow with subtle L4 focal lesion on T1-weighted image (*arrow*). No focal or diffuse signal abnormality is appreciated on sagittal STIR image (**b**). Three-year follow-up shows complete resolution of focal L4 lesion and fatty conversion of bone marrow on T1-weighted (**c**) and STIR (**d**) sagittal images. There is however a compression fracture of L1 superior end plate (*arrowhead*) which is new since prior examination

2.2.2 Myeloma

Chemotherapy leads to a reduction in cellularity and vascularity with eventual normalization of hematopoietic tissue in multiple myeloma. Although likely following the same histologic stages of postchemotherapeutic marrow regeneration as lymphoma and leukemia, imaging characteristics are not always as straightforward. Multiple myeloma may be classified as focal, diffuse, or variegated in bone marrow distribution [18]. The original distribution of neoplastic infiltration as well as the clinical response dictates the imaging characteristics. The use of T1-weighted images before and after the chemotherapy best assesses treatment response [19] (Fig. 2.23). With complete clinical remission, diffuse and variegated patterns usually return to normal bone marrow signal. Even after complete clinical response, focal patterns of involvement are associated with residual signal abnormalities of T1 hypointensity and T2 hyperintensity, as well as absent or peripheral enhancement [20]. These focal abnormalities likely represent inactive disease, as well as irreversible fibrotic changes and bone marrow infarction. However, the evolution of previously identified focal lesions into diffuse infiltrates is concerning for clinical relapse [18].

Insufficiency fractures are a known consequence of multiple myeloma, as neoplastic infiltration weakens and destroys normal trabeculae (Fig. 2.24). In cases of extensive marrow disease, initiation of chemotherapy has been associated with new or progressive compression fractures (Fig. 2.25). These pathologic fractures likely occur as the soft tissue mass regresses and leaves only defective trabecula for support. Even after bone marrow signal characteristics have normalized, compression fractures may demonstrate homogeneous enhancement on postcontrast T1-weighted images, suggesting reactive hyperemia. In patients undergoing treatment for multiple myeloma, back pain which worsens after remission was found to be a good predictor of new or progressive vertebral body compression fractures [18].

Amyloidosis and marrow fibrosis may also be seen as a complication of treatment of multiple myeloma. Amyloidosis is characterized by foci of decreased T1 and STIR signal intensities within bone marrow. Marrow fibrosis is less common [21], with findings of complete marrow conversion to diffusely decreased T1-weighted and STIR signaling [3] (Fig. 2.26) and associated with poor prognosis.

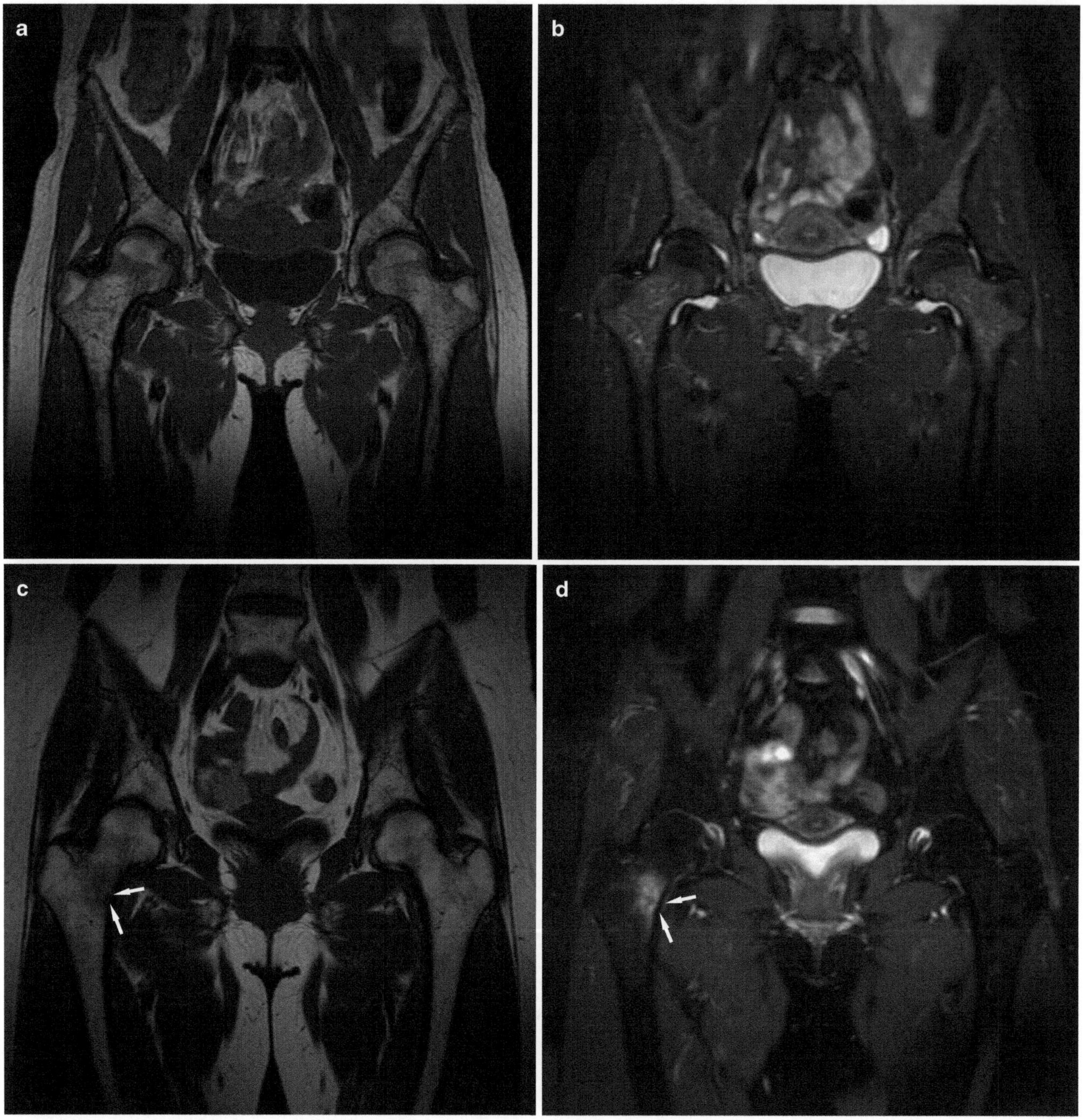

Fig. 2.24 A 56-year-old female with known diagnosis of multiple myeloma. Coronal T1-weighted (**a**) and T2-weighted fat-suppressed images (**b**) at the time of initial diagnosis demonstrate diffuse increase in the marrow vascularity and heterogeneity without discrete lesions. Follow-up MRI 2 years later when patient presented with right hip pain shows conversion to normal marrow vascularity although a nondisplaced fracture of right femoral neck (*arrows*) is evident on T1-weighted image (**c**) with surrounding bone marrow edema on T2-weighted fat-suppressed image (**d**)

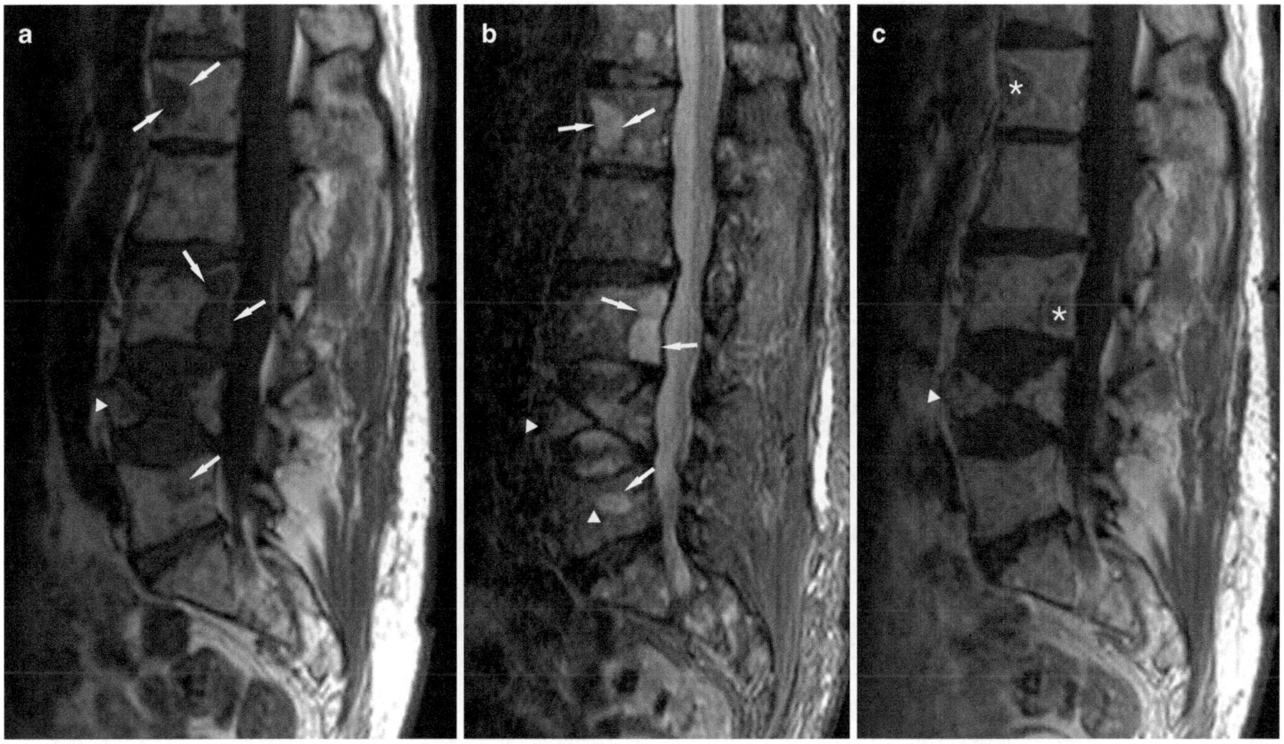

Fig. 2.25 Sagittal T1-weighted (**a**), STIR (**b**), and T1-weighted postcontrast (**c**) images of the thoracolumbar spine in a patient undergoing chemotherapy for multiple myeloma. There are multiple T1-weighted hypointense and inversion recovery hyperintense lesions within the vertebral bodies consistent with focal myelomatous lesions (*arrows*). These lesions demonstrate enhancement on the postcontrast image though large lesions show lack of enhancement centrally (*). In addition, there is a compression fracture of L4 vertebral body (*arrowhead*)

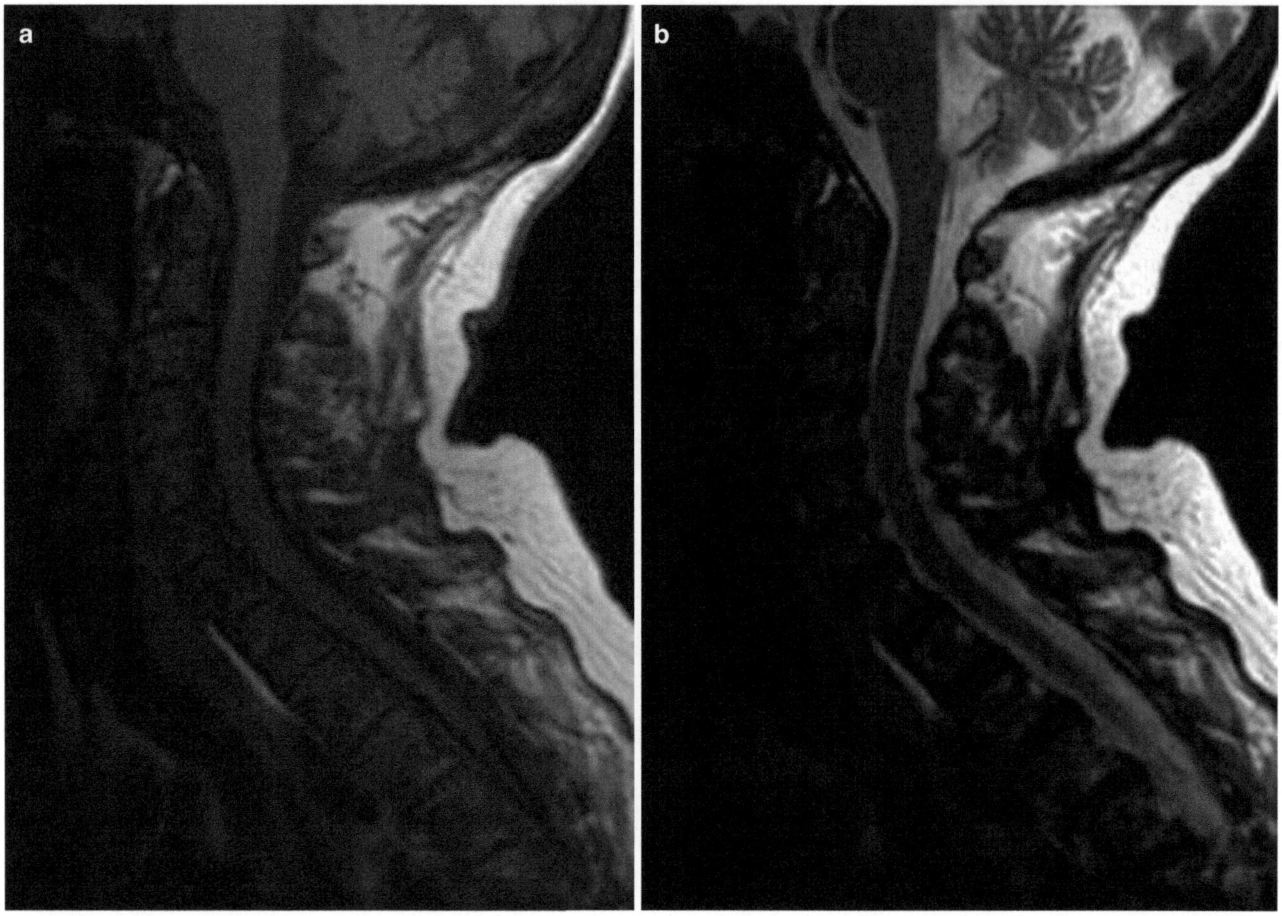

Fig. 2.26 Sagittal T1- (**a**) and T2-weighted (**b**) images of the cervical spine show diffusely decreased T1- and T2-weighted signal throughout the visualized vertebral bone marrow, consistent with myelofibrosis

2.2.3 GCSF

Granulocyte colony-stimulating factor (GCSF) is a hematopoietic growth factor often given as an adjunct to chemotherapy which accentuates bone marrow reconversion. Two forms of GCSF are approved for use in cancer patients in the United States: filgrastim (Neupogen) and pegfilgrastim (Neulasta). Through the stimulation, proliferation, and differentiation of myelogenous cells, these cytokines aid to combat the neutropenic and myelosuppressive effects of chemotherapy. GCSF administration therefore follows MRI signal characteristics of marrow reconversion and hypercellularity, including bone marrow T1 hypointensity and T2/STIR hyperintensity (Fig. 2.27) [6]. An understanding of the patient's clinical prognosis/remission is essential as marrow reconversion and tumor infiltration both share these imaging findings [22]. T1-weighted images are critical showing marrow signal hyperintense to skeletal muscle (Fig. 2.28). In addition, it has been suggested that postcontrast dynamic MRI may aid in the differentiation of tumor from red marrow, as neoplastic cells demonstrate increased enhancement compared to normal hematopoietic marrow [3]. Application of this technique may not be practical in clinical use. Dramatic changes in bone marrow signal after initiation of chemotherapy should alert the radiologist interpreting MR examinations to GCSF administration (Fig. 2.29) rather than diffuse neoplastic marrow infiltration [23].

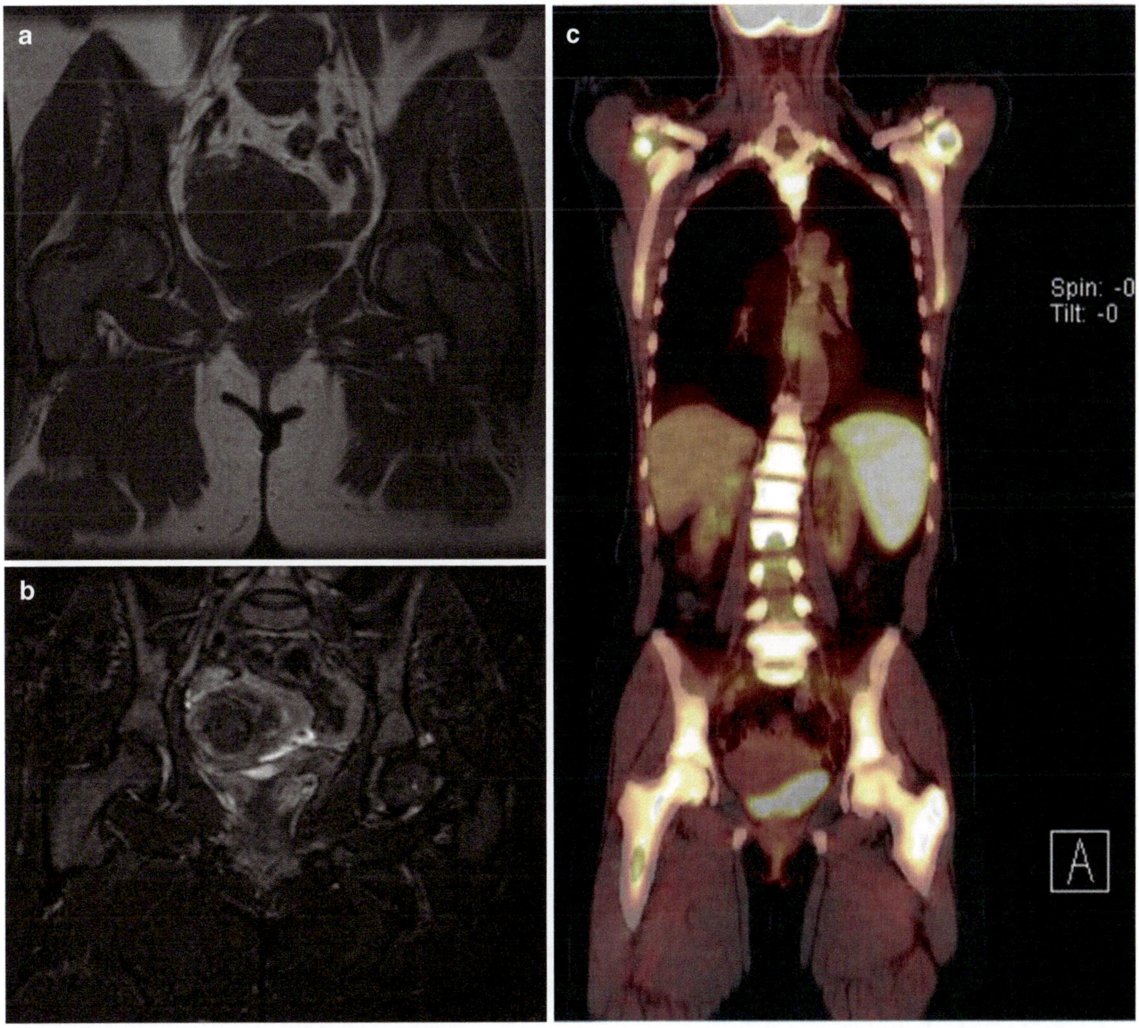

Fig. 2.27 A 47-year-old female undergoing chemotherapy for recently diagnosed breast cancer. Coronal T1-weighted (**a**) and T2-weighted fat-suppressed (**b**) images show diffuse red marrow throughout the visualized skeleton consistent with marrow stimulation with granulocyte colony-stimulating factor treatment. Coronal reconstruction of positron emission tomography (PET)/CT examination 1 week earlier demonstrates diffuse metabolic activity of bone marrow throughout visualized axial and appendicular skeleton (**c**)

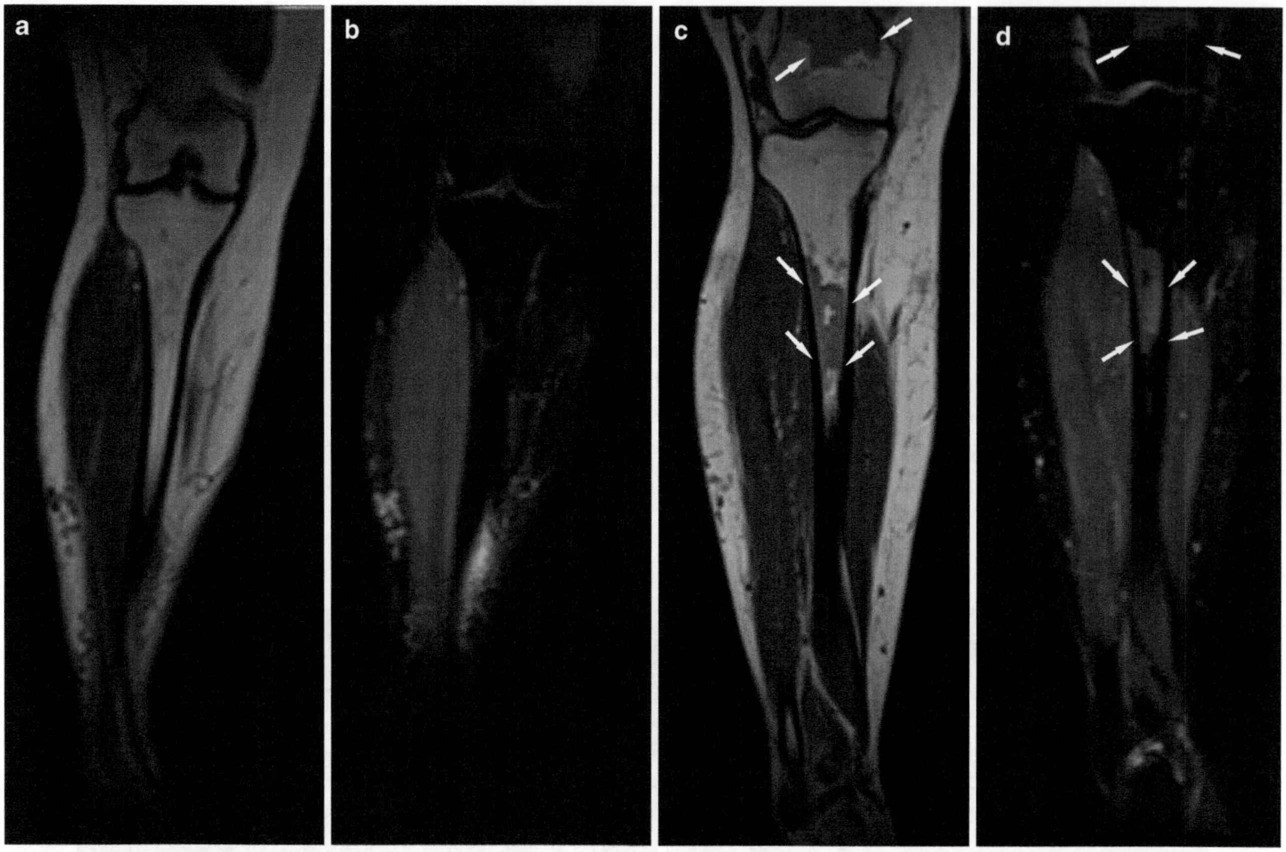

Fig. 2.28 Baseline coronal T1-weighted (**a**) and STIR (**b**) images of the right leg demonstrate minimal patchy red marrow in the proximal tibia. Follow-up MRI obtained 6 weeks after initiation of chemotherapy demonstrates markedly increased red marrow activity (*arrows*) on T1-weighted (**c**) and STIR (**d**) images consistent with marrow stimulation from granulocyte colony-stimulating factor in the chemotherapy regimen

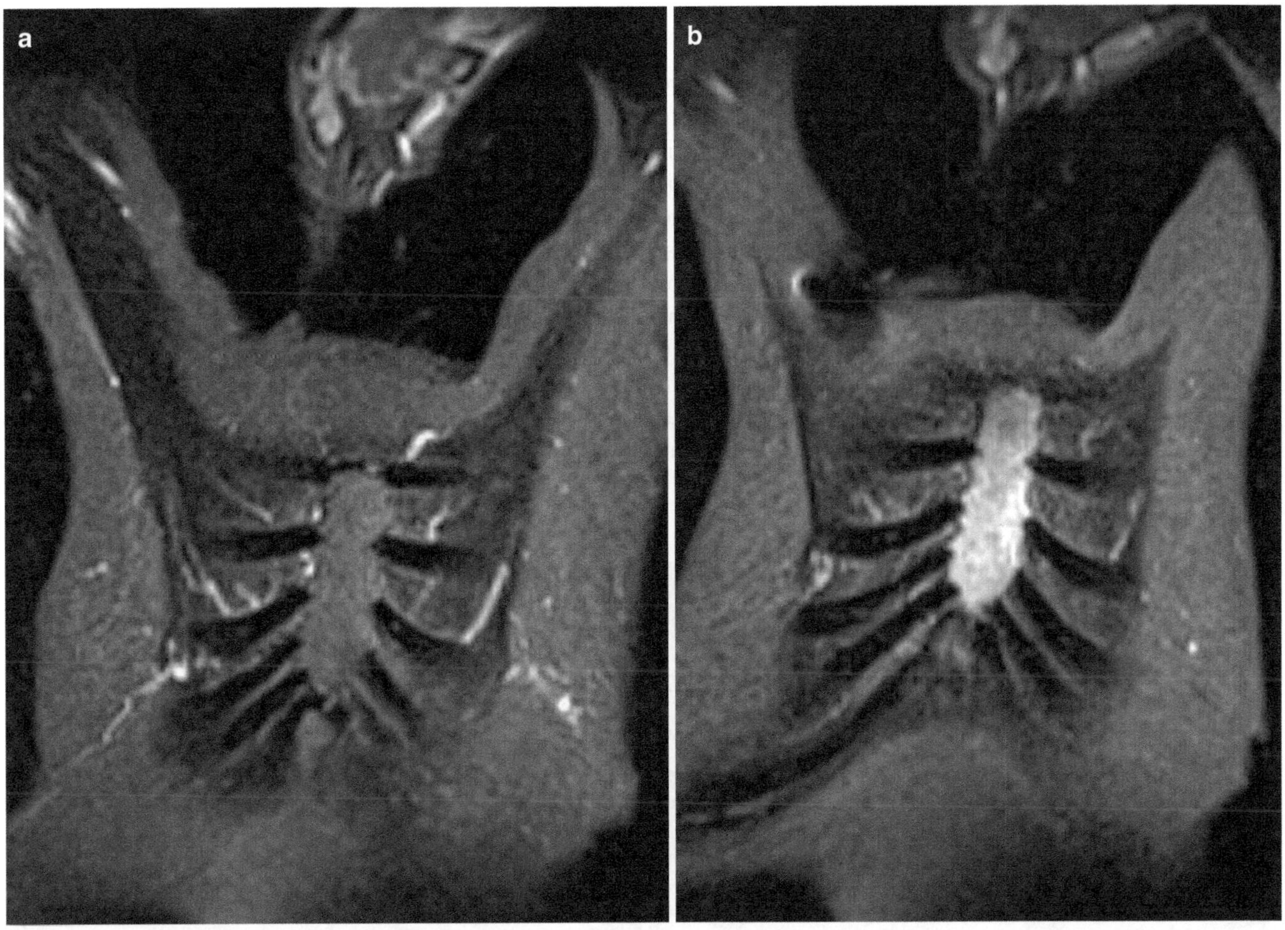

Fig. 2.29 Coronal STIR images of the sternum before (**a**) and 4 weeks following the initiation of chemotherapy regimen for breast cancer (**b**) which included granulocyte colony-stimulating factor. Rapidly progression of STIR signal change is consistent with bone marrow stimulation

2.3 Postoperative

Bone marrow signal changes and trabecular distortion are often visible after surgical intervention particularly following hardware removal (Fig. 2.30). After joint replacements, evidence of surgical reaming may be seen away from the surgical site with lack of normal trabecula and more prominent fatty signal in a linear orientation (Fig. 2.31). In some cases, the marrow edema and hemorrhage could raise suspicion for an infection or neoplasm (Fig. 2.32). Smaller foci of hyperintense STIR or T2-weighted signal may also be seen within surgically manipulated bone marrow with variable T1-weighted imaging appearance. Foci of marrow signal changes are common in posterior iliac crests after bone marrow aspiration (Fig. 2.33). Focal bone marrow signal changes are typically seen at the tip of bony stumps after amputation which may persist for a long period of time and may enhance on postcontrast MRI (Fig. 2.34). Bone graft donor sites also demonstrate bone marrow signal changes. Nearby postoperative changes usually help in determining the etiology such as lumbar spine fixation from iliac crest bone grafting (Fig. 2.35) or scaphoid grafting from the distal radius. Methylmethacrylate used in the surgical augmentation typically appears as signal void, commonly utilized for vertebral compression fractures (Fig. 2.36). Subchondroplasty procedure has recently been introduced to treat bone marrow lesions underlying cartilage defects of the knee which may simulate a neoplasm in the absence of available radiographs or history (Fig. 2.37).

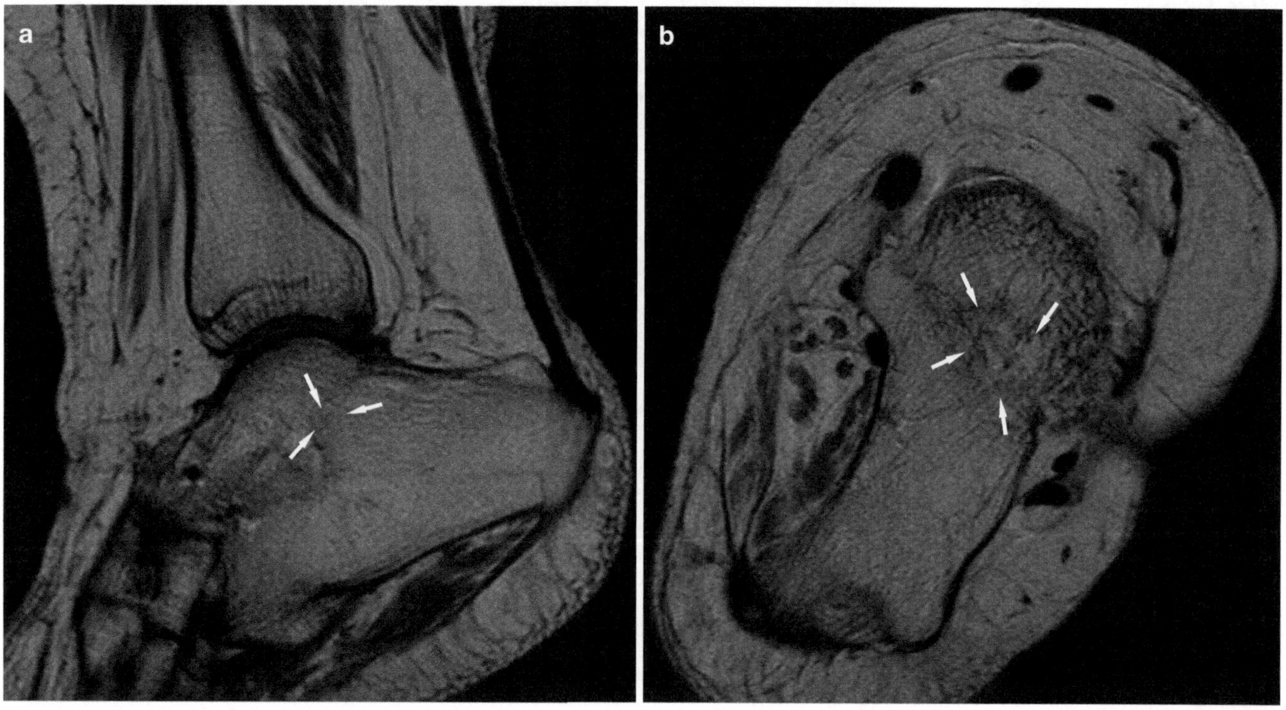

Fig. 2.30 T1-weighted sagittal (**a**) and axial (**b**) images of left ankle show postsurgical changes of subtalar, talonavicular, and calcaneocuboid solid bony fusion with areas of trabecular distortion (*arrows*)

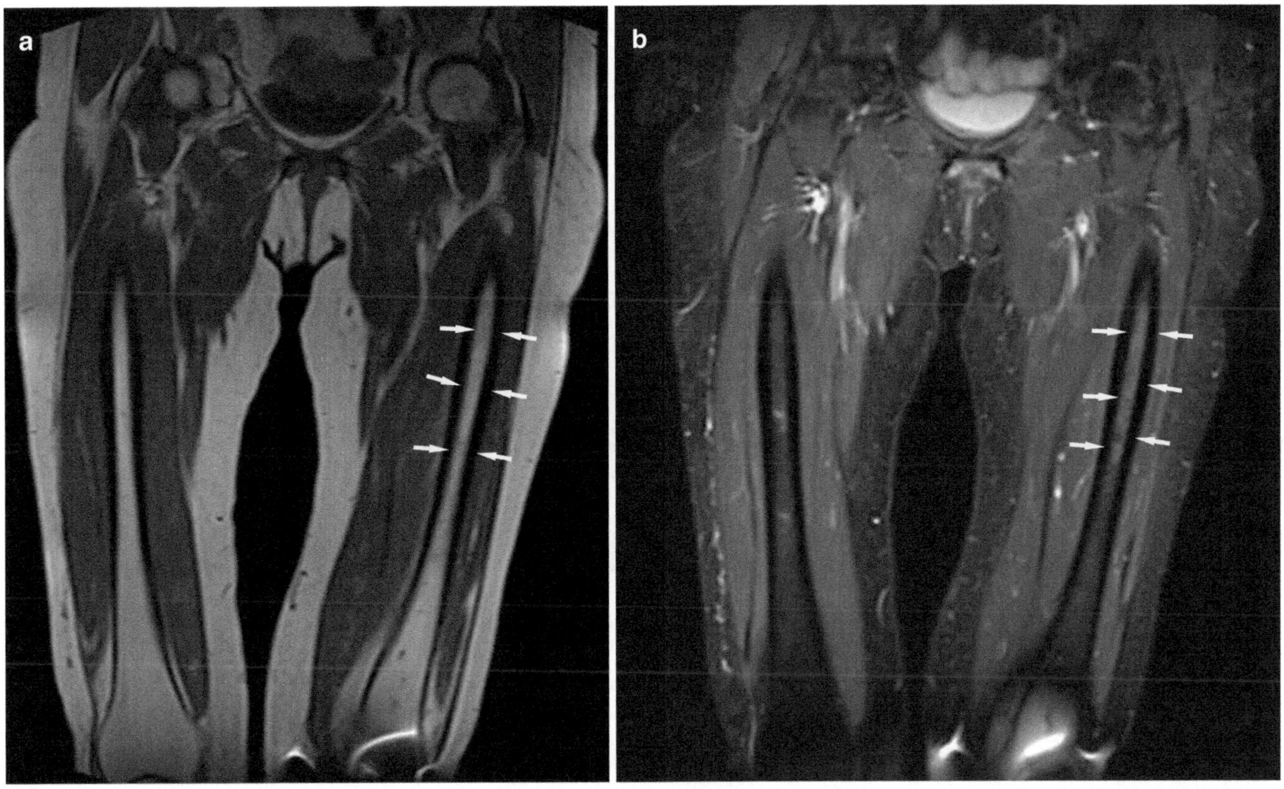

Fig. 2.31 Coronal T1-weighted (**a**) and T2-weighted fat-suppressed (**b**) images of left femur 6 months after total knee arthroplasty show subtle linear marrow signal changes extending to proximal femoral diaphysis (*arrows*) more pronounced on T2-weighted images consistent with residual changes of surgical reaming

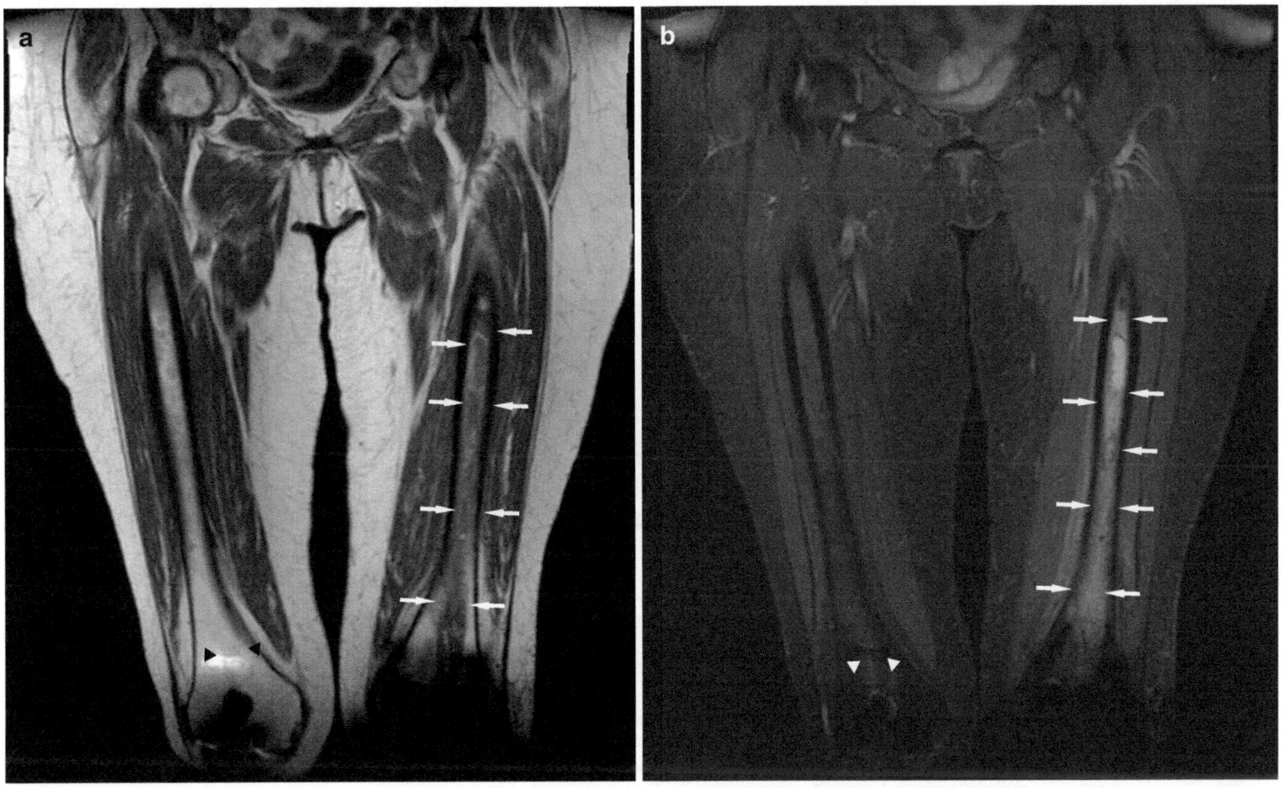

Fig. 2.32 Coronal T1-weighted (**a**) and T2-weighted fat-suppressed (**b**) images of left femur 3 months after total knee arthroplasty show markedly abnormal bone marrow signal in the visualized left femur with small foci of intermixed fatty signal (*arrows*) consistent with surgical reaming-associated trabecular disruption and hemorrhage. Signal changes of the right distal femur appear more subtle in the distal femur (*arrowheads*) close to the femoral component of the arthroplasty which was placed 4 years earlier

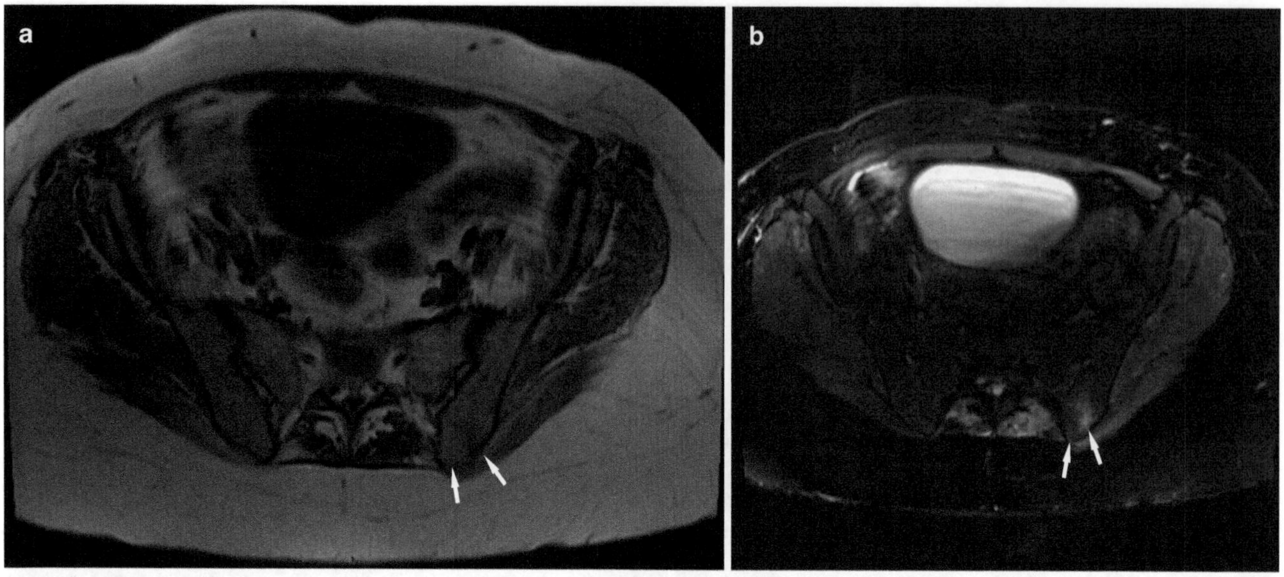

Fig. 2.33 Axial T1-weighted (**a**) and T2-weighted fat-suppressed (**b**) images of the pelvis demonstrate linear subtle signal abnormality of the posterior iliac crest on the left consistent with recent bone marrow aspiration (*arrows*)

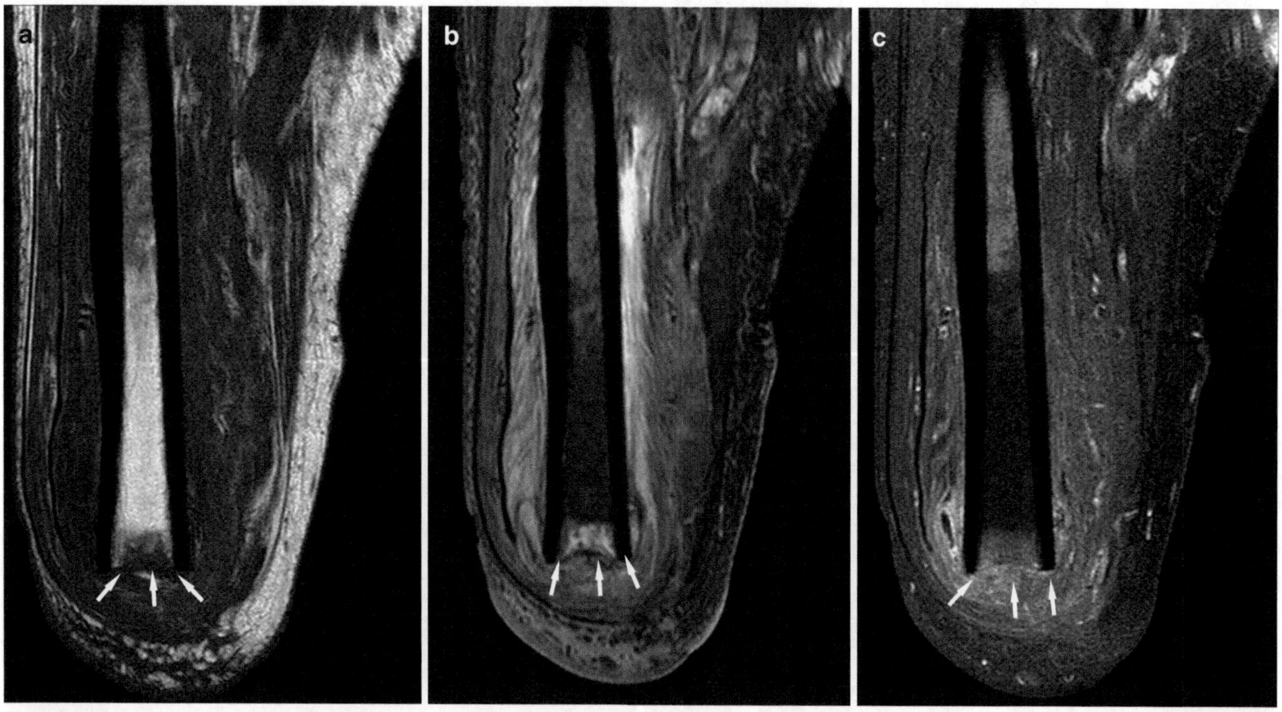

Fig. 2.34 Coronal T1-weighted (**a**), T2-weighted (**b**), and postcontrast T1-weighted fat-saturated (**c**) images of right femur demonstrate post-surgical changes of amputation. There is mild residual marrow infiltration at the tip of the stump (*arrows*) with mild surrounding edema and subtle enhancement

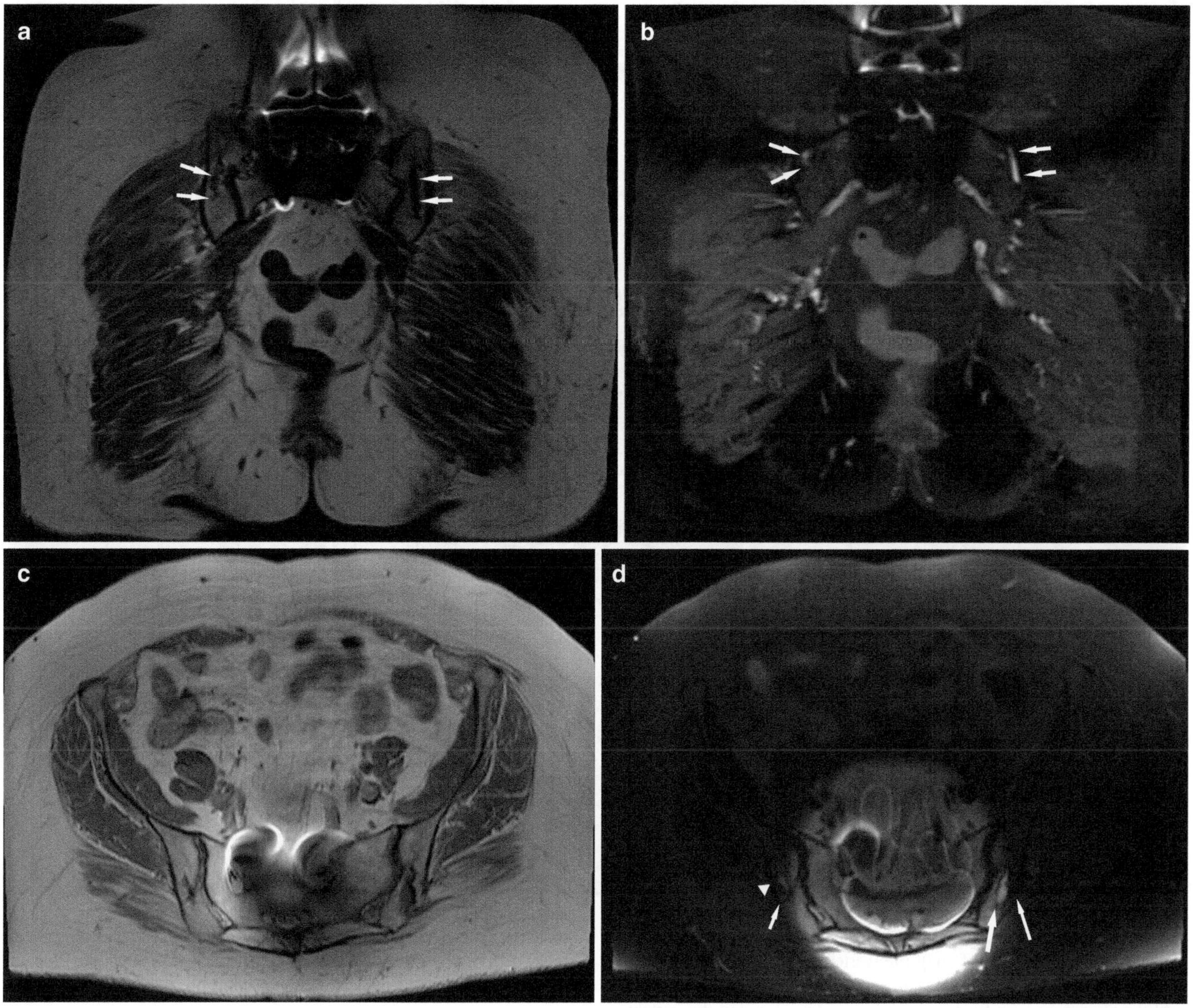

Fig. 2.35 Coronal T1-weighted (**a**) and coronal STIR (**b**) images of the pelvis demonstrate linear areas of abnormal signal in the iliac crests bilaterally simulating fractures (*arrows*). Axial T1-weighted (**c**) and T2-weighted fat-suppressed (**d**) images demonstrate the cortical extension of signal abnormality with widening at the surface on the left (*arrowhead*) consistent with bone graft donor site. Susceptibility artifacts from lower lumbar fixation are helpful in the diagnosis demonstrating location of the bone graft used

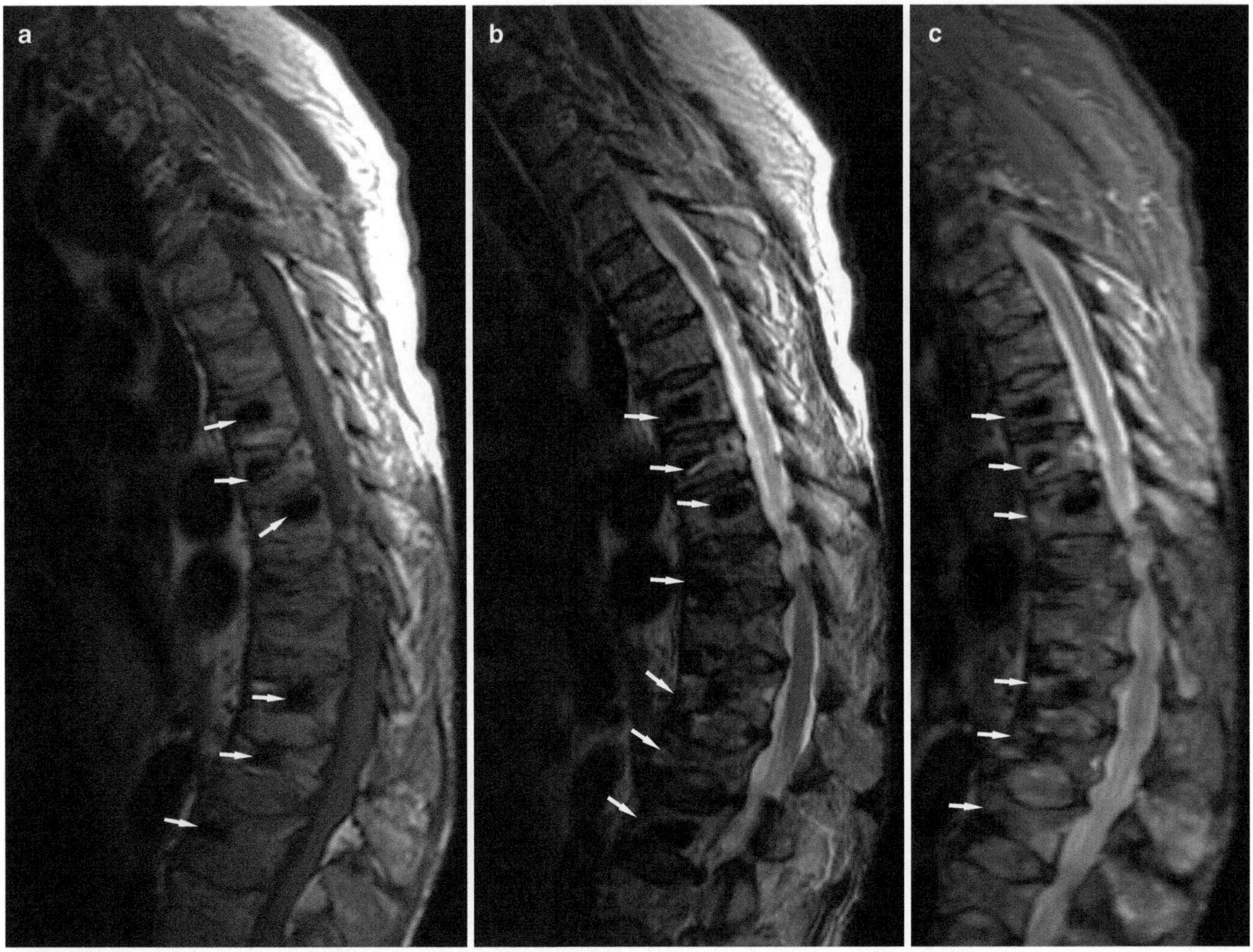

Fig. 2.36 A 51-year-old female with history of multiple myeloma and status post kyphoplasty of multiple vertebrae. Sagittal T1- (**a**) and T2-weighted (**b**) and STIR (**c**) images of the thoracolumbar spine show multilevel compression fractures and foci of low signal in the vertebral bodies (*arrows*) consistent with methylmethacrylate bone cement. Underlying bone marrow is diffusely infiltrated reflecting the changes of multiple myeloma

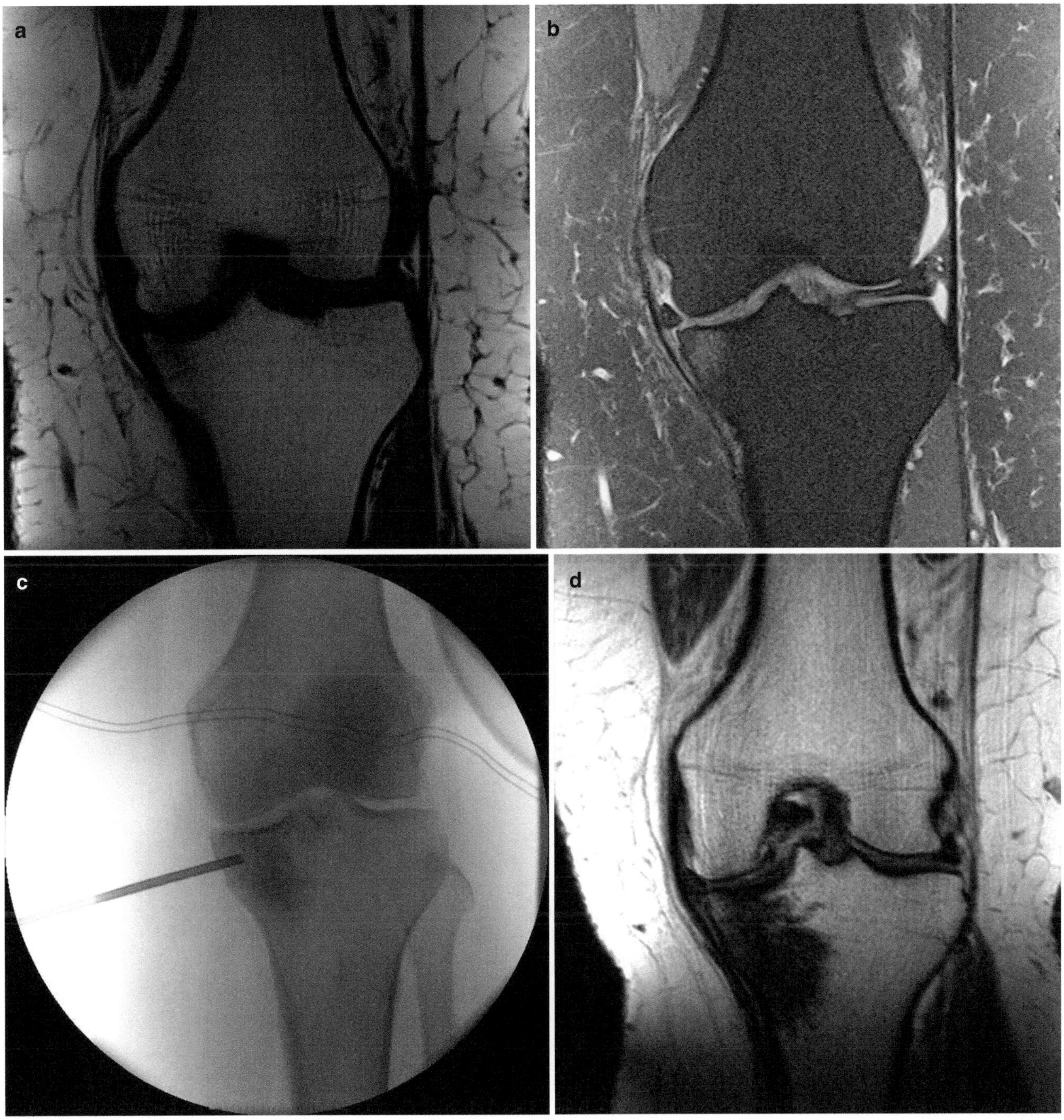

Fig. 2.37 Coronal T1-weighted (**a**) and proton density-weighted fat-suppressed image (**b**) of the left knee demonstrates focal bone marrow edema about the medial tibial plateau. Patient underwent fluoroscopy-guided methylmethacrylate bone cement injection (**c**) consistent with subchondroplasty. Follow-up MRI obtained 4 months after the surgical procedure showed a focus of low signal methylmethacrylate on T1-weighted (**d**) and STIR (**e**) images with a rim of bone marrow edema (*arrows*)

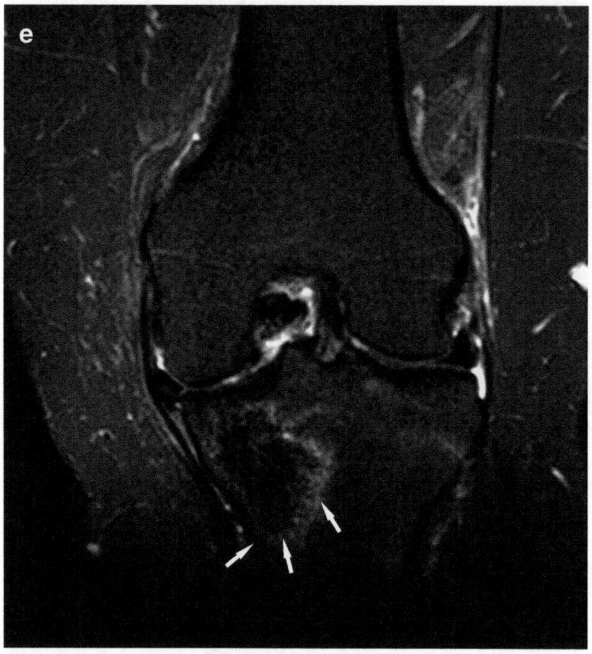

Fig. 2.37 (continued)

References

1. Stevens S, Moore S, Kaplan I. Early and late bone marrow changes after irradiation: MR evaluation. AJR Am J Roentgenol. 1990;154:745–50.
2. Otake S, Mayr N, Ueda T, et al. Radiation-induced changes in MR signal intensity and contrast enhancement of lumbosacral vertebrae: do changes occur only inside the radiation therapy field? Radiology. 2002;222:179–83.
3. Daldrup-Link H, Tobias H, Thomas L. MR imaging of therapy-induced changes of bone marrow. Eur Radiol. 2007;17:743–61.
4. Blomlie V, Rofstad E, Skjonsberg A, et al. Female pelvic bone marrow: serial MR imaging before, during, and after radiation therapy. Radiology. 1995;194:537–43.
5. Mitchell M, Logan P. Radiation-induced changes in bone. Radiographics. 1998;18:1125–36.
6. Fletcher B. Effects of pediatric cancer therapy on the musculoskeletal system. Pediatr Radiol. 1997;27:623–36.
7. O'Donovan DA, Yeung I, Zeman V, et al. Radiation-induced craniofacial bone growth inhibition: development of an animal model. J Craniofac Surg. 2001;12(6):533–43.
8. Rabin B, Meyer J, Berlin J, et al. Radiation-induced changes in the central nervous system and head and neck. Radiographics. 1996;16:1055–72.
9. Iyer R, Jhingran A, Sawaf H, et al. Imaging findings after radiotherapy to the pelvis. AJR Am J Roentgenol. 2001;177:1083–9.
10. Cahan WG, Woodard HQ. Sarcoma arising in irradiated bone; report of 11 cases. Cancer. 1948;1:3–29.
11. Arlen M, Higinbotham NL, Huvos AG, et al. Radiation-induced sarcoma of bone. Cancer. 1971;28:1087–99.
12. Jensen K, Sorensen P, Thomsen C, et al. Magnetic resonance imaging of the bone marrow in patients with acute leukemia during and after chemotherapy. Acta Radiol. 1990;31:361–9.
13. Gerard E, Ferry J, Amrein P, et al. Compositional changes in vertebral bone marrow during treatment for acute leukemia: assessment with quantitative chemical shift imaging. Radiology. 1992;183:39–46.
14. Hwang S, David P. Magnetic resonance imaging of bone marrow in oncology, part 2. Skeletal Radiol. 2007;36:1017–27.
15. O'Neill J, Finlay K, Jurriaans E, et al. Radiological manifestations of skeletal lymphoma. Curr Probl Diagn Radiol. 2009;38:228–36.
16. Kwee T, Kwee R, Verdonck L, et al. Magnetic resonance imaging for the detection of bone marrow involvement in malignant lymphoma. Br J Haematol. 2008;141:60–8.
17. Lien H, Holte H. Fat replacement of Hodgkin disease of bone marrow after chemotherapy: report of three cases. Skeletal Radiol. 1996;25:671–4.
18. Moulopoulos L, Dimopoulos M, Alexanian R, et al. Multiple myeloma: MR patterns of response to treatment. Radiology. 1994;193:441–6.
19. Baur-Melnyk A, Buhmann S, Durr H, et al. Role of MRI for the diagnosis and prognosis of multiple myeloma. Eur J Radiol. 2005;55:56–63.
20. Rahmouni A, Divine M, Mathieu D, et al. MR appearance of multiple myeloma of the spine before and after treatment. AJR Am J Roentgenol. 1993;160:1053–7.
21. Subramanian R, Basu D, Dutta TK. Significance of bone marrow fibrosis in multiple myeloma. Pathology. 2007;39(5):512–5.
22. Fletcher B, Wall J, Hanna S. Effect of hematopoietic growth factors on MR imaging of bone marrow in children undergoing chemotherapy. Radiology. 1993;189:745–51.
23. Hartman RP, Sundaram M, Okuno SH, Sim FH. Effect of granulocyte-stimulating factors on marrow of adult patients with musculoskeletal malignancies: incidence and MRI findings. AJR Am J Roentgenol. 2004;183:645–53.

3 Neoplastic Bone Marrow Infiltration

Hakan Ilaslan and Murali Sundaram

Bone marrow can be replaced by a number of neoplastic disorders, including leukemia, lymphoma, multiple myeloma, and metastases. In the past, evaluation of bone marrow required invasive procedures such as biopsy or aspiration at the time of diagnosis and follow-up after treatment. Magnetic resonance imaging (MRI) is an excellent noninvasive diagnostic modality demonstrating the presence and extent of pathologic bone marrow involvement.

3.1 Plasma Cell Dyscrasias

Multiple myeloma comprises a heterogeneous group of plasma cell neoplasms that primarily involve bone marrow. Radiographs are the most frequently used imaging modality for initial diagnosis and follow-up of these conditions; radiographic findings are incorporated in the Durie–Salmon classification [1]. On radiographs, round, lytic, punched-out lesions of the skull are almost pathognomonic for multiple myeloma and can also be visualized on MRI (Fig. 3.1). MRI is considered the gold-standard imaging method for evaluating bone marrow in these patients. In recent years, whole-body MRI with or without positron emission tomography (PET) has become an important diagnostic tool in the initial staging and follow-up of patients with multiple myeloma [2].

There are five different MRI patterns of marrow involvement in multiple myeloma [3]: normal, focal involvement (lesion(s) >5 mm) (Figs. 3.2 and 3.3), homogeneous diffuse infiltration (Figs. 3.4 and 3.5), combined diffuse infiltration with focal lesions (Fig. 3.6), and variegated (salt-and-pepper) pattern with heterogeneous small foci of bone marrow involvement and interposition of fat islands (Fig. 3.7). Normal bone marrow in patients with multiple myeloma corresponds to a mild plasma cell infiltration (<20 volume % in bone marrow biopsy) [4]. Normal bone marrow signal on MRI does not exclude the diagnosis of multiple myeloma seen in approximately 28 % of cases [4]. In previous studies, the percentage of symptomatic myeloma patients with each of the abnormal MRI bone marrow patterns has ranged from 18 to 50 % for focal pattern, 25 to 43 % for diffuse pattern, and 1 to 5 % for variegated (salt-and-pepper) pattern [4]. The number of MRI focal lesions and the presence of a diffuse pattern correlate with decreased survival of patients with multiple myeloma. MRI of the spine and pelvis may demonstrate approximately 90 % of focal lesions in patients with multiple myeloma and, thus, can be used in cases for which whole-body MRI is not available [3].

Focal myeloma lesions typically show a low to isointense signal intensity compared to skeletal muscle on T1-weighted images (Fig. 3.8), although some myeloma lesions may demonstrate hyperintense signal (Fig. 3.9), unlike most other neoplasms. A hyperintense signal intensity on T2-weighted and short tau inversion recovery (STIR) images is expected (Fig. 3.8), and the lesions typically enhance on postcontrast images. Increased marrow vascularity is a well-known phenomenon that can also be seen on MRI (Fig. 3.10) with or without intravenous contrast administration as prominent tubular structures which should not be mistaken for focal lesions. A decrease in marrow vascularity may be observed on follow-up MRI examinations if the patients are in remission. Distal extremity involvement is unusual in patients with multiple myeloma (Fig. 3.11). Amyloidosis is a known complication of multiple myeloma which may be observed in the hip (Fig. 3.12) or glenohumeral joints (Fig. 3.13). Spinal compression fractures are frequently seen in patients with multiple myeloma which may either be pathologic (Fig. 3.14) or osteoporotic (Fig. 3.15). Extramedullary disease is an uncommon manifestation of multiple myeloma and can either present at the time of diagnosis or develop with disease progression. The most common sites for extramedullary disease are the skin and soft tissues (Fig. 3.16), although myeloma can infiltrate any organ in the body. Presence of extramedullary disease is often associated with poor prognosis [5].

The diagnosis of solitary plasmacytoma (Fig. 3.17) of the bone is based on the presence of a solitary bone lesion, with a

H. Ilaslan, M. Sundaram, *Pediatric and Adult MRI Atlas of Bone Marrow: Normal Appearances, Variants and Diffuse Disease States*, DOI 10.1007/978-3-642-02740-6_3

confirmed infiltration by plasma cells on biopsy of the lesion in the absence of clonal plasma cells on bone marrow biopsy. The spine, pelvis, and proximal femurs are common locations for plasmacytomas. MRI signal characteristics for plasmacytomas are similar to those seen with myeloma lesions. Although treatment with radiation is usually sufficient for local cure of plasmacytomas, most patients with this condition will eventually develop multiple myeloma, likely because of the growth of previously occult lesions. Smoldering, or asymptomatic, myeloma is considered a precursor to multiple myeloma. Some signs of the disease are present, such as plasma cells in the bone marrow or elevated blood protein levels, although smoldering myeloma patients do not have typical symptoms associated with active symptomatic multiple myeloma, such as anemia, excessive calcium in the blood, kidney disease, or bone involvement. Nearly all smoldering myeloma patients progress to symptomatic or active multiple myeloma with a median time to progression of 5 years. The current standard of care for smoldering myeloma patients is the so-called "watch and wait" approach. These patients are followed clinically and by imaging until progression to symptomatic multiple myeloma occurs.

Monoclonal gammopathy of undetermined significance (MGUS) is the most common variety of plasma cell dyscrasia. This condition is characterized by the presence of a monoclonal immunoglobulin (M-protein), in the serum or urine of patients who do not meet the diagnostic criteria for multiple myeloma, Waldenström macroglobulinemia, amyloidosis, or other lymphoproliferative disorders. Patients with MGUS have higher incidences of osteoporosis and vertebral fractures than are seen in the healthy population. MRI may demonstrate osteoporotic fractures in patients with MGUS and is able to demonstrate focal lesions in patients who progress to multiple myeloma.

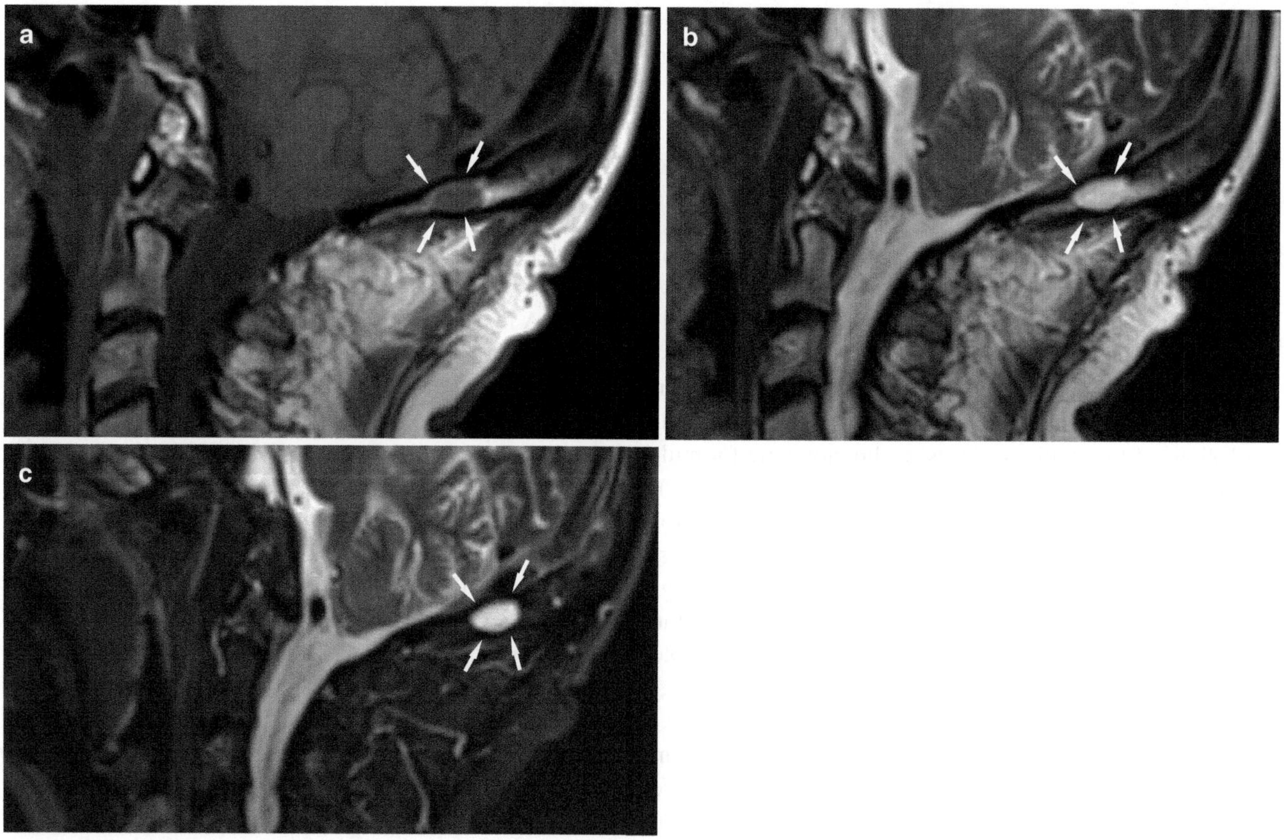

Fig. 3.1 Sagittal T1-weighted (**a**), T2-weighted (**b**), and T2-weighted fat-suppressed (**c**) MRI of the skull base demonstrate a focal ovoid lesion (*arrows*) in the occipital bone consistent with patient's known multiple myeloma

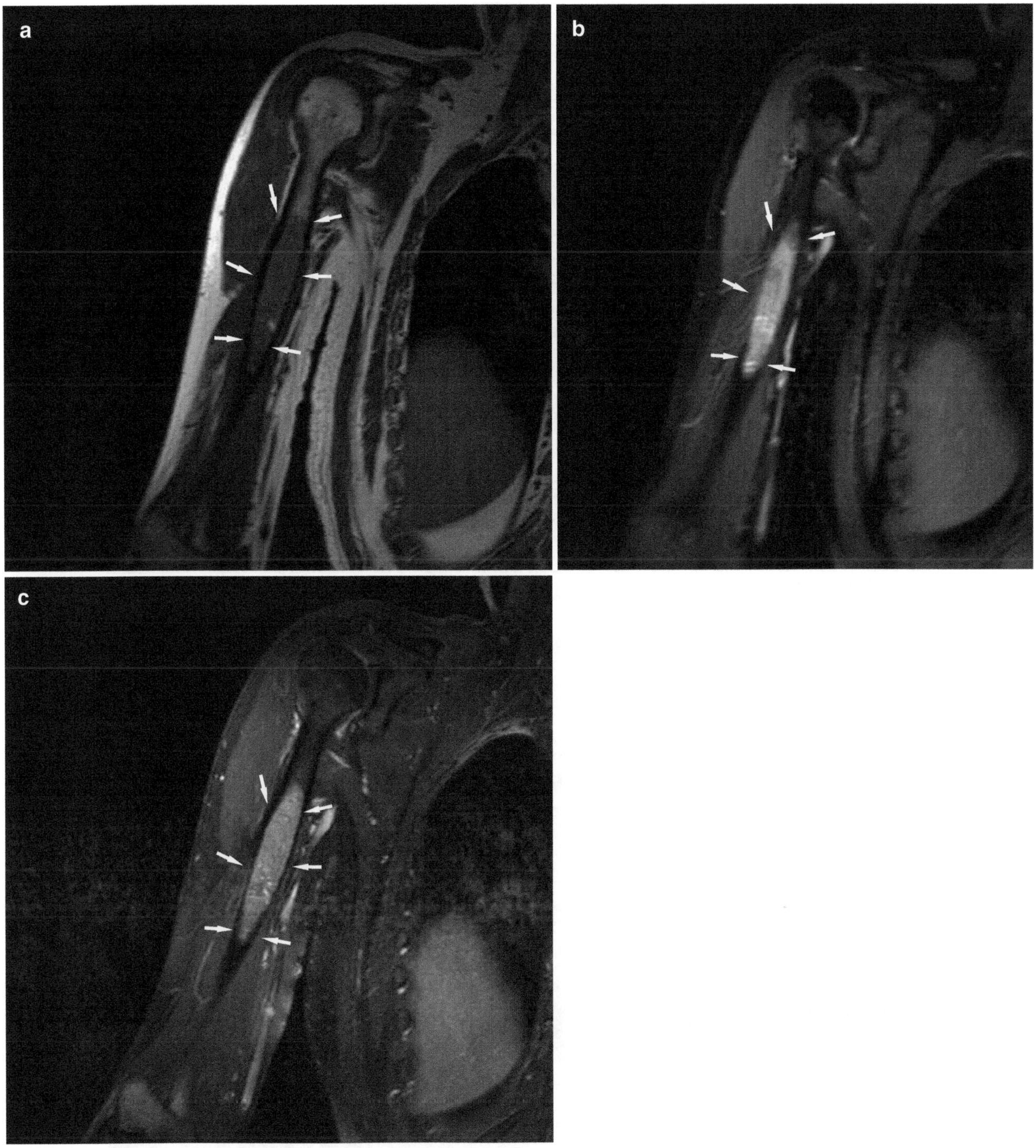

Fig. 3.2 A 49-year-old male multiple myeloma patient. Coronal T1-weighted (**a**), coronal STIR (**b**), and coronal T1-weighted fat-saturated postcontrast images of the right humerus demonstrate a large marrow-infiltrating tumor in the diaphysis (*arrows*) consistent with focal myeloma lesion. Please note the homogeneously diffuse enhancement of the myeloma lesion on postcontrast images (**c**)

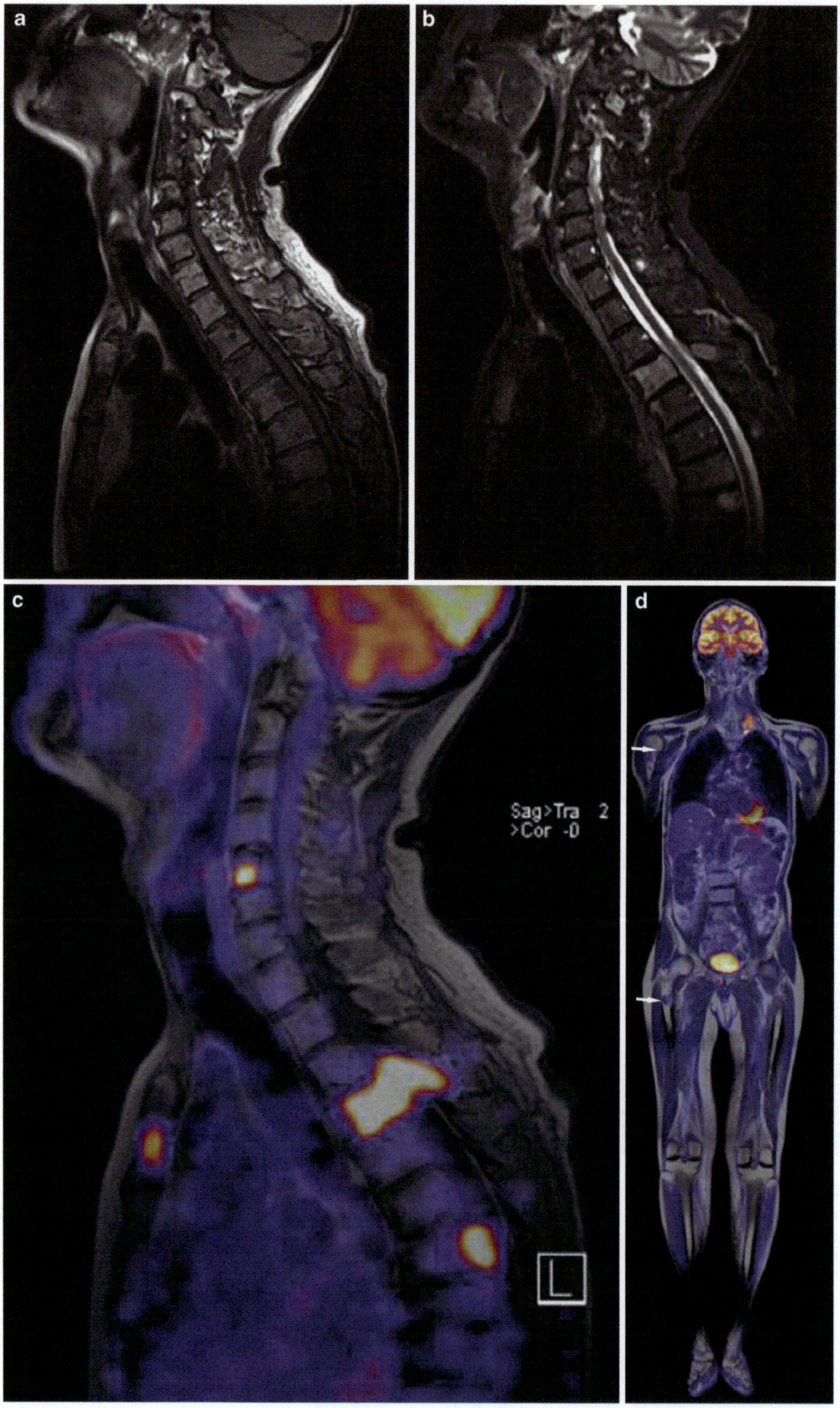

Fig. 3.3 A 57-year-old man with recent multiple myeloma diagnosis. Sagittal T1-weighted (**a**) and STIR (**b**) sequence images demonstrate several marrow-infiltrating myeloma lesions in the spine and sternal manubrium. T1-weighted PET-MRI fused (**c**) image demonstrate increased metabolic activity in these lesions. Whole-body coronal T2-weighted fused at MR image (**d**) demonstrates additional lesions in the right proximal femur and right proximal humerus (*arrows*)

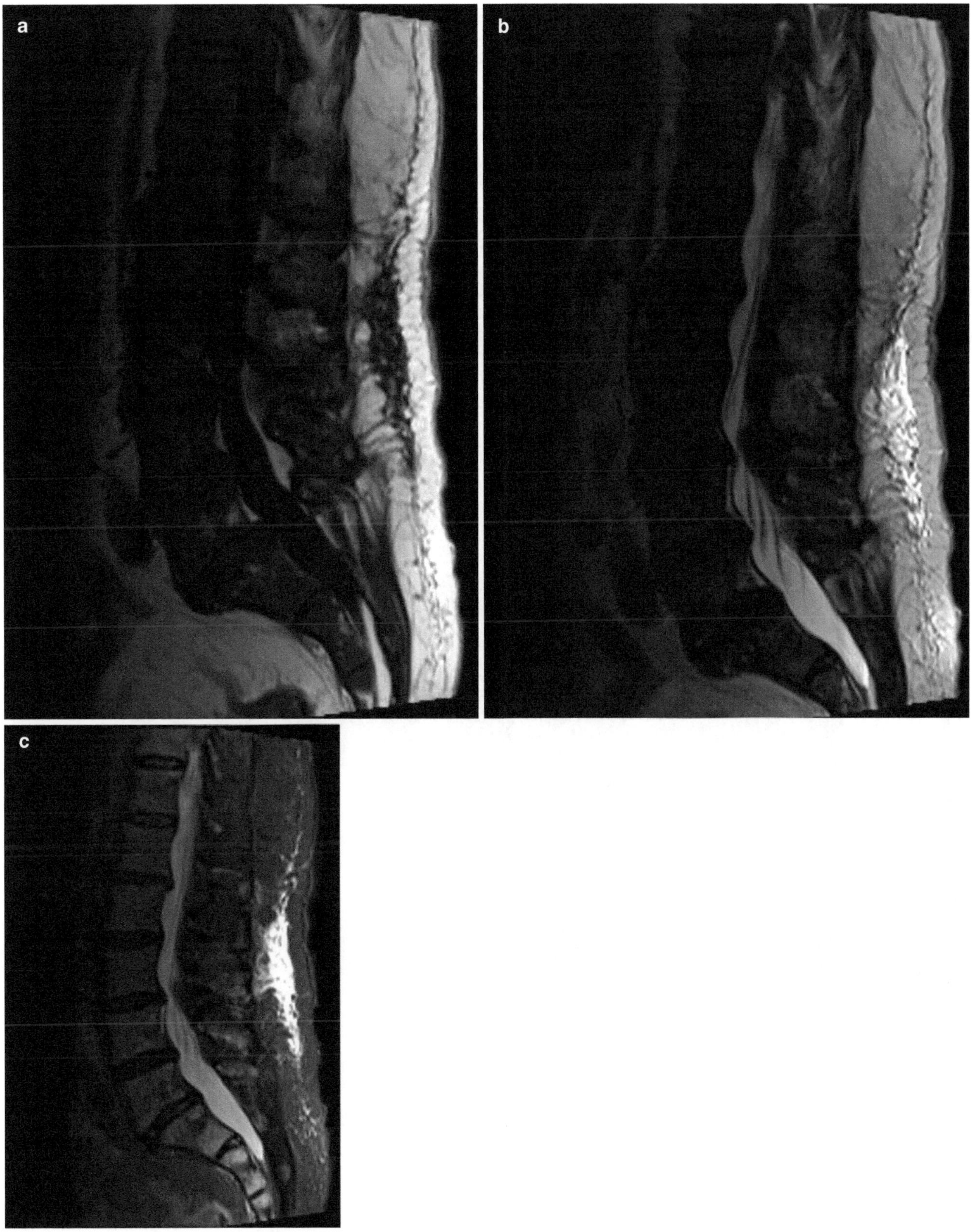

Fig. 3.4 A 65-year-old male with known multiple myeloma. T1-weighted sagittal (**a**), T2-weighted sagittal (**b**), and STIR sagittal (**c**) images show diffuse myelomatous infiltration of the bone marrow with minimal scattered fatty signal

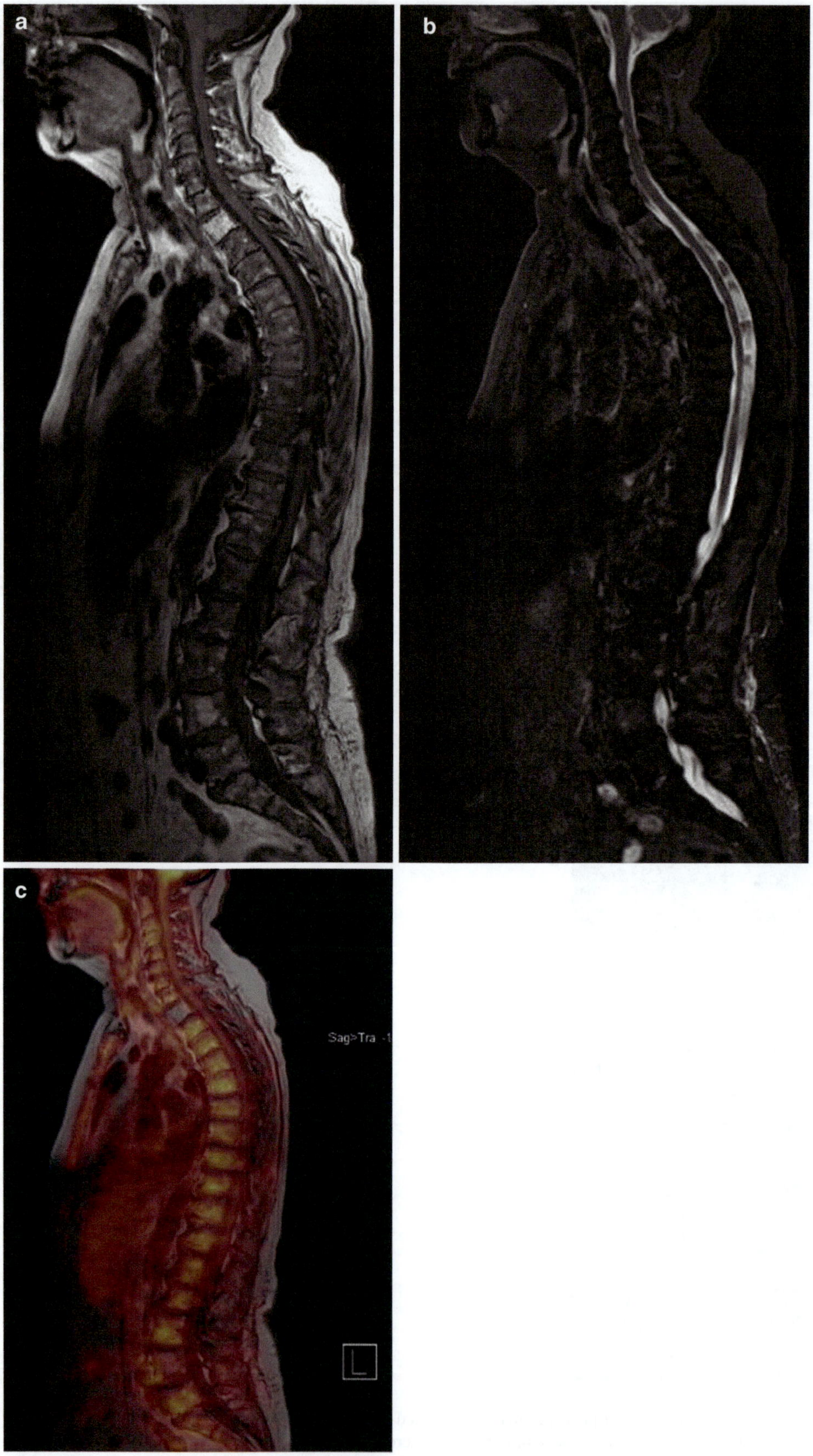

Fig. 3.5 An 89-year-old female with known multiple myeloma. Diffuse infiltration of the bone marrow is visualized on T1-weighted sagittal (**a**) and STIR sagittal (**b**) MR images with fatty signal at T2 and L4 vertebral bodies consistent with hemangiomas. T1-weighted fused PET-MRI image on sagittal plane (**c**) demonstrates the bone marrow to be diffusely avid with the exception of T2 and L4 hemangiomas

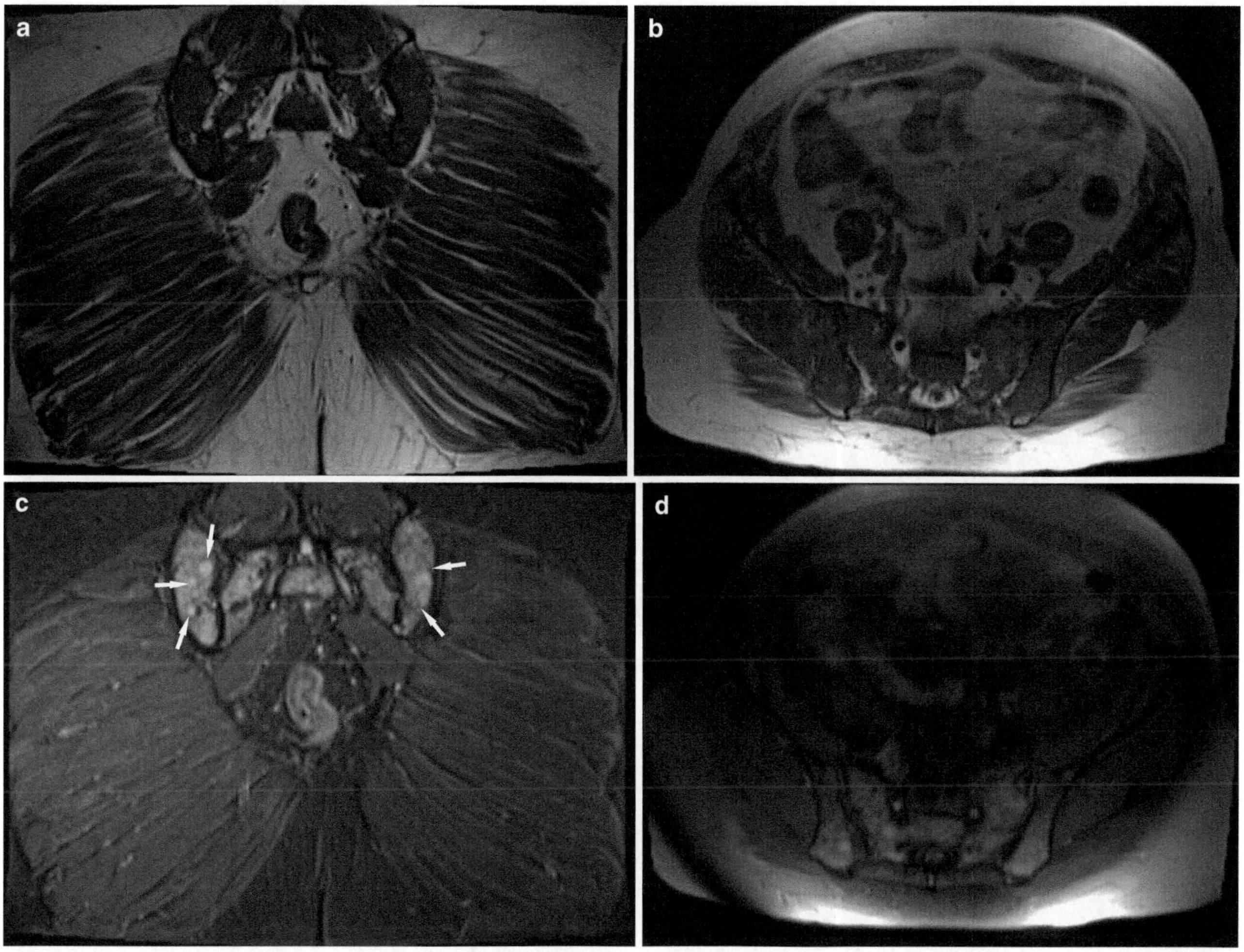

Fig. 3.6 A 65-year-old male with history of multiple myeloma. T1-weighted coronal (**a**) and axial (**b**) images of the pelvis demonstrate diffuse marrow infiltration. Coronal STIR (**c**) and axial T2-weighted (**d**) images show multiple small focal lesions (*arrows*) which are difficult to visualize on T1-weighted images due to diffuse marrow infiltration

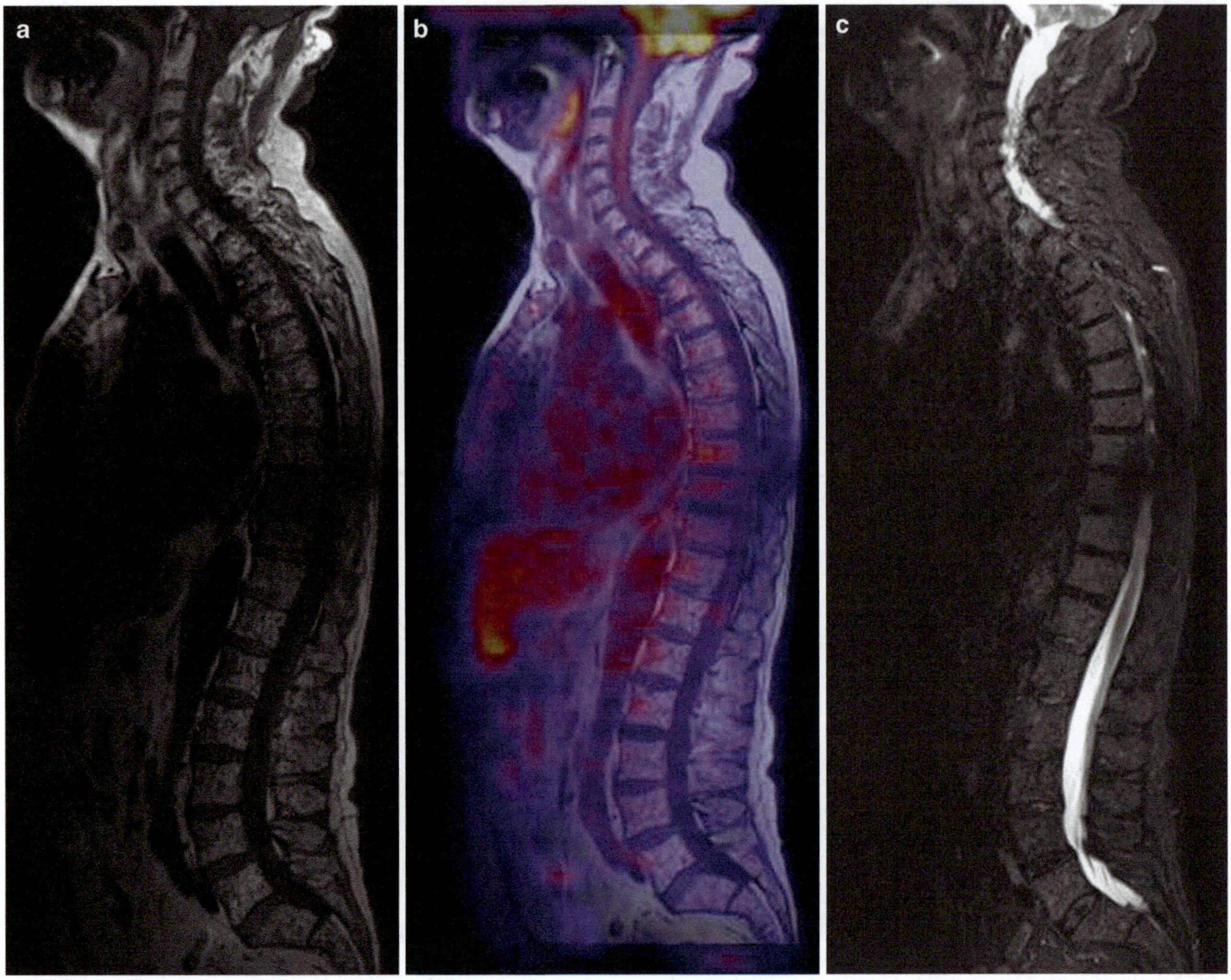

Fig. 3.7 An 80-year-old male with recent multiple myeloma diagnosis. Sagittal T1-weighted (**a**) demonstrates innumerable small myeloma lesions intermixed with fatty marrow background consistent with variegated or salt-and-pepper pattern. T1-weighted fused PET-MRI image (**b**) demonstrates mild FDG avidity of small myeloma lesions. Lesions are difficult to appreciate on sagittal STIR image (**c**)

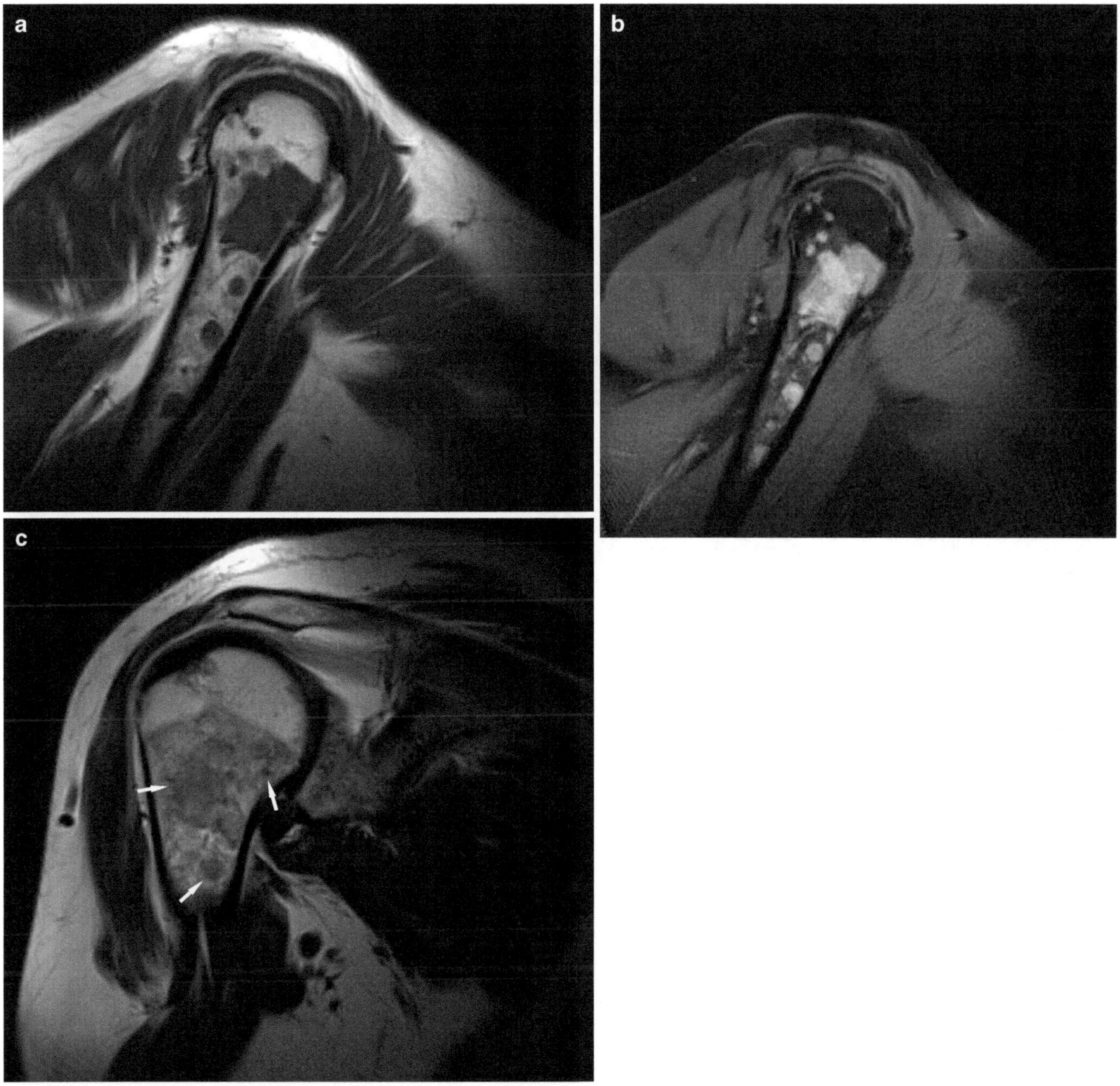

Fig. 3.8 A 61-year-old male with known multiple myeloma. Multiple lesions with varying sizes are noted in the humerus which demonstrate hypointense signal on T1-weighted sagittal image (**a**) compared to adjacent skeletal muscle. These lesions demonstrate hyperintense signal on T2-weighted fat-suppressed sagittal image (**b**). Lesions appear more subtle on T2-weighted coronal image (**c**) without fat suppression (*arrows*)

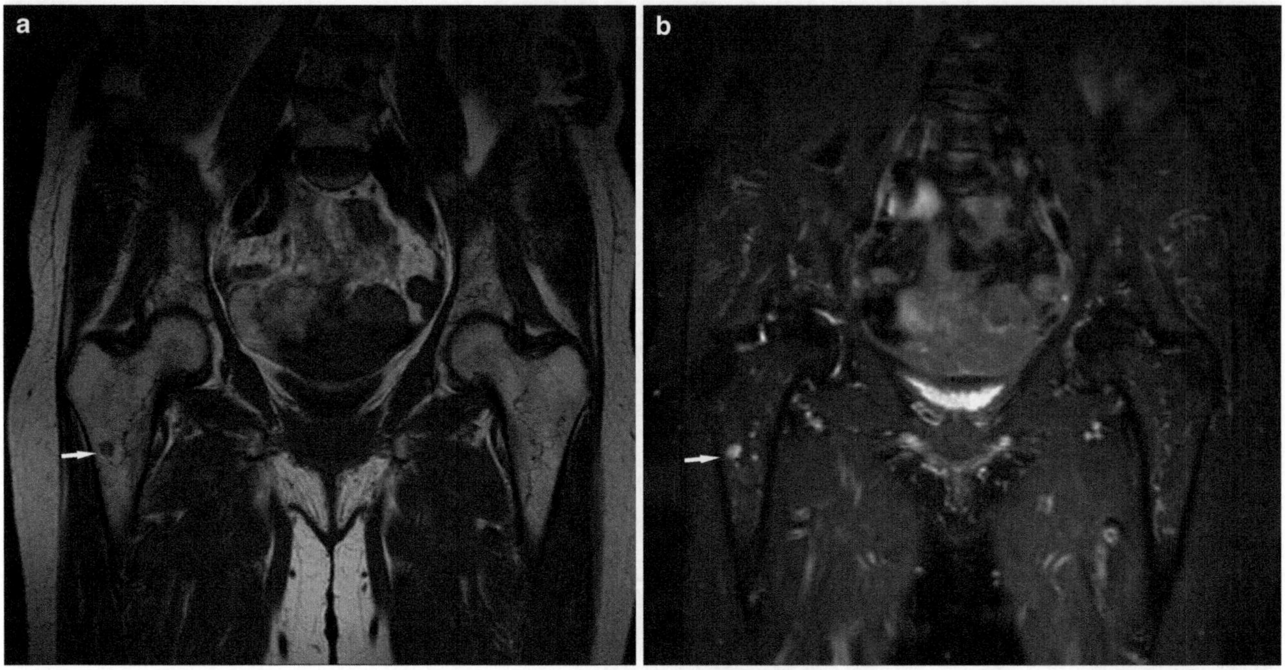

Fig. 3.9 A 74-year-old female with known multiple myeloma. Coronal T1-weighted (**a**) image demonstrates a focal myeloma lesion in the right subtrochanteric femur (*arrows*) which appears slightly hyperintense to skeletal muscle on T1-weighted images. This lesion is hyperintense on coronal STIR image (**b**). Please note the hypervascularity of underlying bone marrow, quite typical of multiple myeloma

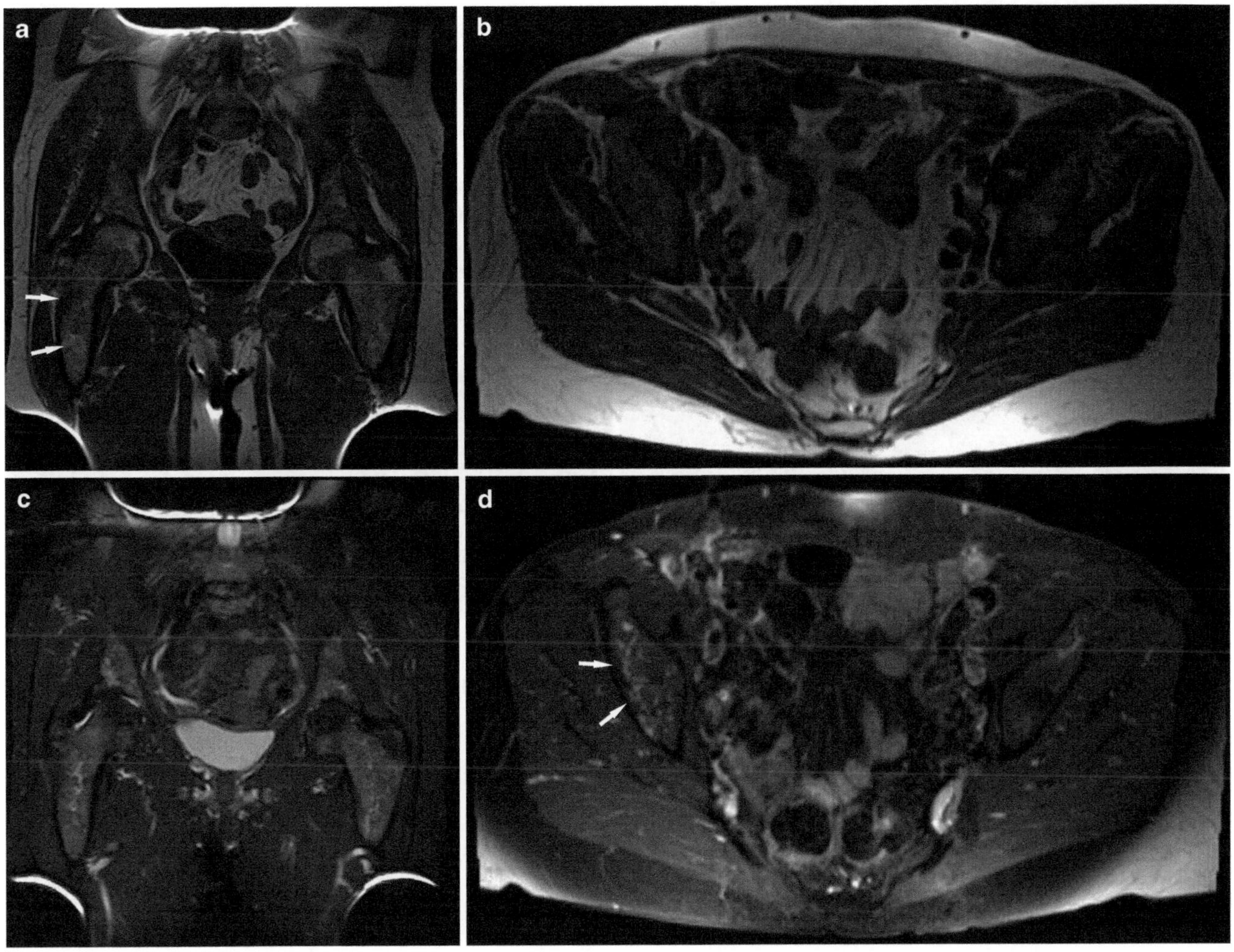

Fig. 3.10 A 72-year-old female with known multiple myeloma. Coronal (**a**) and axial (**b**) T1-weighted precontrast images of the pelvis demonstrate prominent red marrow signal without discrete lesions. On STIR coronal (**c**) and postcontrast T1-weighted fat-suppressed (**d**) images, prominent marrow vascularity is seen, particularly on the right side (*arrows*)

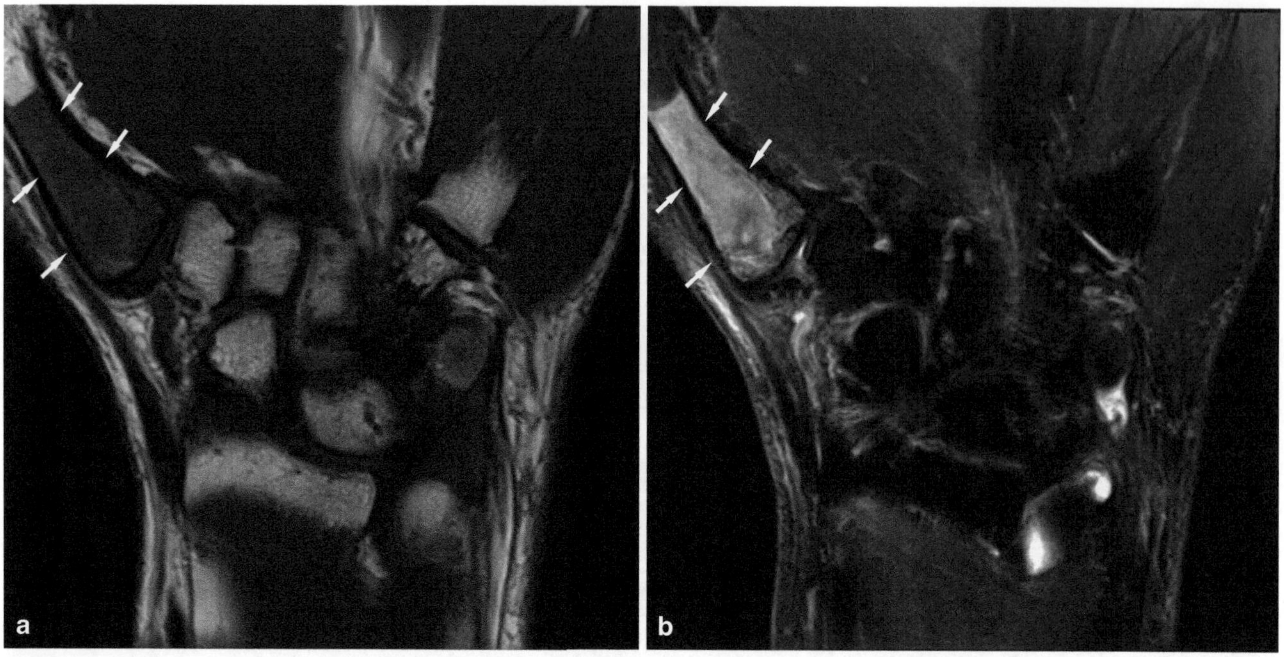

Fig. 3.11 A 70-year-old male with known multiple myeloma. Coronal T1-weighted (**a**) and T2-weighted fat-suppressed (**b**) images of the left wrist demonstrate a large marrow-infiltrating myeloma lesion involving the first metacarpal (*arrows*)

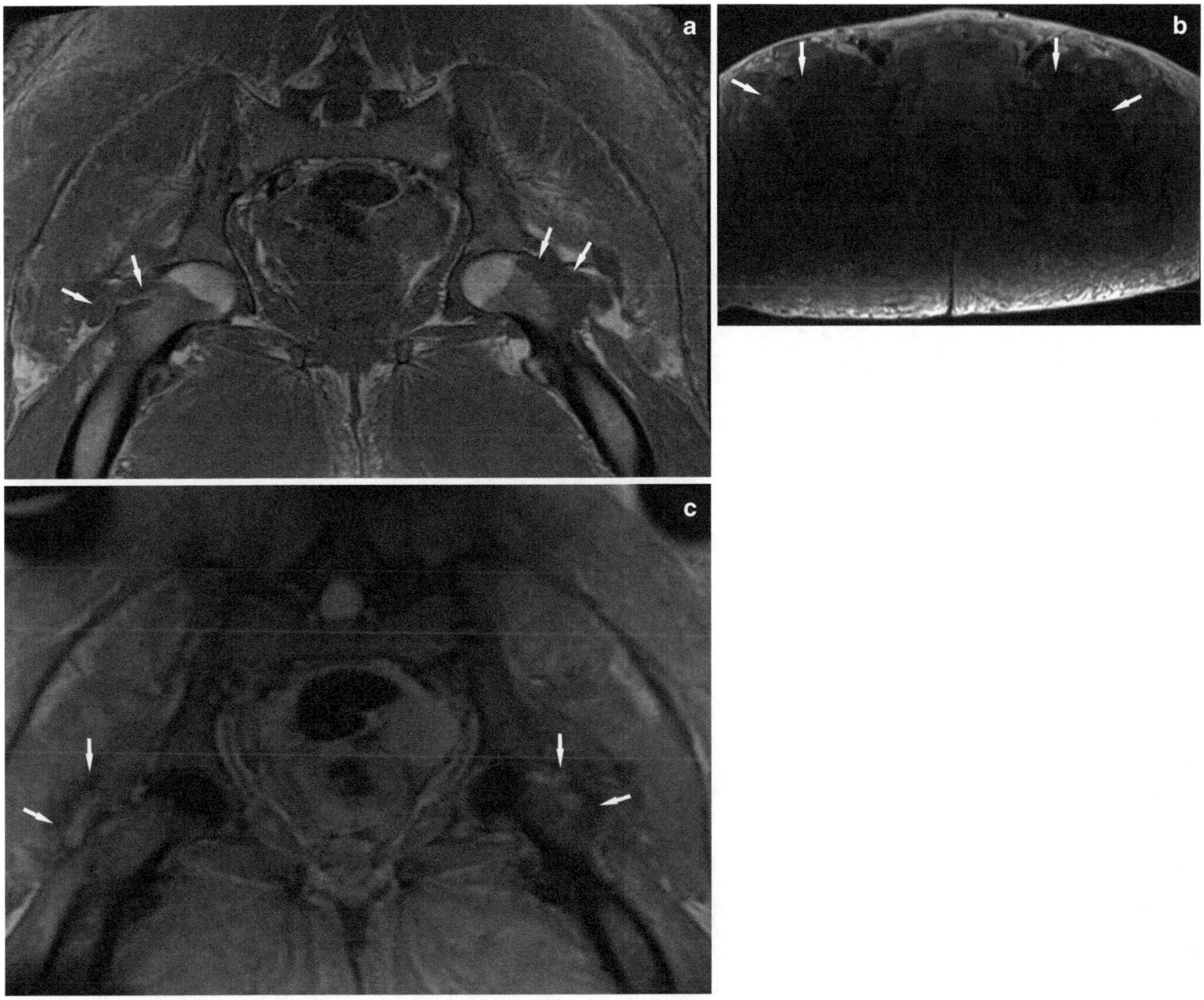

Fig. 3.12 A 49-year-old female with known multiple myeloma. T1-weighted coronal (**a**), T2-weighted axial (**b**) and STIR coronal (**c**) images of the pelvis demonstrate prominent bone marrow signal and bilateral hip joint masses with hypointense signal eroding femoral necks laterally. These intra-articular hip joint masses demonstrate predominantly hypointense on all pulse sequences consistent with amyloidosis (*arrows*)

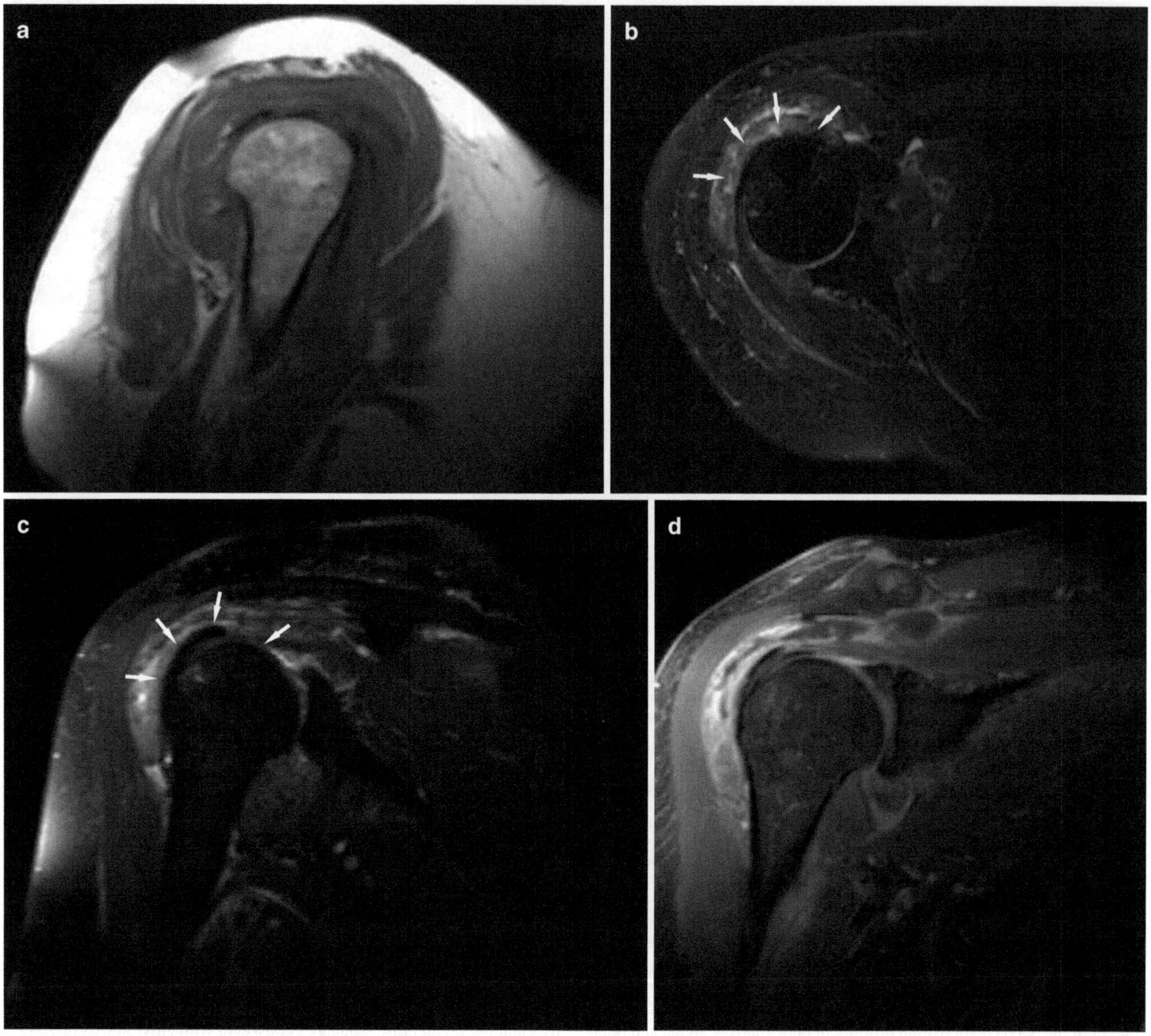

Fig. 3.13 A 52-year-old female with known multiple myeloma presented with right shoulder pain. T1-weighted sagittal image (**a**) shows heterogeneous bone marrow signal with multiple tiny myeloma lesions. T2-weighted fat-suppressed axial (**b**) and coronal images (**c**) demonstrate large synovial masses with predominantly low signal in axillary pouch and subacromial-subdeltoid bursa (*arrows*). Postcontrast T1-weighted fat-suppressed image (**d**) shows synovial enhancement particularly in the periphery. A synovial biopsy revealed amyloid deposition

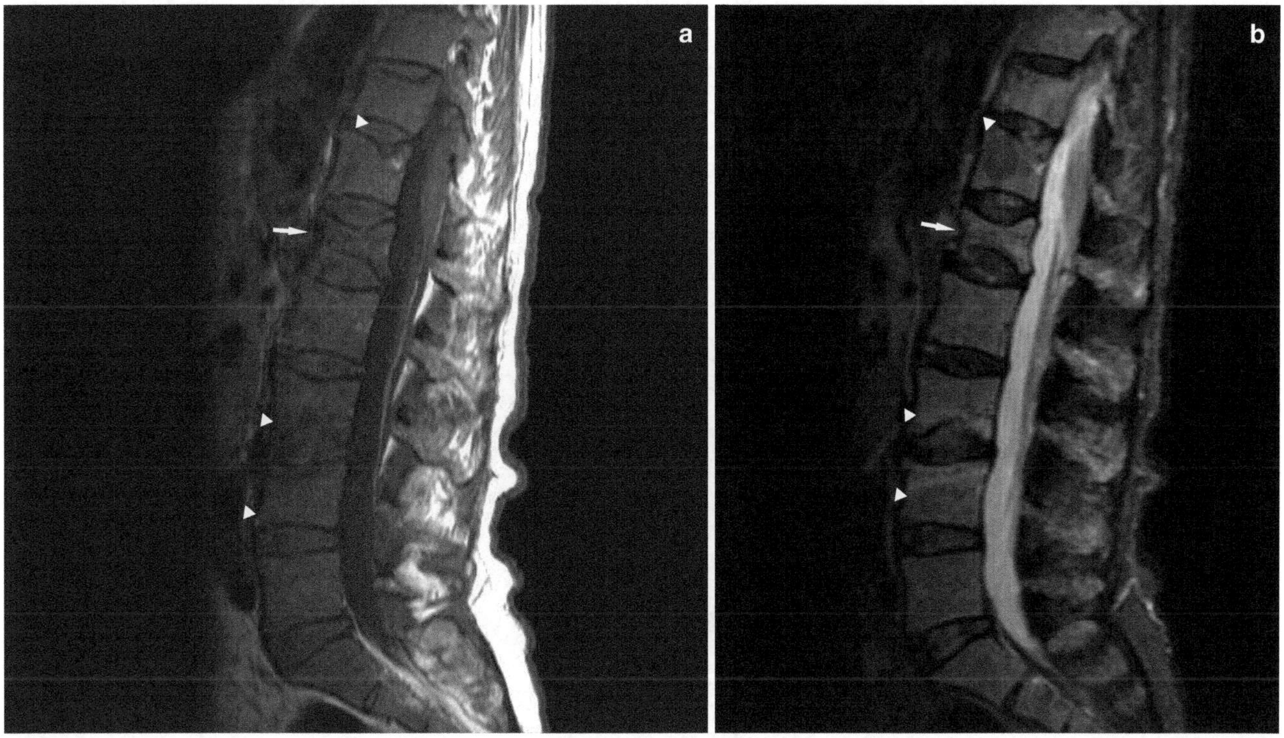

Fig. 3.14 A 71-year-old female with known multiple myeloma. Sagittal T1-weighted (**a**) and sagittal STIR (**b**) sequence images demonstrate diffuse marrow infiltration and pathologic compression deformity of L1 (*arrows*). Mild compression deformities of T12, L3, and L4 are also noted (*arrowheads*)

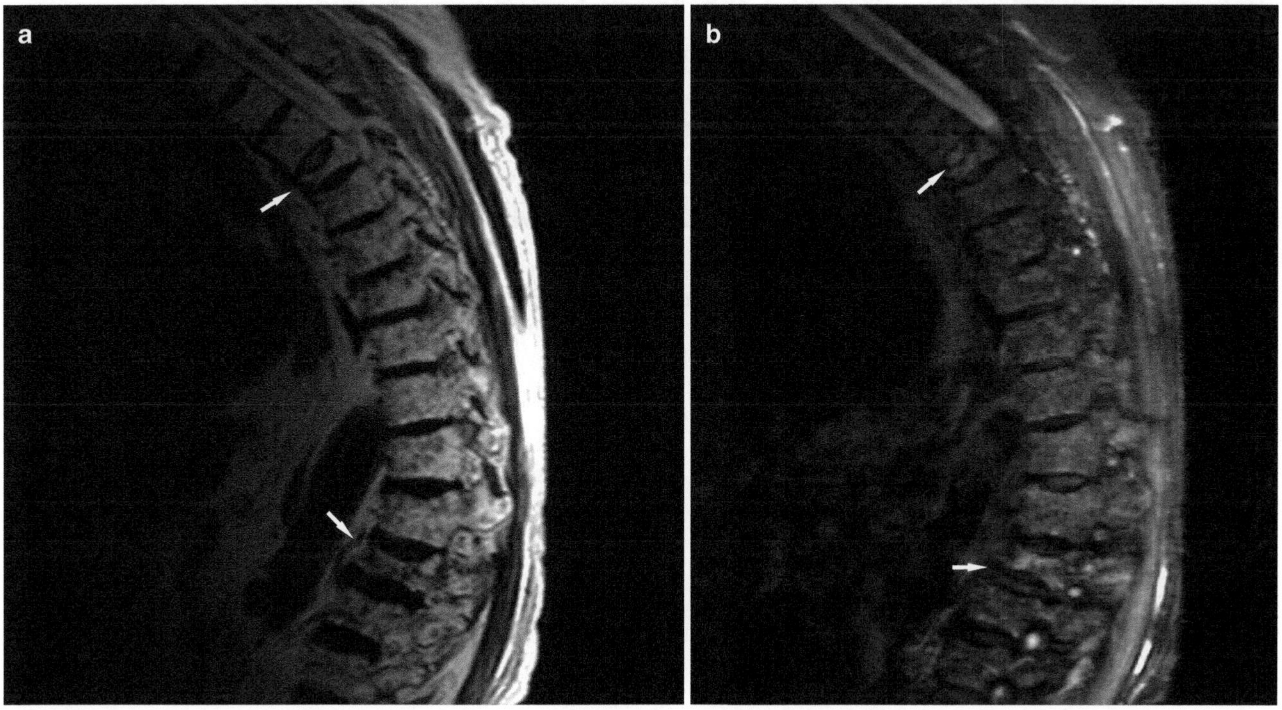

Fig. 3.15 68-year-old male with known multiple myeloma. Osteoporotic compression fractures of T5 and L1 (*arrows*) are noted on sagittal T1-weighted (**a**) and STIR (**b**) sequences with mild associated bone marrow edema. No underlying focal myelomatous lesions are identified

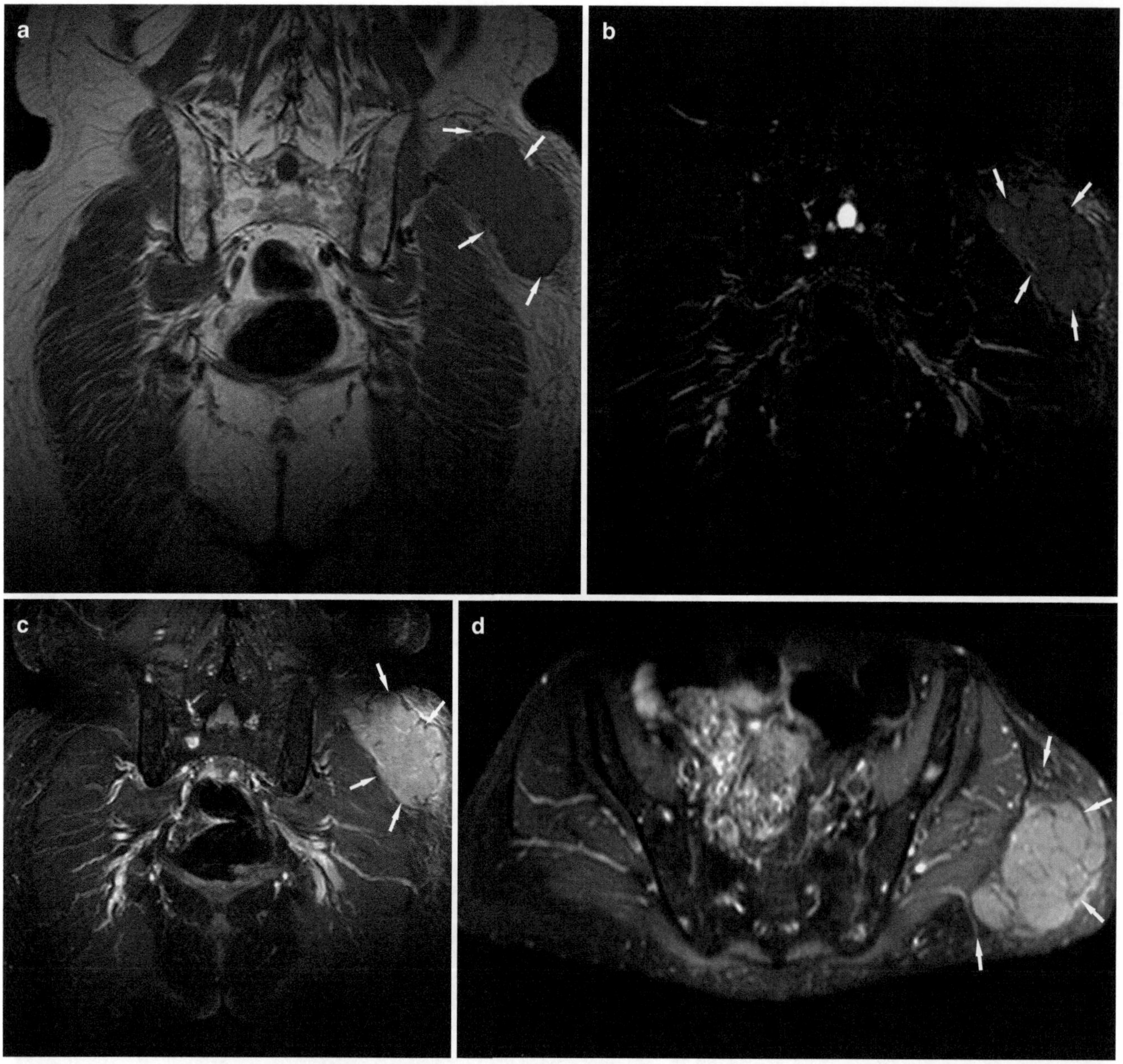

Fig. 3.16 A 61-year-old patient with known multiple myeloma. Coronal T1-weighted (**a**) and coronal STIR (**b**) images demonstrate bone marrow lesions and large lobulated subcutaneous mass overlying the left gluteal musculature (*arrows*). T1-weighted fat-saturated coronal (**c**) and axial (**d**) images demonstrate diffuse enhancement of this mass (*arrows*) (Image-guided biopsy revealed an extramedullary multiple myeloma lesion)

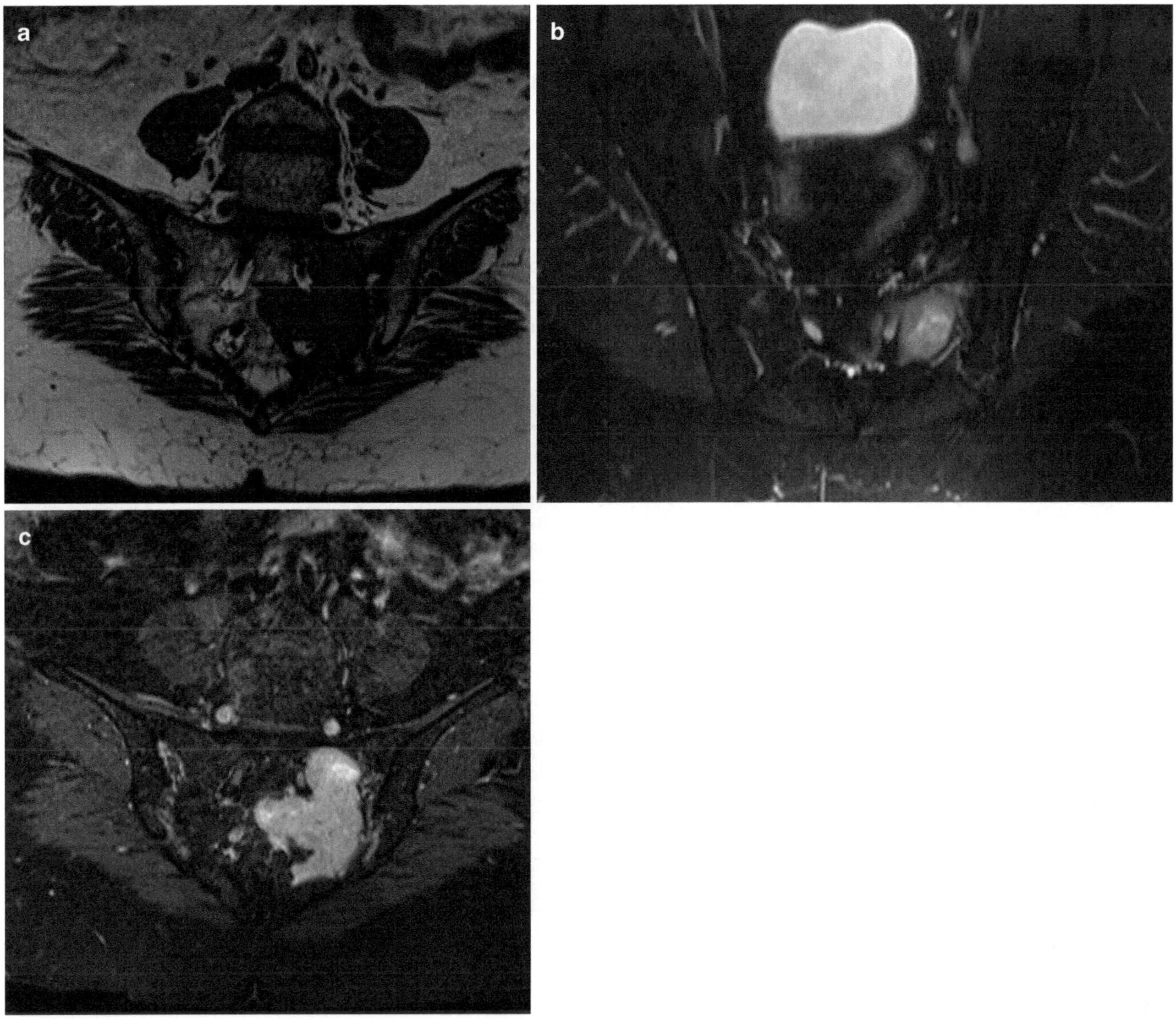

Fig. 3.17 A 70-year-old female with low back pain. T1-weighted coronal (**a**) image demonstrates a large hypointense marrow infiltrating lesion of the left sacral ala and sacral body. Hyperintense signal is noted on T2-weighted fat-suppressed axial image (**b**) and STIR coronal image (**c**). T1-weighted fat-saturated coronal postcontrast image demonstrates diffuse enhancement of the lesion. An image-guided biopsy was performed which showed a plasmacytoma. The patient developed multiple myeloma 1 year after the diagnosis of plasmacytoma

3.2 Lymphoma

Lymphomas are malignant neoplasms arising from lymphatic cells. Lymphomas are divided into two categories: Hodgkin's lymphoma and non-Hodgkin's lymphoma. Lymphoma of the bone marrow is often due to secondary involvement from disseminated disease but can occasionally present as primary extranodal disease. Malignant lymphoma of the bone and bone marrow comprises approximately 7 % of all bone malignancies and 5 % of extranodal lymphomas [6]. Musculoskeletal lymphomas are typically classified into four subtypes: primary bone lymphoma, multifocal primary bone lymphoma, disseminated lymphoma with secondary osseous and marrow involvement within 6 months of lymphoma diagnosis, and disseminated lymphoma with secondary osseous and marrow involvement more than 6 months after diagnosis [7]. Bone and bone marrow involvement is more frequently seen in patients with non-Hodgkin's lymphoma (Fig. 3.18). Bone marrow involvement is unusual in patients with Hodgkin's lymphoma, occurring only in 4–14 % of cases [8] (Fig. 3.19).

MRI may be used to detect focal bone lesions, monitor treatment effects, and evaluate the overall status of the bone

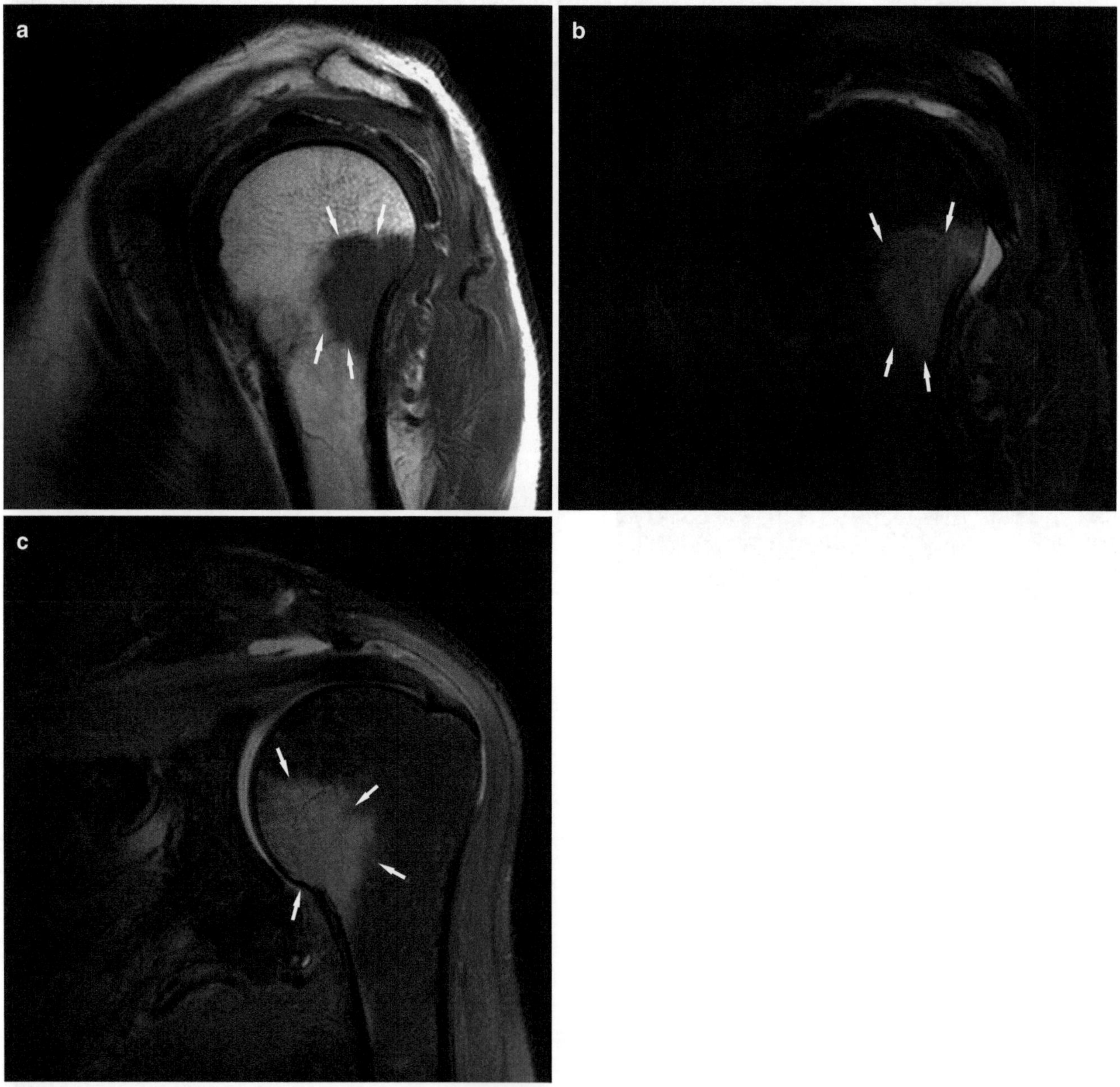

Fig. 3.18 A 63-year-old male with left shoulder pain. Sagittal T1-weighted (**a**) image demonstrates a hypointense marrow-infiltrating lesion in the humeral head and neck medially (*arrows*). T2-weighted fat-suppressed sagittal (**b**) and coronal plane (**c**) images show hyperintense signal within the lesion (*arrows*). An image-guided biopsy revealed primary non-Hodgkin's lymphoma

marrow in patients with lymphoma. When clinicians are evaluating bone marrow abnormalities in patients with suspected lymphoma, comparison of bone marrow signal and the signal of nearby skeletal muscle is crucial. When diffuse or focal areas of bone marrow are hypointense to skeletal muscle on T1-weighted images in a patient after the neonatal period, a neoplastic etiology should be suspected (Fig. 3.20). Bone marrow involvement is important to recognize because it signifies upstaging to stage IV disease, requiring modifications in the treatment in most patients. Contrast enhancement of lymphomatous lesions is also typically seen; however, when large tumors are encountered, an absence of central enhancement is suggestive of necrosis (Fig. 3.21). Permeation of the tumor through the cortex into surrounding soft tissues without obvious cortical destruction is not unusual in cases of lymphoma (Fig. 3.22). Primary bone lymphoma is commonly found in the long bones, frequently arising from the metadiaphysis of the femur, tibia, and humerus [7]. Axial skeletal involvement, including the pelvis, scapula, ribs, and vertebral bodies, is less frequently seen. Multifocal primary bone lymphoma can have both axial and appendicular lesions, commonly in the distal femur, proximal tibia, and spine. Secondary osseous lymphoma typically affects the axial skeleton, including the spine, pelvis (Fig. 3.23), skull, ribs, and facial bones [7]. Associated large soft tissue masses are common in patients with secondary osseous lymphomas (Fig. 3.24). When diffuse bone marrow involvement is present, leukemia is often considered in the differential diagnosis (Fig. 3.25).

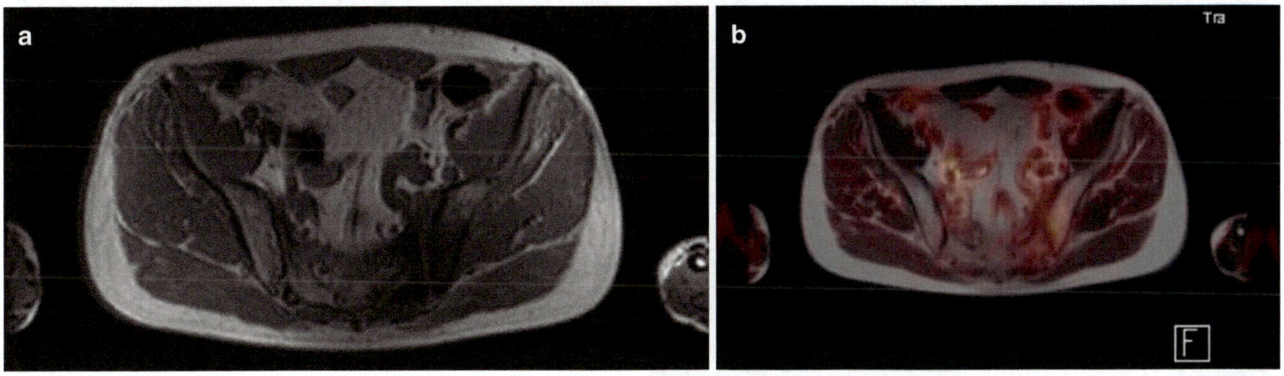

Fig. 3.19 A 69-year-old female with Hodgkin's lymphoma. Axial T1-weighted image (**a**) of the pelvis demonstrates a large marrow-infiltrating hypointense lesion centered around the left SI joint with involvement of the sacrum and ilium. Fused PET-MRI T2-weighted axial image (**b**) demonstrates FDG avidity of the lesion

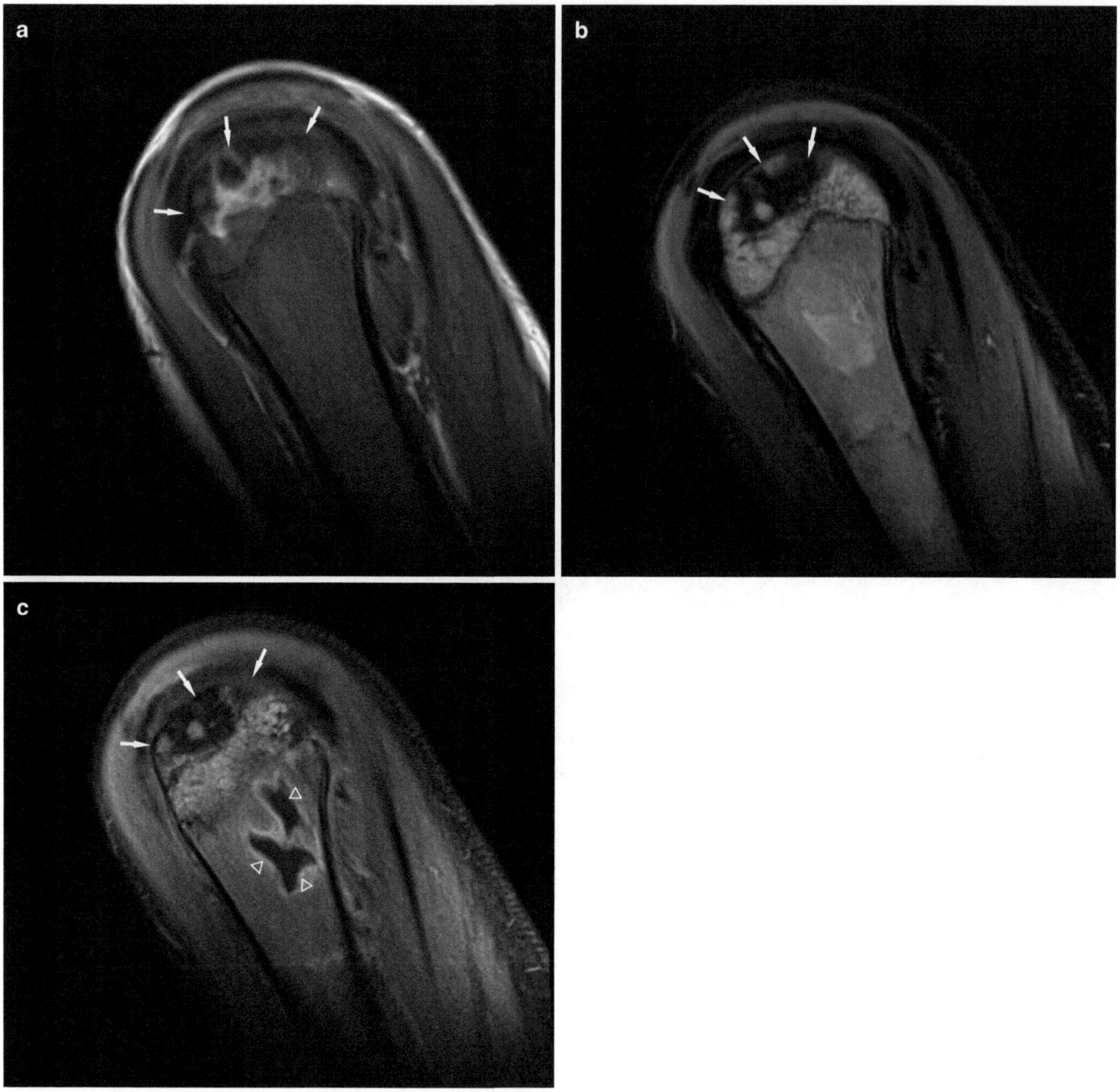

Fig. 3.20 A 17-year-old male with right shoulder pain. T1-weighted sagittal image (**a**) demonstrates infiltrated bone marrow which appears iso- to hypointense compared to skeletal muscle with nearly absent fat in the epiphysis (*arrows*). Findings are more subtle on T2-weighted fat-suppressed sagittal image (**b**), and postcontrast T1-weighted fat-suppressed image (**c**) shows lack of enhancement in the humeral neck (*arrow heads*). An image-guided biopsy revealed non-Hodgkin's lymphoma

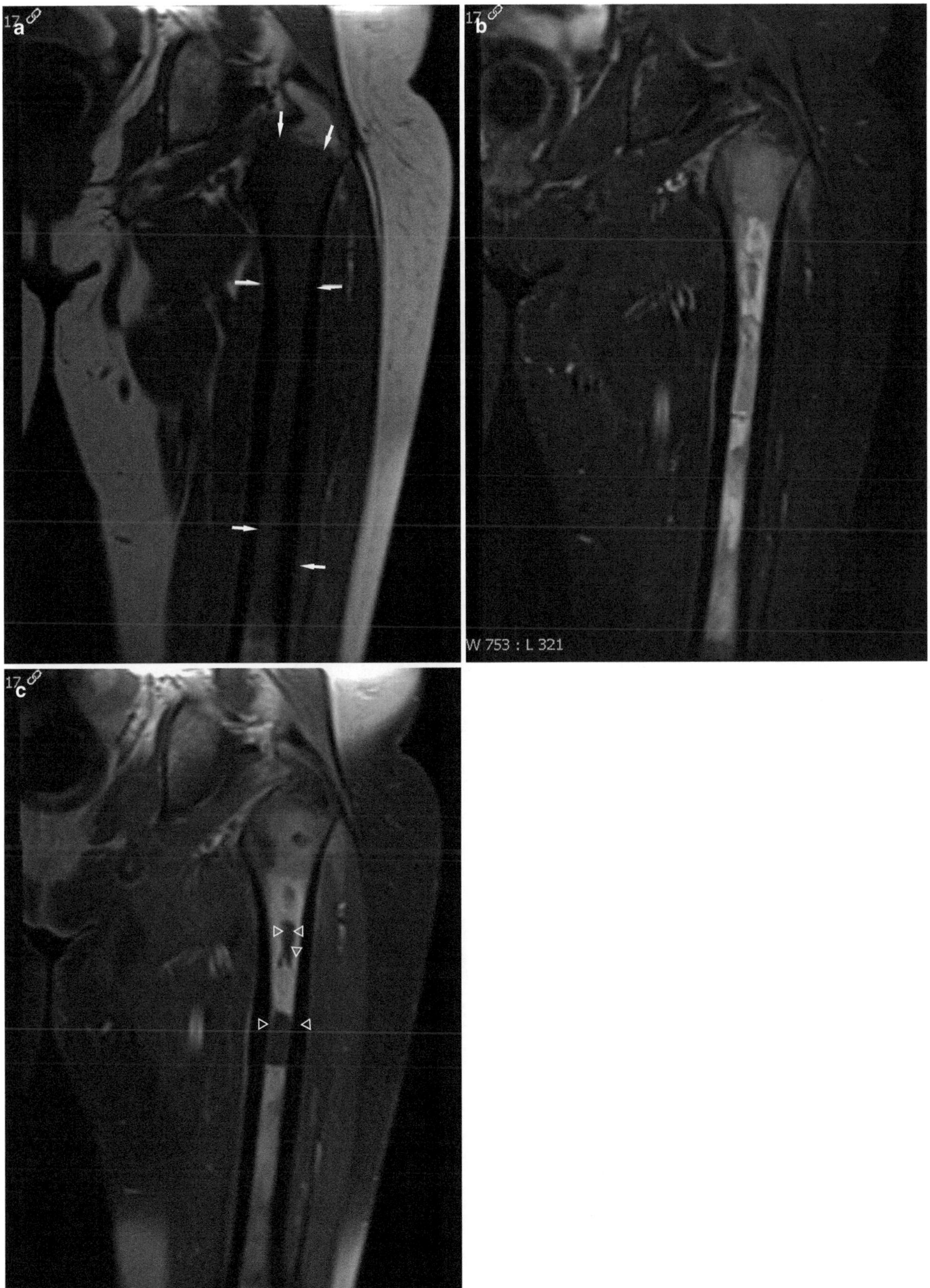

Fig. 3.21 64-year-old female with non-Hodgkin's lymphoma. T1-weighted coronal image of the left femur (**a**) demonstrates a long segment homogeneously hypointense marrow-infiltrating process consistent with patient's known lymphoma (*arrows*). T2-weighted fat-suppressed coronal image (**b**) shows heterogeneous appearance of the lesion with areas of hypointensity more centrally and hyperintensities mostly in the periphery. Postcontrast T1-weighted fat-suppressed coronal image (**c**) demonstrates enhancement in the majority of the lesion with central and proximal areas which lack enhancement, suggestive of necrotic changes (*arrowheads*)

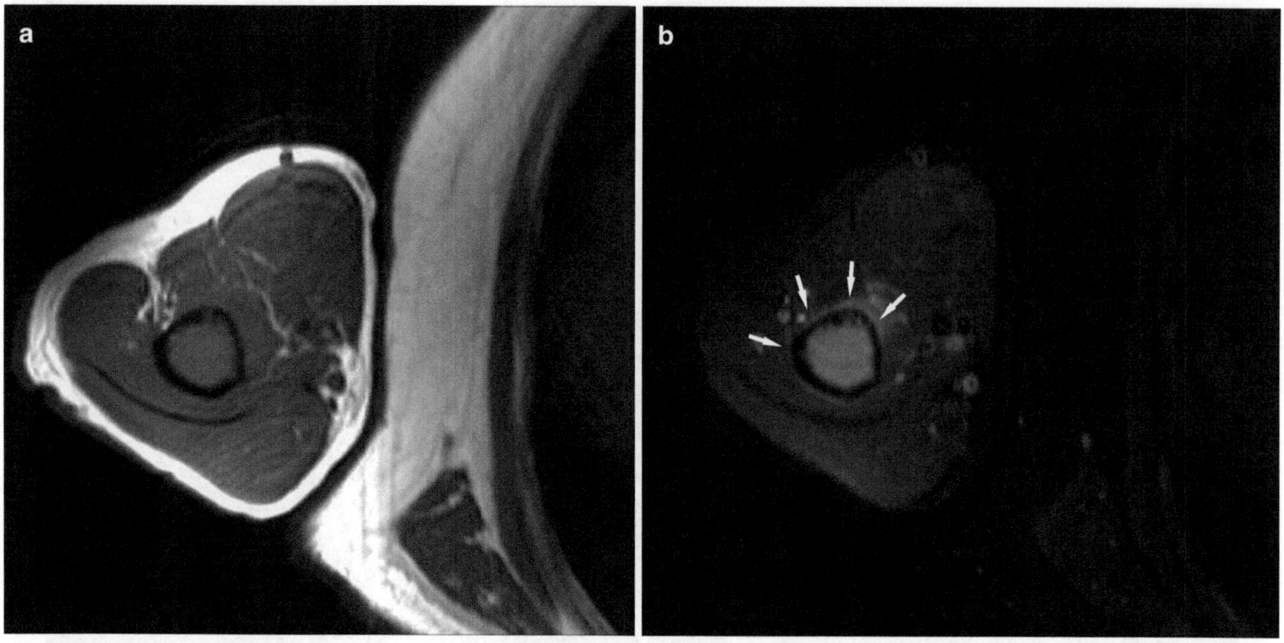

Fig. 3.22 An 83-year-old female with diffuse large B-cell lymphoma. Axial T1-weighted (**a**) and T2-weighted fat-suppressed (**b**) images of the right humerus demonstrate bone marrow infiltration consistent with a lymphoma lesion. Subtle linear areas of cortical permeation are better visualized on T2-weighted images with associated small soft tissue mass anteriorly (*arrows*)

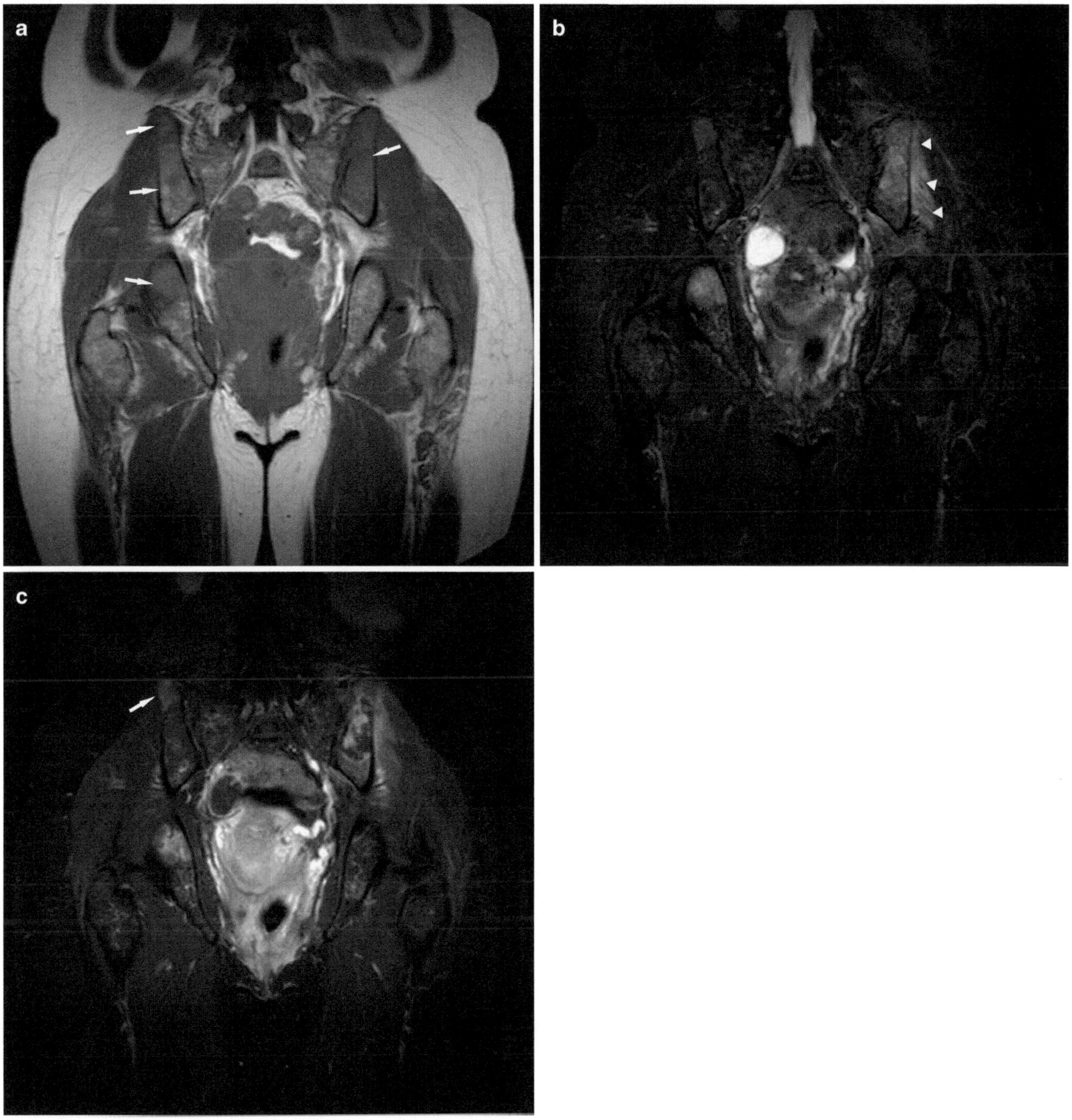

Fig. 3.23 A 49-year-old female with B-cell non-Hodgkin's lymphoma. Coronal T1-weighted (**a**), T2-weighted fat-suppressed (**b**), and post-contrast T1-weighted fat-suppressed (**c**) images demonstrate several foci of bone marrow infiltration and abnormal enhancement consistent with lymphoma lesions (*arrows*). Soft tissue extension is noted about the left iliac crest (*arrowheads*)

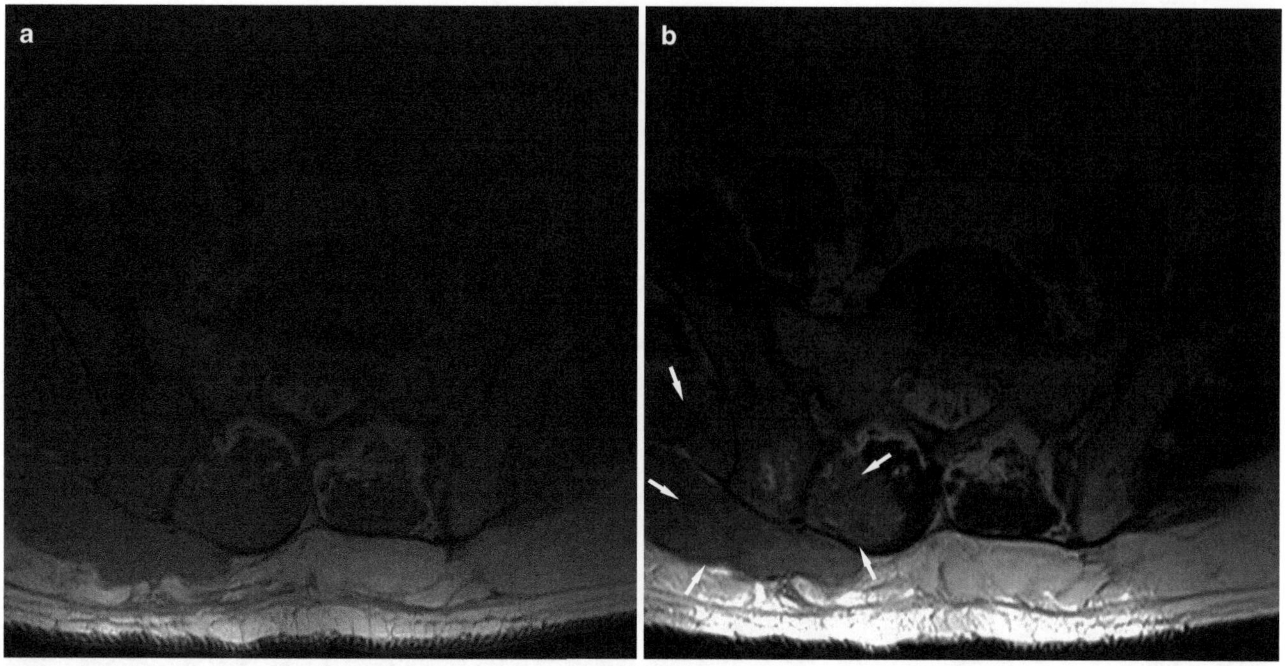

Fig. 3.24 A 61-year-old patient with diffuse large B-cell lymphoma. Axial T1-weighted (**a**) and T2-weighted (**b**) images of the pelvis demonstrate a marrow-infiltrating lesion of the right posterior iliac crest with associated large soft tissue mass (*arrows*)

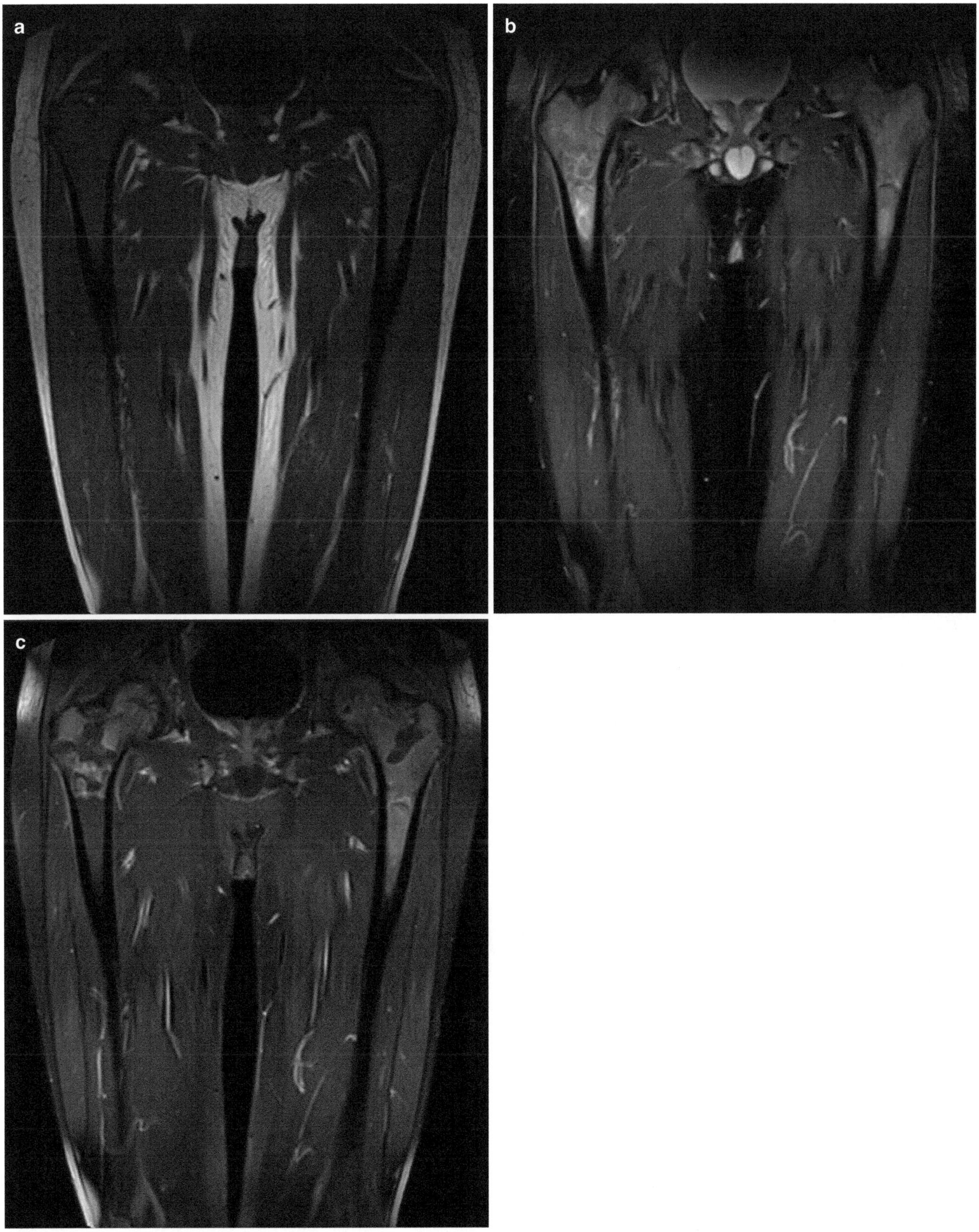

Fig. 3.25 A 19-year-old male with weakness and weight loss. Coronal T1-weighted (**a**) and T2- weighted fat-suppressed (**b**) images of the femurs demonstrate diffuse bone marrow infiltration. Heterogeneous enhancement pattern is noted on postcontrast T1-weighted fat-saturated coronal image (**c**). An image-guided biopsy showed diffuse large B-cell lymphoma

3.3 Leukemia

Leukemias are a group of heterogeneous neoplastic bone marrow disorders involving white blood cells. Leukemias have been recognized as acute or chronic, based on their untreated disease course. Leukemias may also be divided into myeloid or lymphoid types according to their cell origin.

MRI is known to be very sensitive for showing bone marrow changes in patients with leukemia [9]. The diffuse MR pattern of marrow involvement in leukemia is typical (Fig. 3.26) but not specific for the disease, as this pattern may be seen in other systemic diseases such as lymphomas. Additionally, recognition of diffuse marrow infiltration can be difficult, especially in younger children who have an abundance of hematopoietic bone marrow. On T1-weighted images, bone marrow signal should be compared to the signal of nearby skeletal muscle. Hematopoietic bone marrow should be hyperintense to skeletal muscle except in neonates. After the neonatal period, bone marrow signal that is hypointense compared to skeletal muscle should be considered suspicious for a diffuse marrow-infiltrating neoplasm such as leukemia (Fig. 3.27). On T2-weighted images and STIR images, hyperintense signal is frequently seen in patients with acute leukemia (Fig. 3.28), and intermediate to low signal is frequently seen in patients with chronic leukemias (Fig. 3.29). In postcontrast images, acute leukemia-related bone marrow infiltrates tend to enhance, although foci of absent enhancement could be seen suggestive of necrosis (Fig. 3.27).

In acute leukemias, the evaluation of response to treatment requires serial bone marrow biopsies during the course of therapy. MRI has been shown to be an important noninvasive modality for assessing the posttreatment status of the bone marrow, either detecting new lesions or demonstrating normal signal intensity. As with lymphomatous involvement of the bone marrow, extraosseous soft tissue extension of the tumor (or "permeation") may occur without obvious cortical destruction. In patients with acute leukemia, local relapse may be seen in the form of focal disease called "chloroma" or "myeloid sarcoma," which can be easily recognized on MR images as a focus of bone marrow infiltration with or without soft tissue extension (Fig. 3.30). Chloromas are more frequently seen in the setting of treated acute myeloid leukemia; although rare, they can also be seen in patients with acute lymphoblastic leukemia (Fig. 3.31).

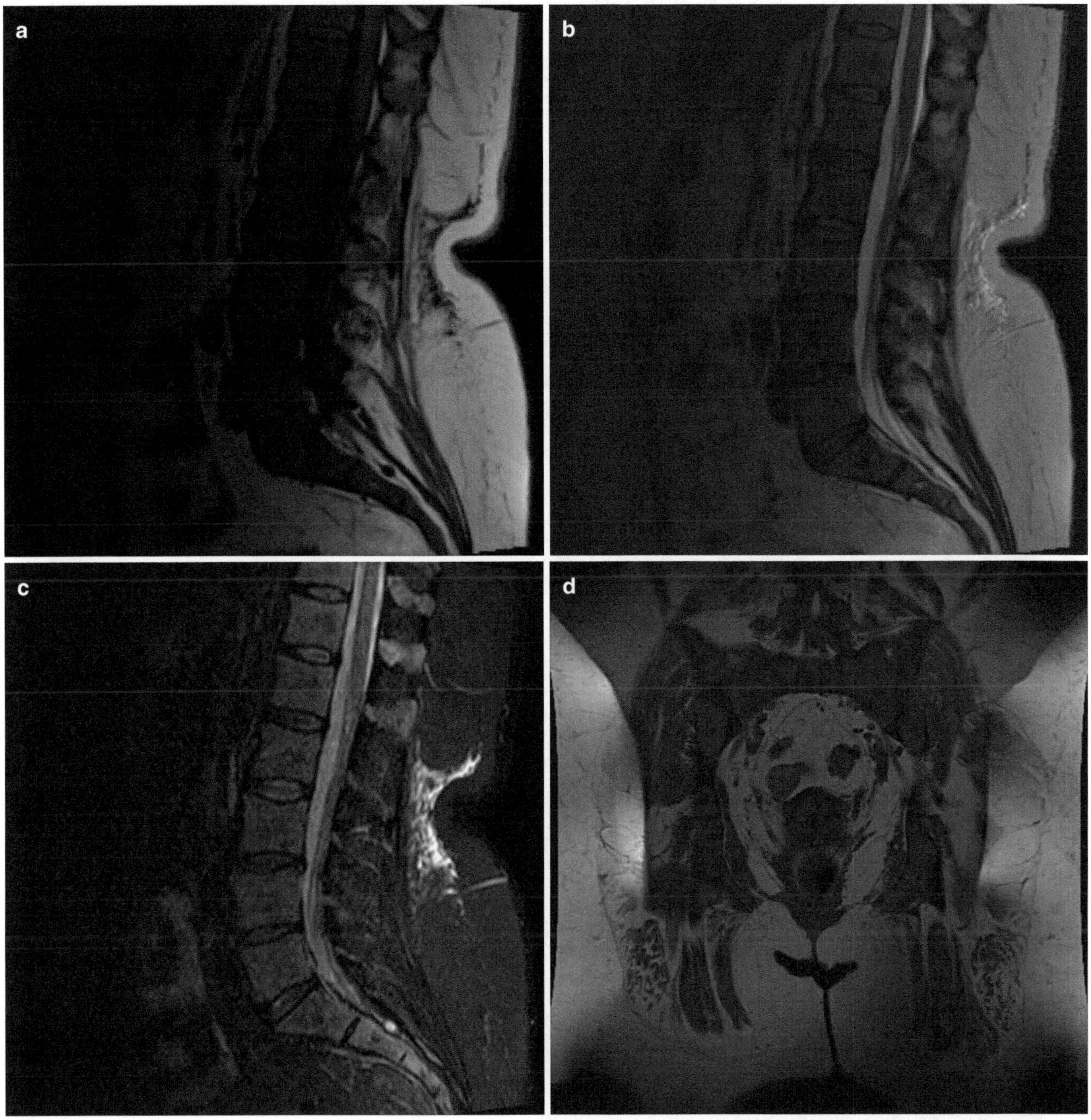

Fig. 3.26 A 52-year-old female with acute lymphoblastic leukemia. Diffuse leukemic infiltration of the bone marrow is visualized on T1-weighted sagittal image (**a**) of the lumbar spine. Bone marrow signal abnormality is difficult to appreciate on sagittal T2-weighted (**b**) and STIR (**c**) images of the lumbar spine. T1-weighted coronal image (**d**) of pelvis also shows diffuse marrow infiltration

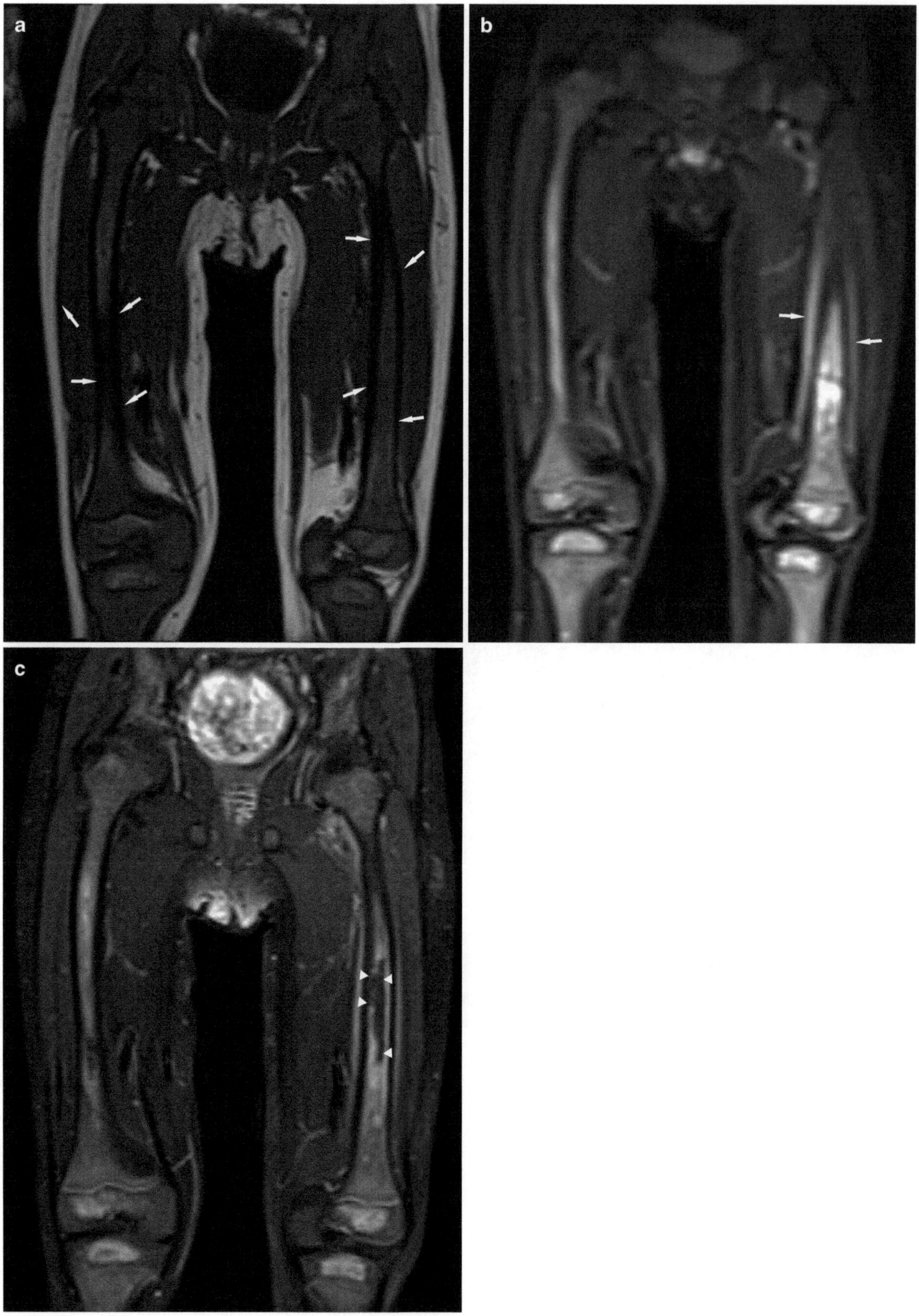

Fig. 3.27 A 3-year-old boy presented with failure to grow. T1-weighted coronal image (**a**) of the bilateral femurs demonstrates diffuse marrow abnormality most intense in the distal femoral diaphyses (*arrows*) which appear to be hypointense to skeletal muscle consistent with leukemic infiltrates. Diffusely hyperintense signal on T2-weighted coronal image corresponding to T1 signal abnormalities (**b**) periostitis along the left femur (*arrowheads*). Postcontrast T1-weighted fat-saturated image (**c**) demonstrates lack of enhancement in the femoral diaphysis greater on the left side, suggestive of bone marrow necrosis. Bone marrow aspiration was performed which revealed acute myelogenous leukemia

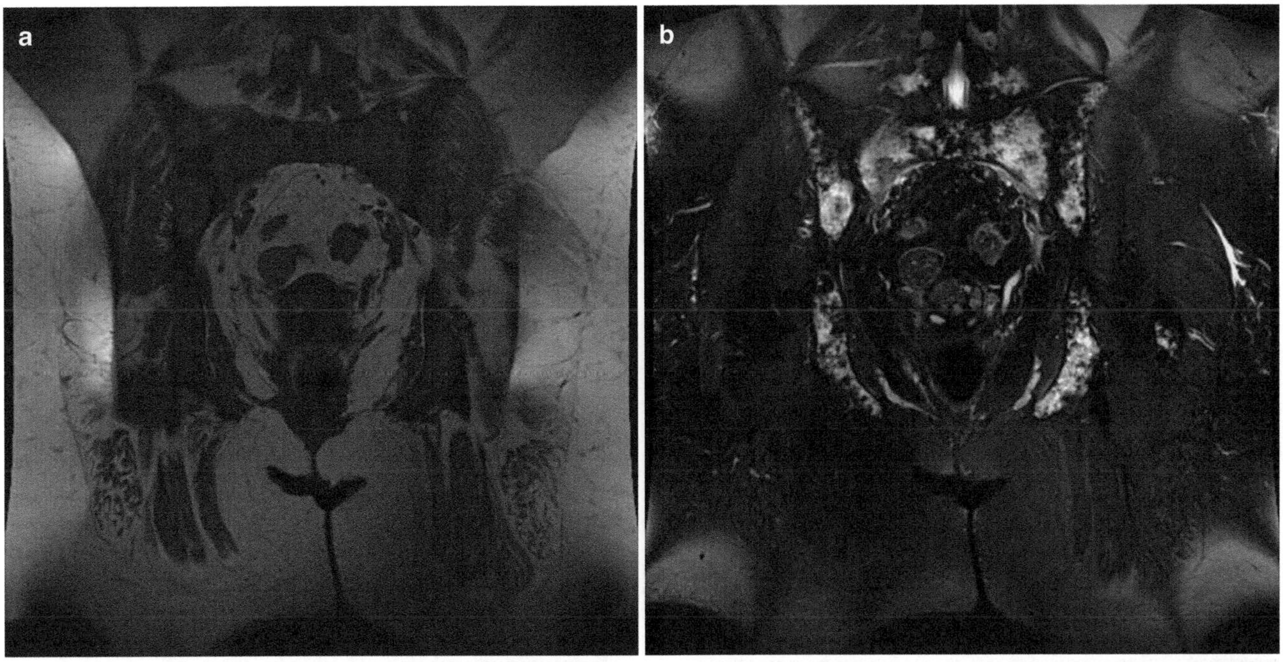

Fig. 3.28 A 49-year-old female with acute lymphoblastic leukemia. Diffuse leukemic infiltration of the bone marrow is present throughout pelvis on T1-weighted coronal image (**a**). Markedly hyperintense signal of leukemic infiltrates is noted on T2-weighted fat-suppressed image (**b**)

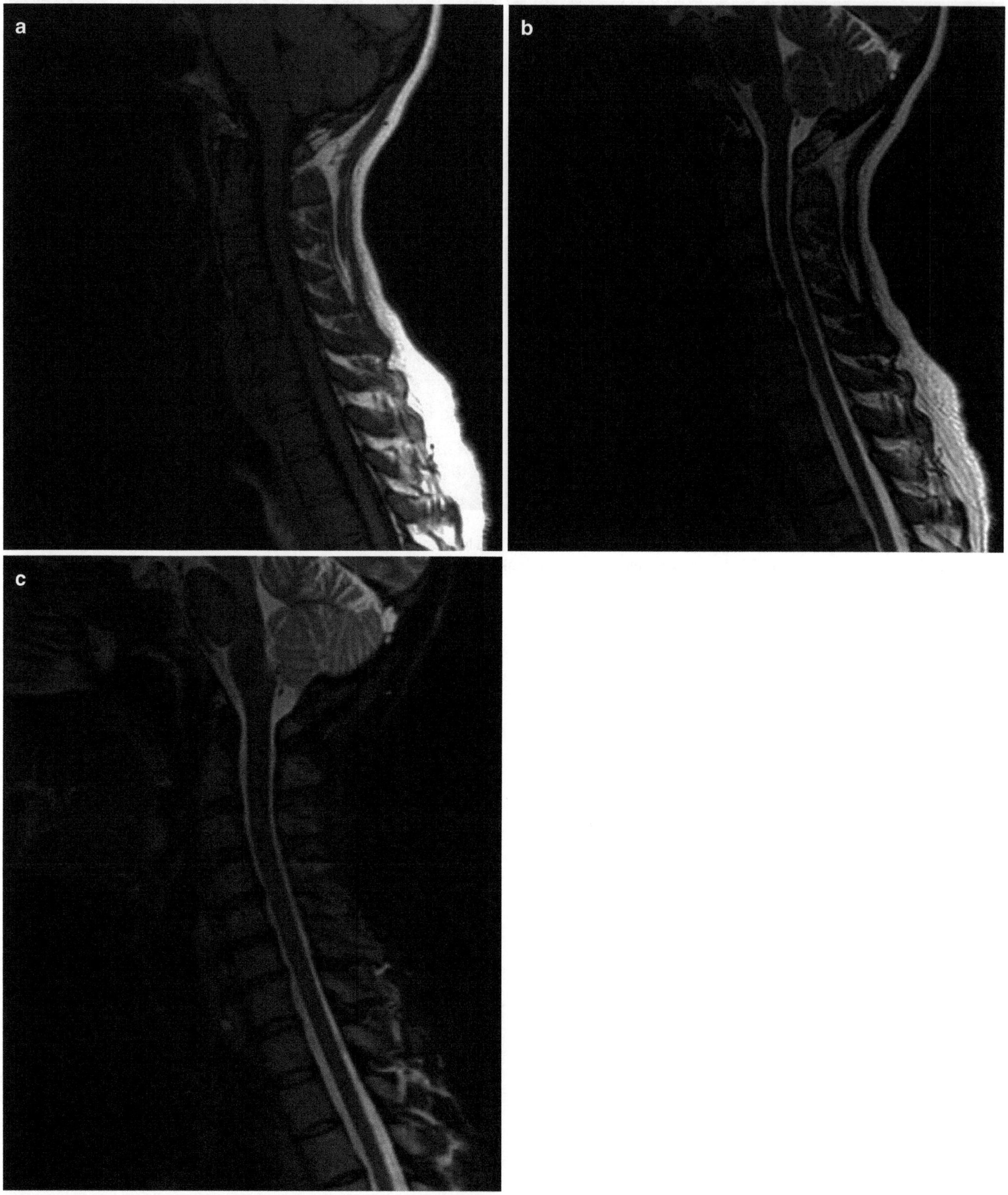

Fig. 3.29 A 56-year-old female with chronic lymphoblastic leukemia. Diffuse hypointensity of the visualized bone marrow is noted on sagittal T1-weighted (**a**), T2-weighted (**b**), and STIR (**c**) sequences

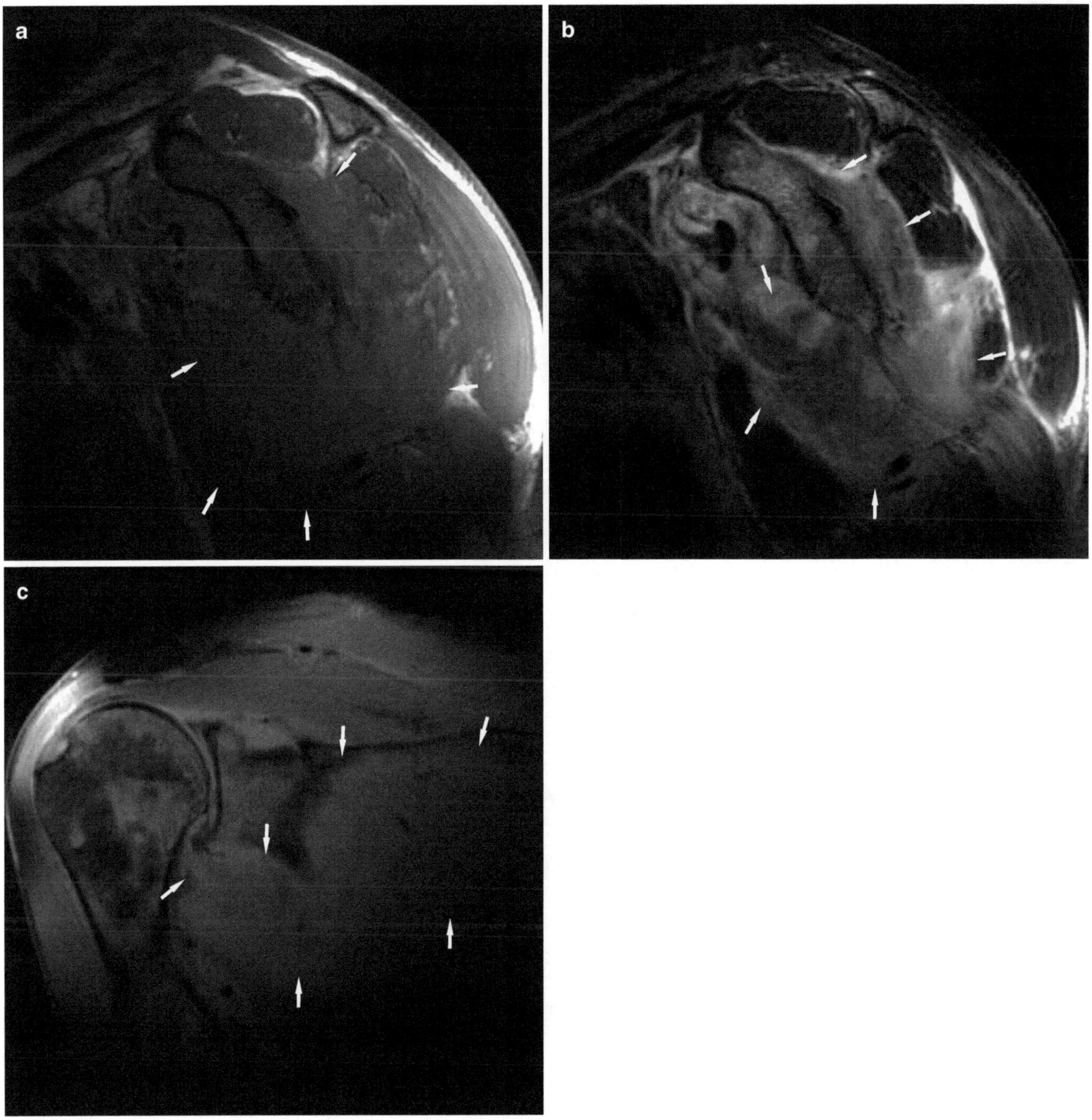

Fig. 3.30 A 59-year-old male with history of treated acute myeloid leukemia. Patient presented with shoulder pain and MRI was obtained. T1-weighted sagittal (**a**), T2-weighted sagittal (**b**), and proton density-weighted fat-suppressed coronal (**c**) images demonstrate a large soft tissue mass and underlying abnormal marrow involving the scapula (*arrows*). A biopsy of the mass showed leukemic infiltrates consistent with a chloroma

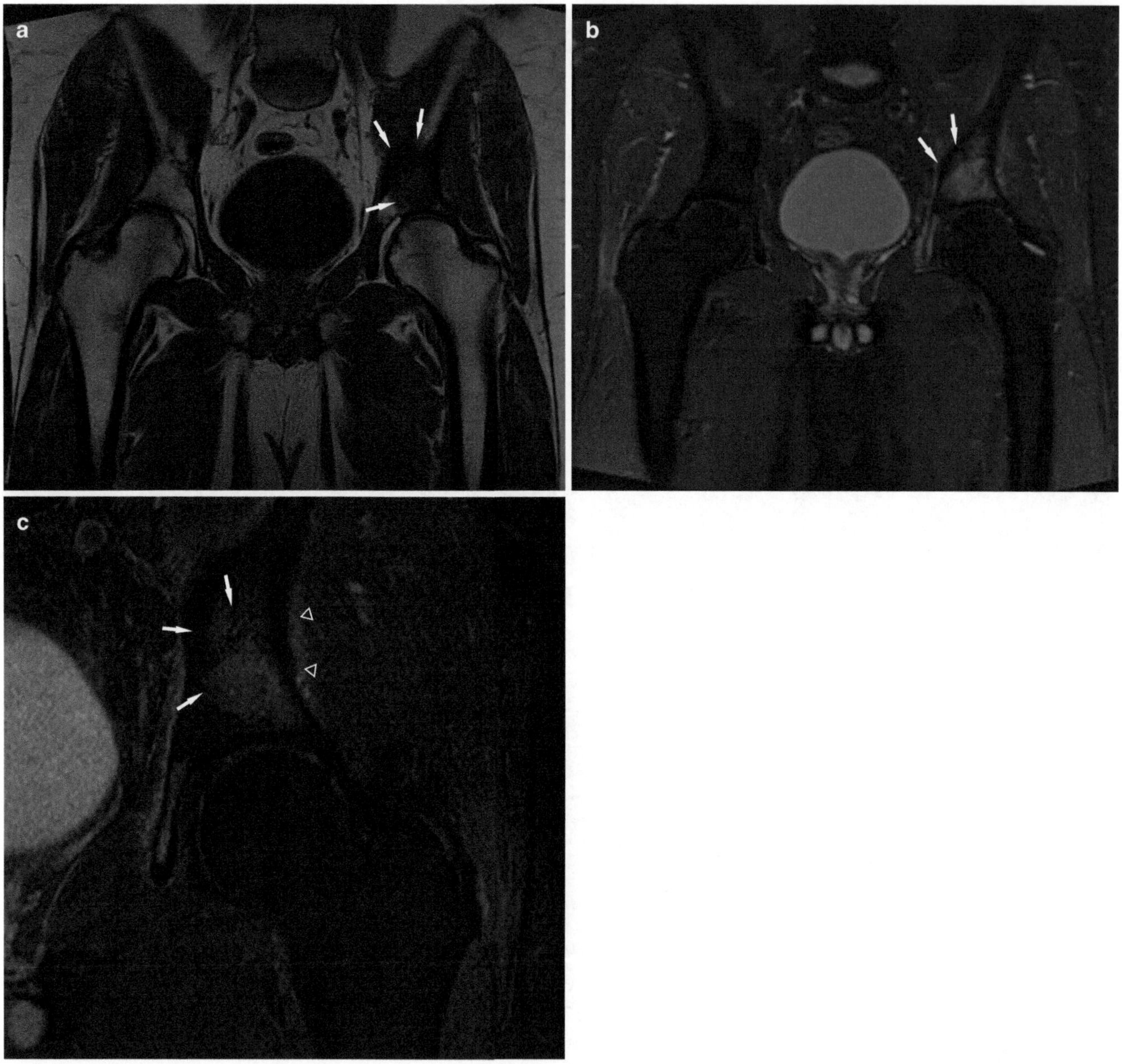

Fig. 3.31 42-year-old patient with history of treated acute lymphoblastic leukemia, in remission. Patient presented with left hip pain and an MRI was obtained showing focal bone marrow infiltration about the left acetabulum (*arrows*) on T1-weighted (**a**) and T2-weighted (**b**) coronal images consistent with a chloroma. Small field of view T2-weighted image (**c**) of the left hip shows subtle leukemic infiltrates in the adjacent soft tissues (*arrowheads*)

3.4 Myeloproliferative Neoplasms

3.4.1 Myelodysplastic Syndromes

Myelodysplastic syndromes are a heterogeneous group of clonal hematological stem cell disorders. Myelodysplastic syndromes are considered a premalignant condition in a subgroup of patients who progress to acute myelogenous leukemia. MRI is helpful for follow-up imaging in these patients, detecting early bone marrow changes related to the development of leukemia and offering clinicians the information they need to change treatment strategies [10]. These patients receive blood transfusions due to pancytopenia, which can lead to iron deposition in the bone marrow. MRI findings often reflect different stages of the disease and degree of iron deposition in the bone marrow (Fig. 3.32) [11]. Prominent hematopoietic bone marrow signal is present in most of these patients even in the absence of iron deposition (Fig. 3.33). The development of focal or diffuse hypointense T1-weighted and hyperintense T2-weighted/STIR signal should raise suspicion for the presence of leukemia (Fig. 3.34).

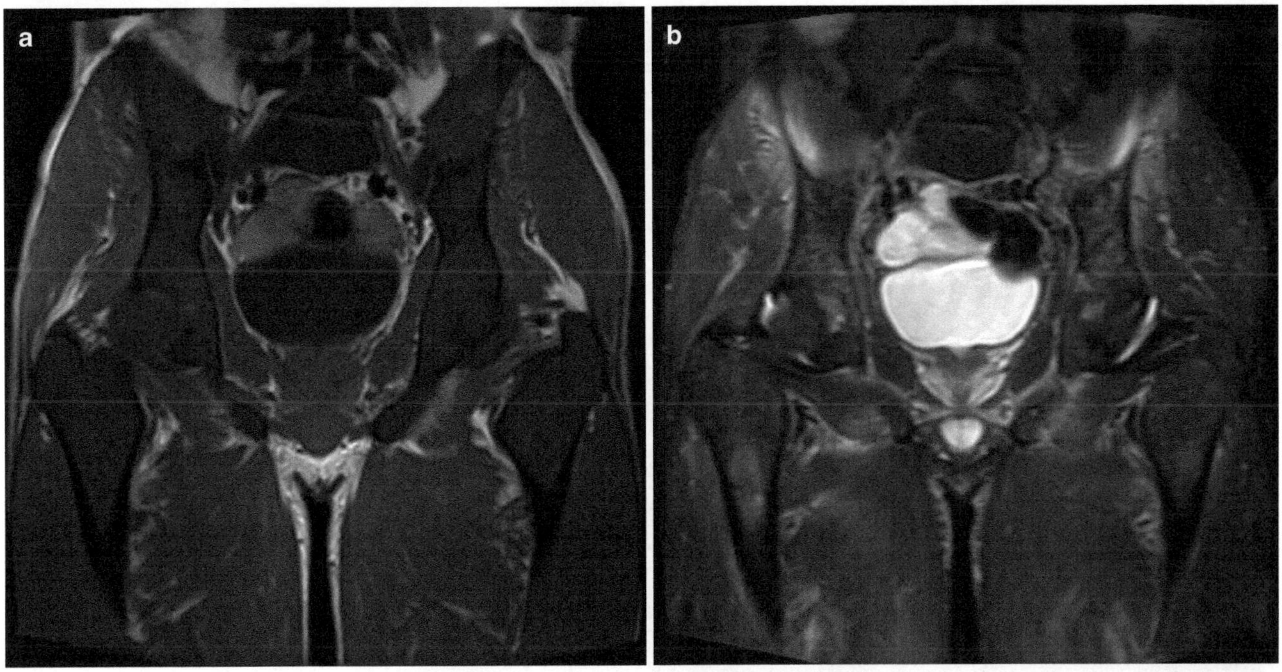

Fig. 3.32 A 39-year-old male with a long-standing history of myelodysplastic syndrome. Coronal T1-weighted (**a**) and STIR (**b**) images demonstrate hypointense bone marrow signal throughout the pelvis and proximal femurs likely due to iron deposition

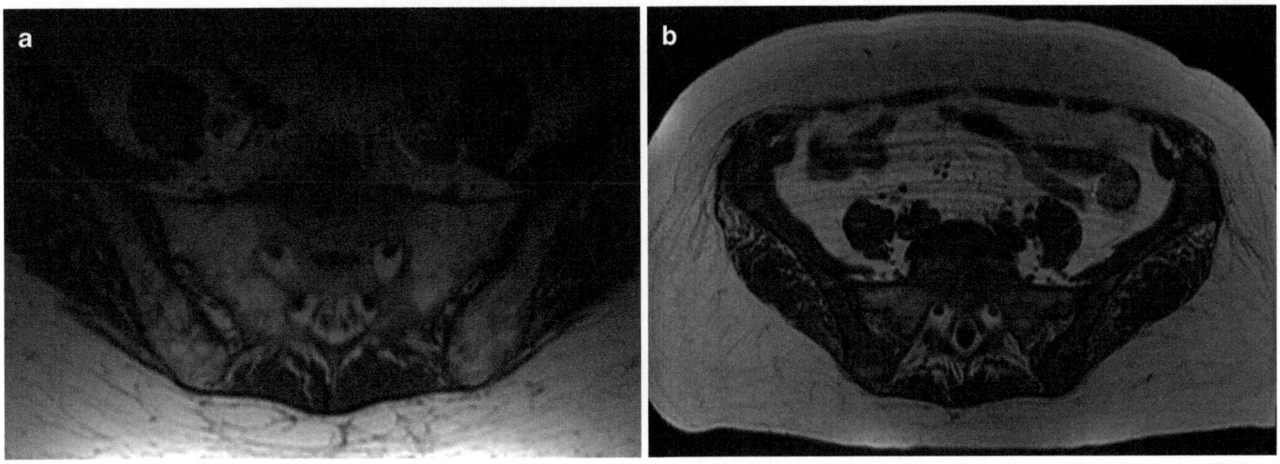

Fig. 3.33 A 66-year-old female with history of myelodysplastic syndrome. Axial T1-weighted image of the pelvis (**a**) demonstrates normal appearing bone marrow signal. A 6-year follow-up shows hypointense bone marrow on T1-weighted axial image (**b**) likely due to iron deposition

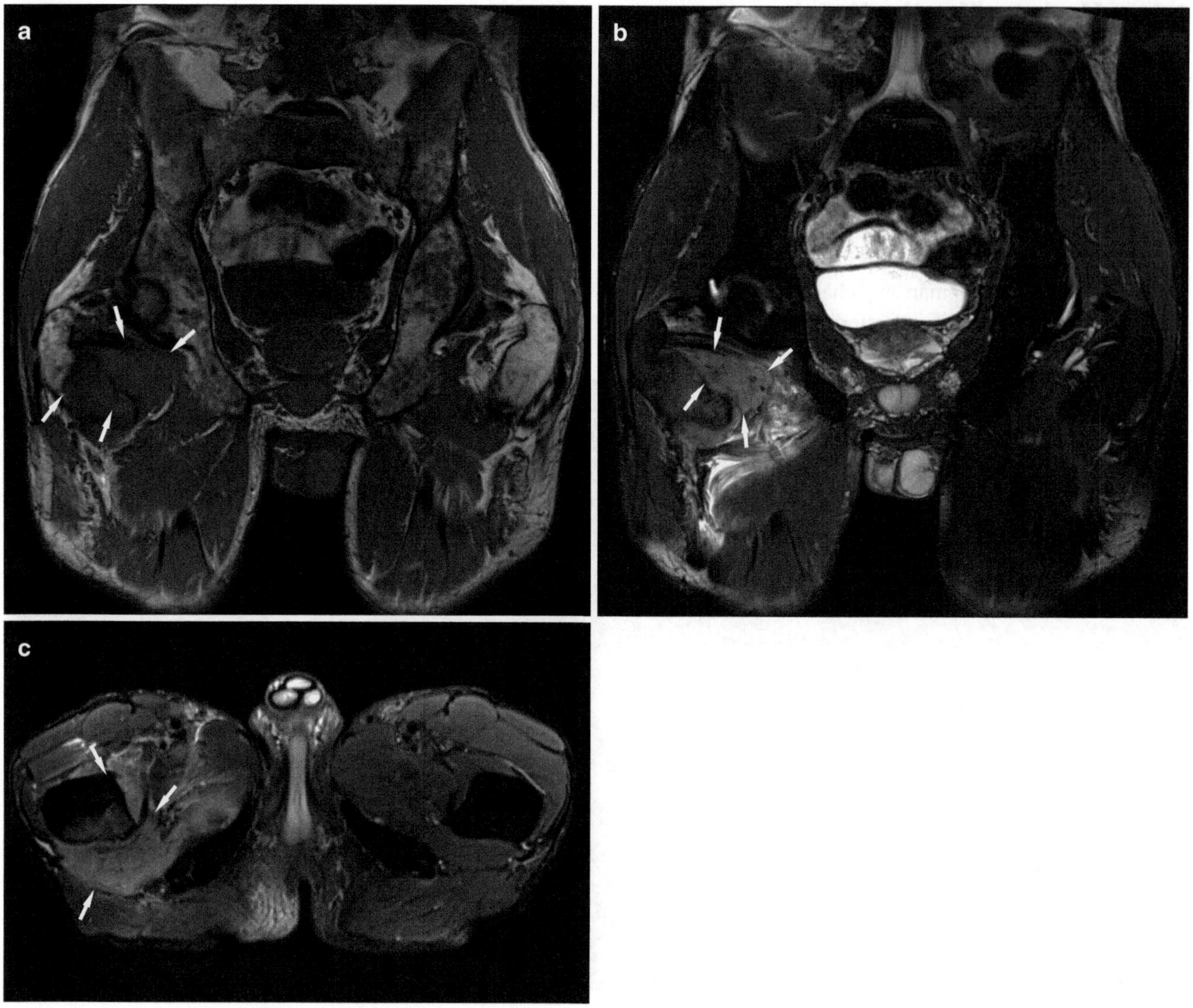

Fig. 3.34 A 36-year-old male with history of myelodysplastic syndrome and recent right hip pain. Coronal T1-weighted (**a**), coronal STIR (**b**), and axial T2-weighted fat-suppressed (**c**) images of the pelvis demonstrate a large soft tissue mass (*arrows*) associated with right proximal femur with underlying bone marrow signal abnormality. An image-guided biopsy showed progression to leukemia

3.4.2 Polycythemia Vera

Polycythemia vera is a neoplastic myeloproliferative bone marrow stem cell disorder that is characterized as a panhyperplastic red blood cell disorder. The most prominent feature of this disease is an elevation of absolute red blood cell mass due to uncontrolled red blood cell production. MRI in these patients typically shows nonspecific patchy or diffuse hematopoietic red marrow (Fig. 3.35). The appearance of the bone marrow might change if chemotherapy is being administered (Fig. 3.36).

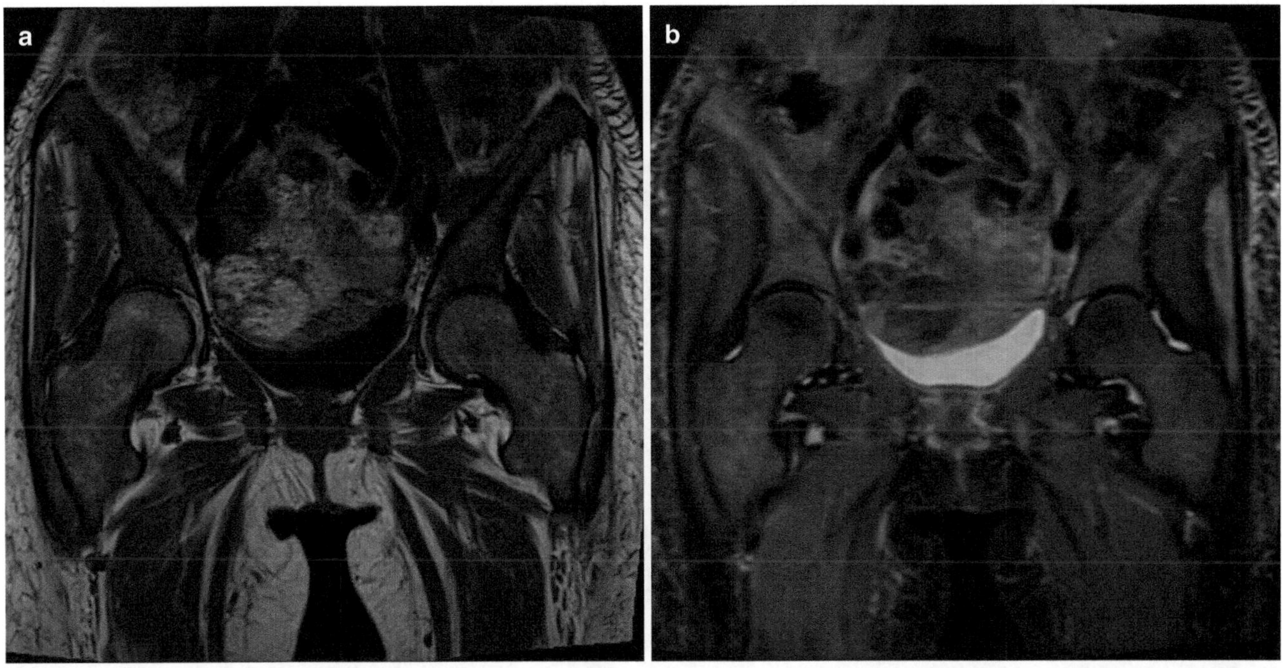

Fig. 3.35 A 65-year-old female with recently diagnosed polycythemia vera. Coronal T1-weighted (**a**) and coronal STIR (**b**) sequences through pelvis demonstrate moderate prominence of hematopoietic red marrow

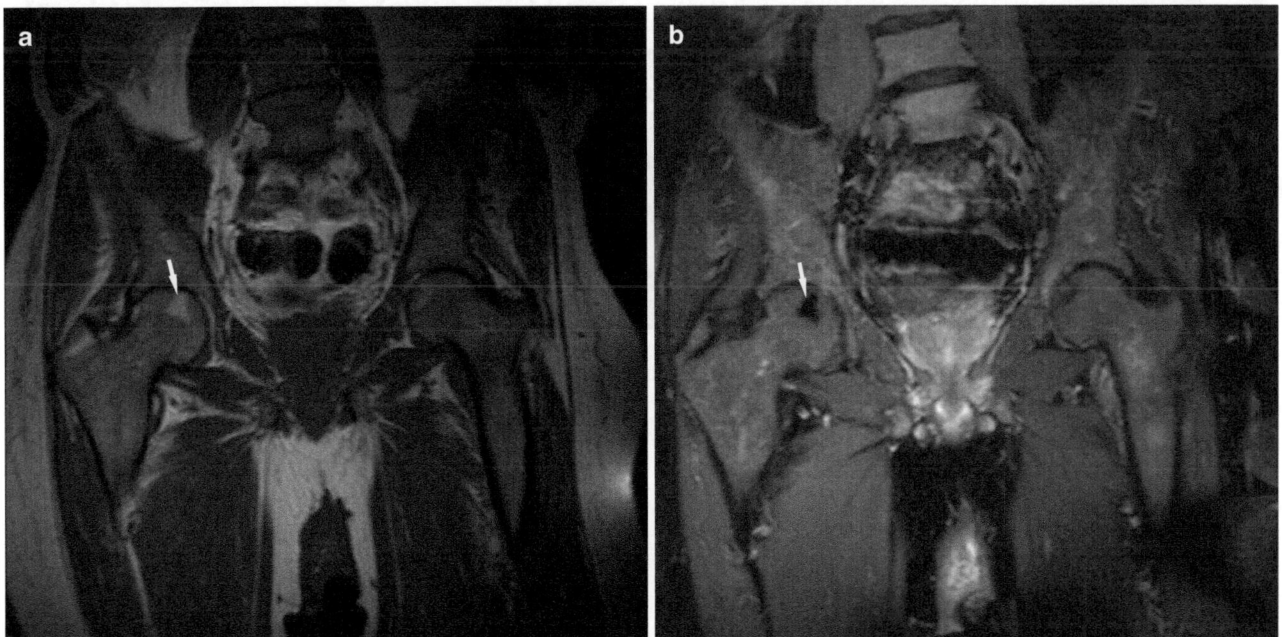

Fig. 3.36 A 67-year-old male with history of polycythemia vera undergoing chemotherapy. Coronal T1-weighted (**a**) and coronal STIR (**b**) images demonstrate mild diffuse red marrow signal with a focus of preserved fatty marrow signal at the right femoral epiphysis (*arrows*)

3.4.3 Myelofibrosis

Primary myelofibrosis is a clonal infiltrative disorder of the bone marrow caused by neoplastic transformation of early hematopoietic stem cells. This disorder is characterized by anemia, extramedullary hematopoiesis, hepatosplenomegaly, abnormal morphology of the red blood cells and peripheral blood, and excessive collagen and reticulin fiber accumulation in bone marrow causing fibrosis. Primary myelofibrosis is categorized as a chronic myeloproliferative disorder, along with chronic myelogenous and polycythemia vera. Secondary myelofibrosis is caused by underlying chronic myeloproliferative disorders and other chronic diseases such as systemic lupus erythematosus, nephrotic syndrome, lymphoma, leukemia, and myeloma [12]. On MRI, bone marrow is typically hypointense compared to skeletal muscle on both T1- and T2-weighted images in varying degrees, reflecting marrow fibrosis [13] (Figs. 3.37 and 3.38). Contrast enhancement of the bone marrow with gadolinium-based contrast agents is typically seen [13] (Fig. 3.38).

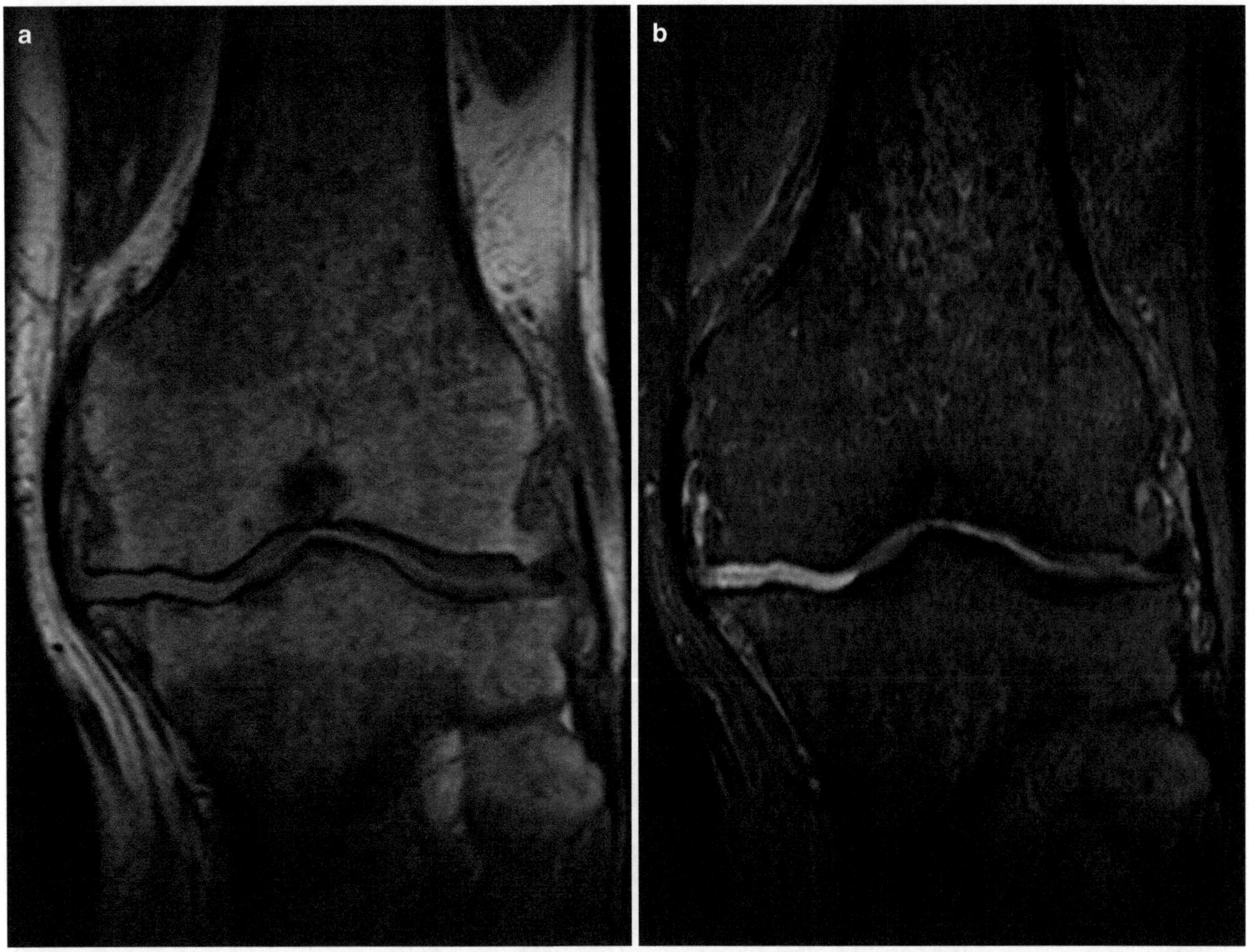

Fig. 3.37 A 79-year-old male. Predominantly low-signal-intensity bone marrow signal is noted on both T1-weighted (**a**) and T2-weighted (**b**) images of the left knee, consistent with patient's known myelofibrosis

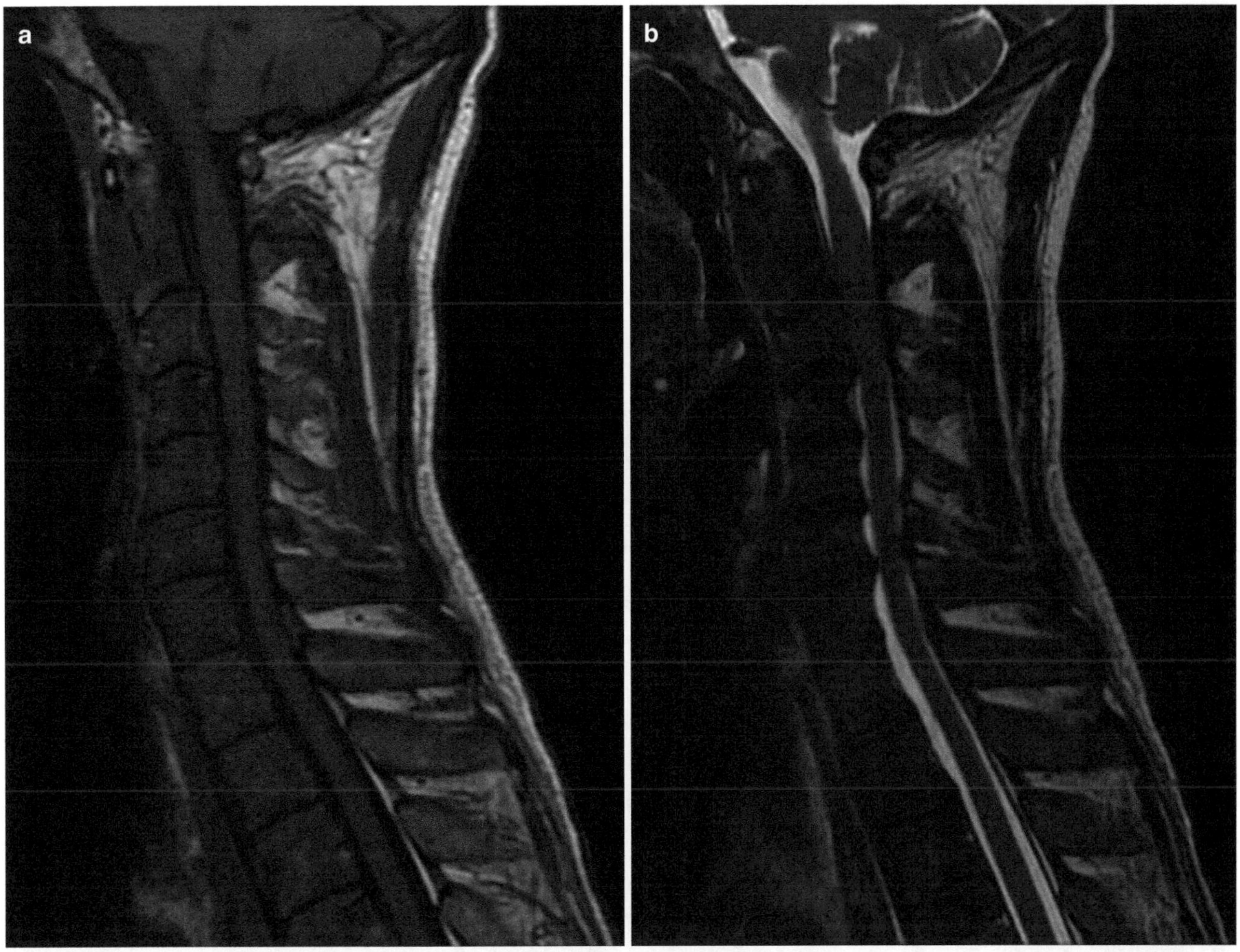

Fig. 3.38 A 56-year-old male. Sagittal T1-weighted (**a**) and T2-weighted (**b**) images of the cervical spine demonstrate diffuse hypointense signal of the bone marrow consistent with patient's known myelofibrosis

3.5 Metastatic Disease

Diffuse infiltration of the bone marrow due to metastatic disease is unusual except in the terminal stages of cancer. When diffuse infiltration of the bone marrow is seen on T1-weighted images in adult patients with known metastatic disease, the etiology is often breast carcinoma in women (Fig. 3.39) and prostate carcinoma in men (Fig. 3.40). In the pediatric population, diffuse bone marrow metastatic disease (Fig. 3.41) is often due to neuroblastoma or, less frequently, rhabdomyosarcoma [14]. It is important to differentiate between diffuse marrow infiltration and hematopoietic marrow hypertrophy, as most of these patients are receiving bone marrow-stimulating agents as part of their chemotherapy regimens. Preservation of some bone marrow fat is almost invariably present in patients with hematopoietic marrow stimulation, whereas patients with diffuse metastatic disease will demonstrate complete bone marrow infiltration (Fig. 3.42). When complete metastatic infiltration of the bone marrow is present, underlying avascular necrosis can be difficult to recognize unless subarticular collapse is present (Fig. 3.43).

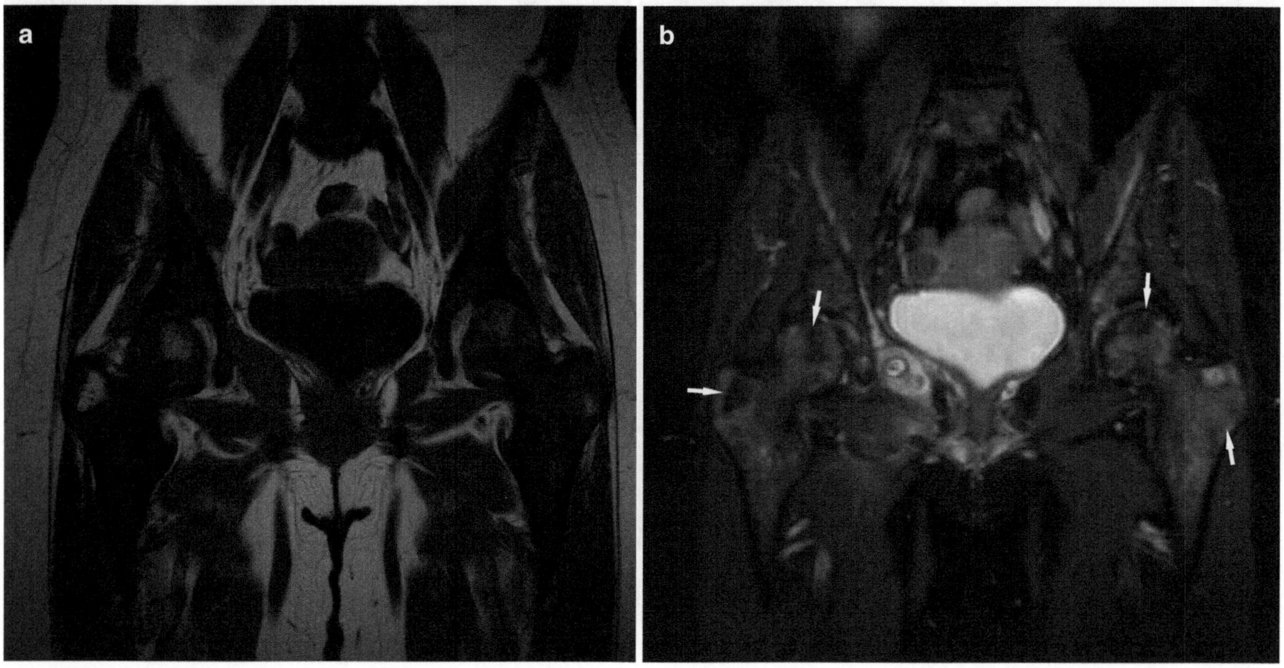

Fig. 3.39 A 57-year-old female with history of breast cancer. Coronal T1-weighted (**a**) and STIR (**b**) images of the pelvis demonstrate hypointense marrow infiltration consistent with diffuse metastatic disease. Small foci of preserved normal fatty marrow signal in the femoral head epiphyses and apophyses bilaterally (*arrows*)

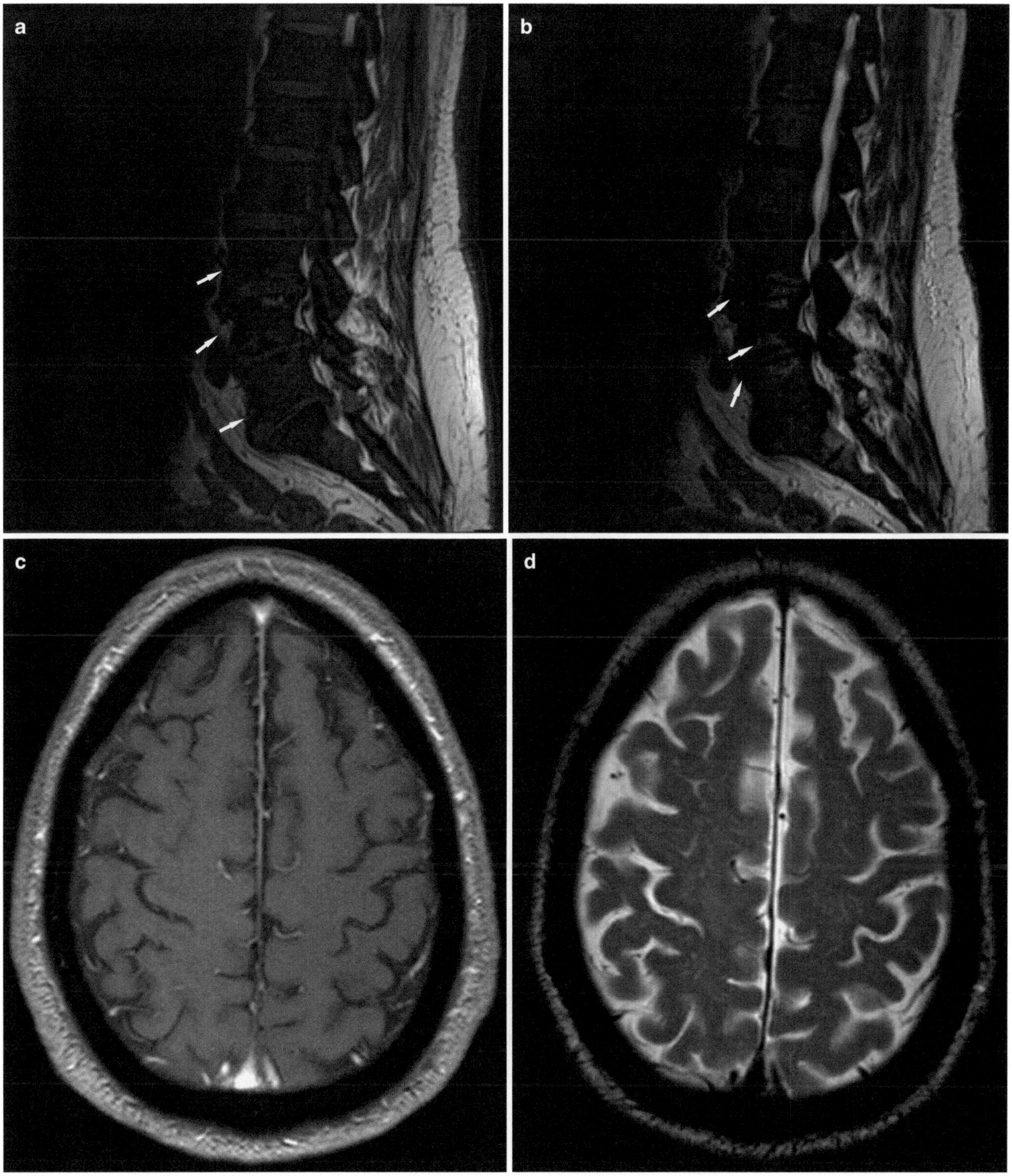

Fig. 3.40 An 81-year-old male with history of metastatic prostate cancer. Diffuse hypointense marrow infiltrative process is noted throughout lumbar spine on T1-weighted (**a**) and T2-weighted (**b**) images. Small amount of preserved fatty bone marrow signal noted in the endplates of lower lumbar spine, secondary to degenerative disc disease (*arrows*). Axial T1-weighted postcontrast (**c**) and T2-weighted (**d**) images of the skull also demonstrate diffuse hypointense bone marrow signal consistent with metastatic disease

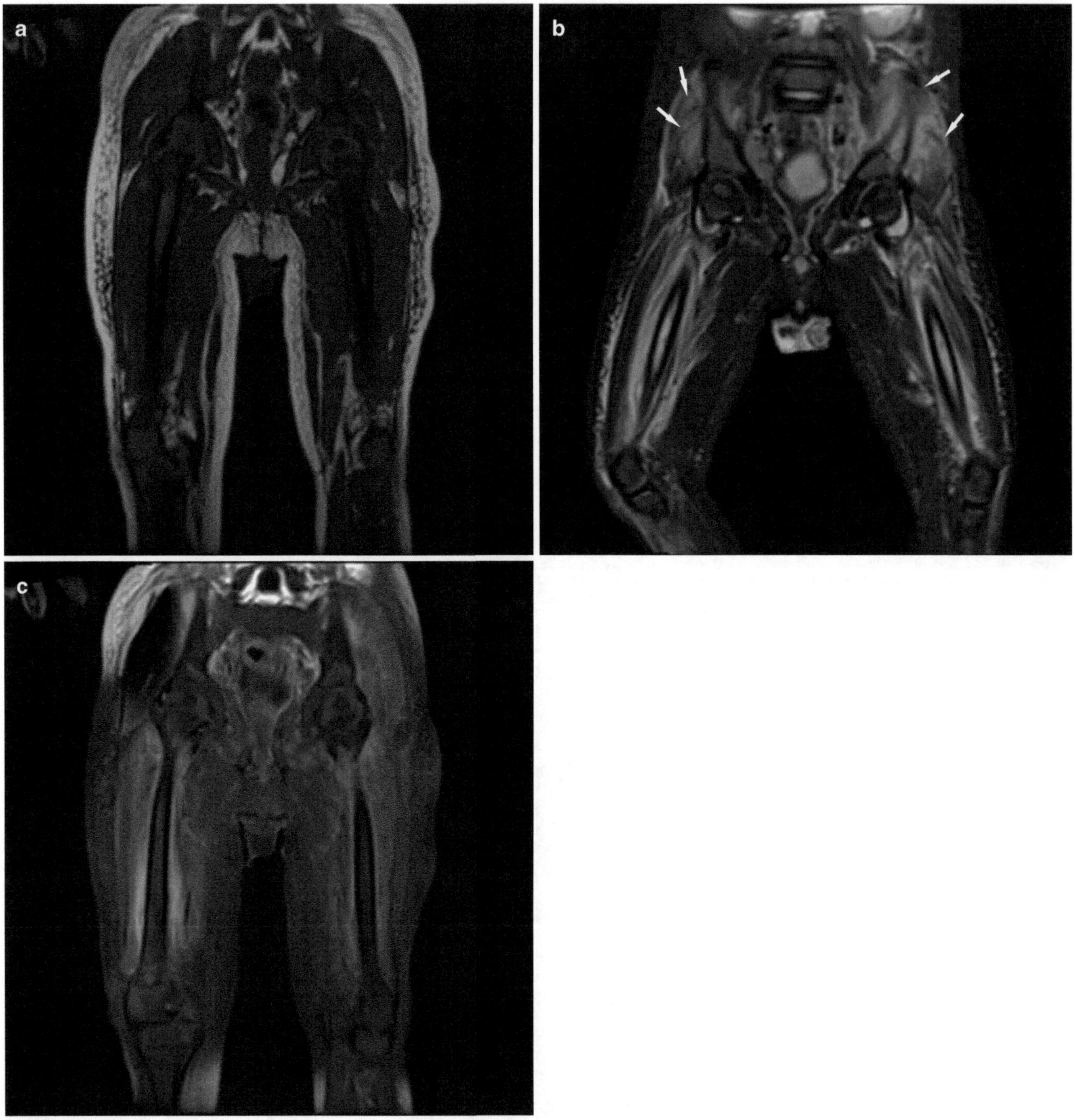

Fig. 3.41 A 2-year-old male was brought to hospital for not weight bearing on his right side. Coronal T1-weighted (**a**), coronal STIR (**b**), and coronal T1-weighted fat-saturated postcontrast (**c**) images of the lower extremities demonstrate diffuse bone marrow infiltration throughout the visualized skeleton with soft tissue extension about the pelvis (*arrows*). Further workup including a biopsy showed metastatic neuroblastoma

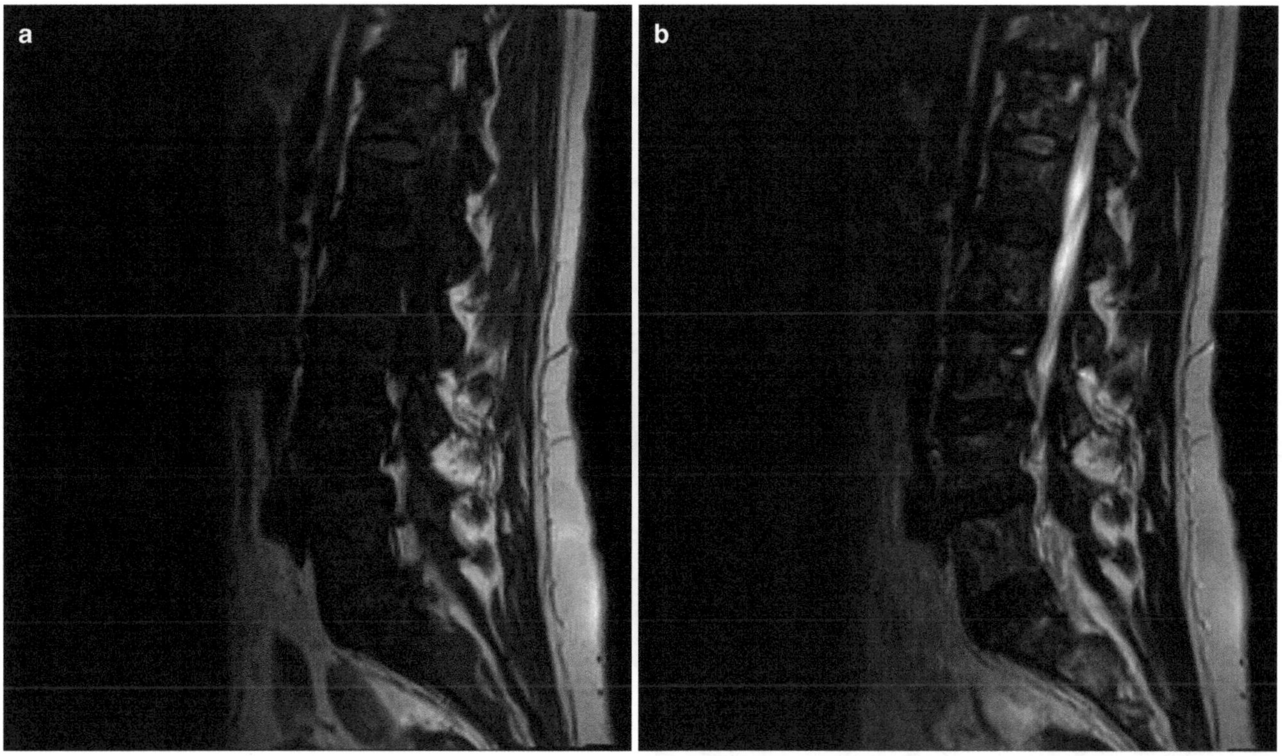

Fig. 3.42 A 49-year-old female with breast cancer. Sagittal T1-weighted (**a**) and T2-weighted (**b**) images of the lumbar spine demonstrate diffuse hypointense bone marrow signal consistent with metastatic disease

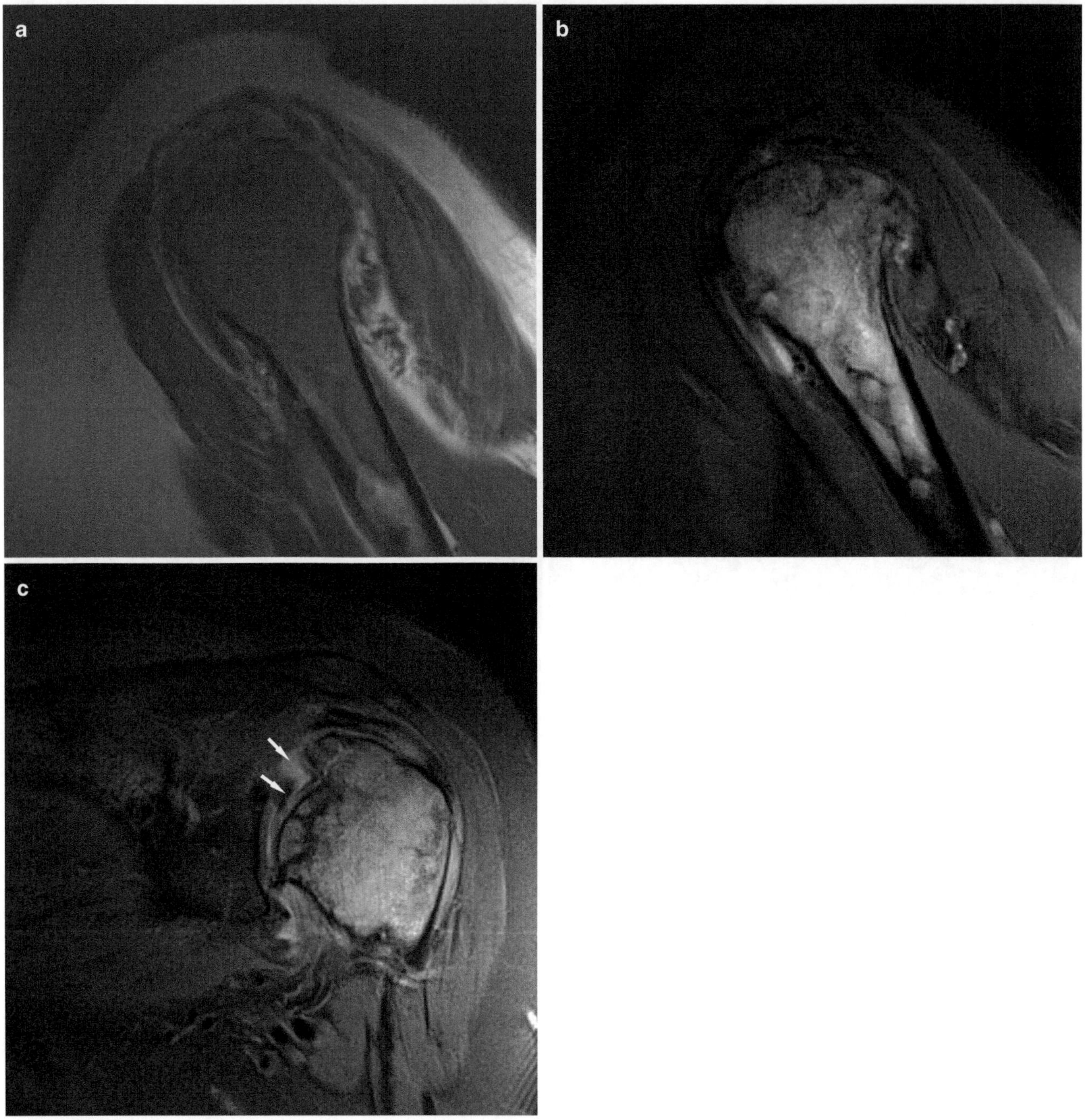

Fig. 3.43 52-year-old female with history of breast cancer presented with gradually worsening left shoulder pain. Sagittal T1-weighted (**a**) and T2-weighted fat-suppressed (**b**) images of the left shoulder demonstrate a large metastatic lesion in the proximal humerus. Coronal T2-weighted fat-suppressed image (**c**) demonstrates subchondral collapse from avascular necrosis involving the humeral head (*arrows*)

References

1. Durie BG, Salmon SE. A clinical staging system for multiple myeloma. Correlation of measured myeloma cell mass with presenting clinical features, response to treatment, and survival. Cancer. 1975;36(3):842–54.
2. Moulopoulos LA, Varma DG, Dimopoulos MA, et al. Multiple myeloma: spinal MR imaging in patients with untreated newly diagnosed disease. Radiology. 1992;185(3):833–40.
3. Dimopoulos MA, Hillengass J, Usmani S, Zamagni E, Lentzsch S, Davies FE, Raje N, Sezer O, Zweegman S, Shah J, Badros A, Shimizu K, Moreau P, Chim C-S, Lahuerta JJ, Hou J, Jurczyszyn A, Goldschmidt H, Sonneveld P, Palumbo A, Ludwig H, Cavo M, Barlogie B, Anderson K, Roodman GD, Rajkumar SV, Durie BGM, Terpos E, et al. Role of magnetic resonance imaging in the management of patients with multiple myeloma: a consensus statement. J Clin Oncol. 2015;33(6):657–64.
4. Hillengass J, Landgren O. Challenges and opportunities of novel imaging techniques in monoclonal plasma cell disorders: imaging "early myeloma.". Leuk Lymphoma. 2013;54(7):1355–63.
5. Usmani SZ, Heuck C, Mitchell A, Szymonifka J, Nair B, Hoering A, Alsayed Y, Waheed S, Haider S, Restrepo A, Van Rhee F, Crowley J, Barlogie B. Extramedullary disease portends poor prognosis in multiple myeloma and is over-represented in high-risk disease even in the era of novel agents. Haematologica. 2012;97(11):1761–7.
6. Fletcher CDM, Unni KK, Mertens F, editors. Pathology and genetics of tumours of soft tissue and bone. Lyon: IARC Press; 2002; 2002 International Agency for Research on Cancer; 2002. Pathology and genetics of tumours of soft tissue and bone: World Health Organization classification of tumours; pp: 306–8.
7. Ostrowski ML, Unni KK, Banks PM, Shives TC, Evans RG, O'Connell MJ, Taylor WF, et al. Malignant lymphoma of bone. Cancer. 1986;58(12):2646–55.
8. Vassilakopoulos TP, Angelopoulou MK, Constantinou N, Karmiris T, Repoussis P, Roussou P, Siakantaris MP, Korkolopoulou P, Kyrtsonis M-C, Kokoris SI, Dimopoulou MN, Variamis E, Viniou N-A, Konstantopoulos K, Dimitriadou EM, Androulaki A, Patsouris E, Doussis-Anagnostopoulou IA, Panayiotidis P, Boussiotis VA, Kittas C, Pangalis GA, et al. Development and validation of a clinical prediction rule for bone marrow involvement in patients with Hodgkin lymphoma. Blood. 2005;105(5):1875–80.
9. Vande Berg BC, Schmitz PJ, Scheiff JM, Filleul BJ, Michaux JL, Ferrant A, Jamart J, Malghem J, Maldague BE, et al. Acute myeloid leukemia: lack of predictive value of sequential quantitative MR imaging during treatment. Radiology. 1995;197(1):301–5.
10. Takagi S, Tanaka O, Origasa H, Miura Y. Prognostic significance of magnetic resonance imaging of femoral marrow in patients with myelodysplastic syndromes. J Clin Oncol. 1999;17(1):277–83.
11. Lewis S, Wainscoat JS, Moore NR, Golding SJ. Magnetic resonance imaging in myelodysplastic syndromes. Br J Radiol. 1995;68(806):121–7.
12. McCarthy DM. Annotation. Fibrosis of the bone marrow: content and causes. Br J Haematol. 1985;59(1):1–7.
13. Amano Y, Onda M, Amano M, Kumazaki T. Magnetic resonance imaging of myelofibrosis. STIR and gadolinium-enhanced MR images. Clin Imaging. 1997;21(4):264–8.
14. Ruzal-Shapiro C, Berdon WE, Cohen MD, Abramson SJ. MR imaging of diffuse bone marrow replacement in pediatric patients with cancer. Radiology. 1991;181(2):587–9.

Anemias

4

Hakan Ilaslan and Murali Sundaram

4.1 Introduction

Anemia occurs when there is lower than normal red blood cells, resulting in diminished quantity of hemoglobin. Anemia can be caused by various etiologies such as blood loss, destruction of red blood cells, and decreased or faulty red blood cell production. In response to anemia, erythropoietin secreted by the kidneys stimulates the bone marrow to increase total red blood cell mass. When the bone marrow is stimulated, increased hematopoietic marrow can be visualized on the Magnetic Resonance Imaging (MRI) examination demonstrating normal distribution and signal intensity.

4.2 Physiologic Red Marrow Hyperplasia

Physiologic hypertrophy of the hematopoietic marrow can be seen in patients with iron- or vitamin-deficiency anemia (Fig. 4.1), smokers, obese individuals (Fig. 4.2), and marathon runners. Heavy smokers tend to have a 20–25 % increase in the number of peripheral blood and leukocytes [1], which may explain the increased red marrow seen in these patients compared to light smokers or nonsmokers. Increased prevalence of hematopoietic bone marrow hyperplasia in marathon runners has been postulated to develop as a response to "sports anemia," which is frequently seen in aerobically trained athletes (Fig. 4.3) [2]. On MRI, physiologic red marrow hypertrophy appears as hyperintense foci compared to skeletal muscle on T1-weighted images (Figs. 4.1 and 4.2), showing normal distribution (i.e., involvement of the metaphysis and diaphysis rather than the epiphysis, although partial involvement of the epiphysis or apophysis may be seen). On T2-weighted and Short Tau Inversion Recovery (STIR) sequences, a corresponding hyperintense signal is expected. Mild diffuse enhancement of red marrow is typical (Fig. 4.1).

H. Ilaslan, M. Sundaram, *Pediatric and Adult MRI Atlas of Bone Marrow: Normal Appearances, Variants and Diffuse Disease States*, DOI 10.1007/978-3-642-02740-6_4

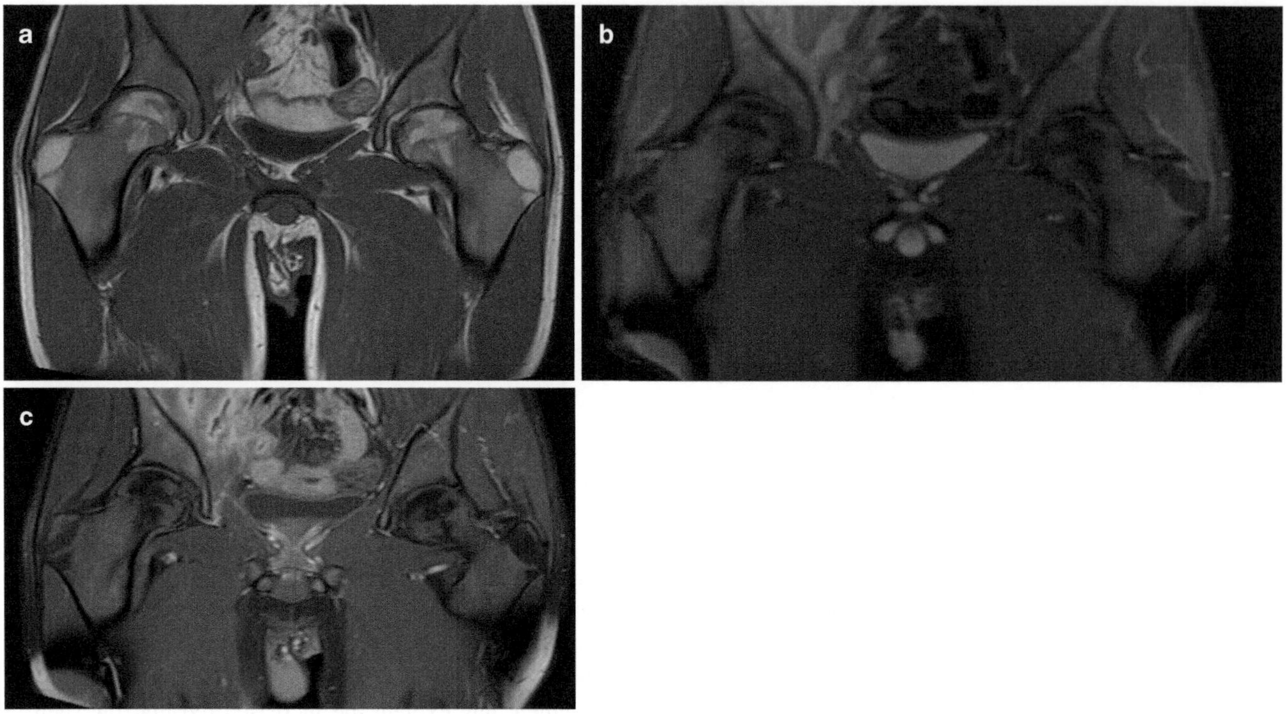

Fig. 4.1 A 19-year-old male with recently diagnosed inflammatory bowel disease and iron deficiency anemia (hemoglobin 9.4 g/dL and hematocrit 31 %). Coronal T1-weighted (**a**) and STIR (**b**) images demonstrate prominent red marrow signal partially extending into proximal femoral epiphyses bilaterally. Postcontrast T1-weighted fat-saturated image (**c**) demonstrates mild diffuse enhancement of red marrow as expected

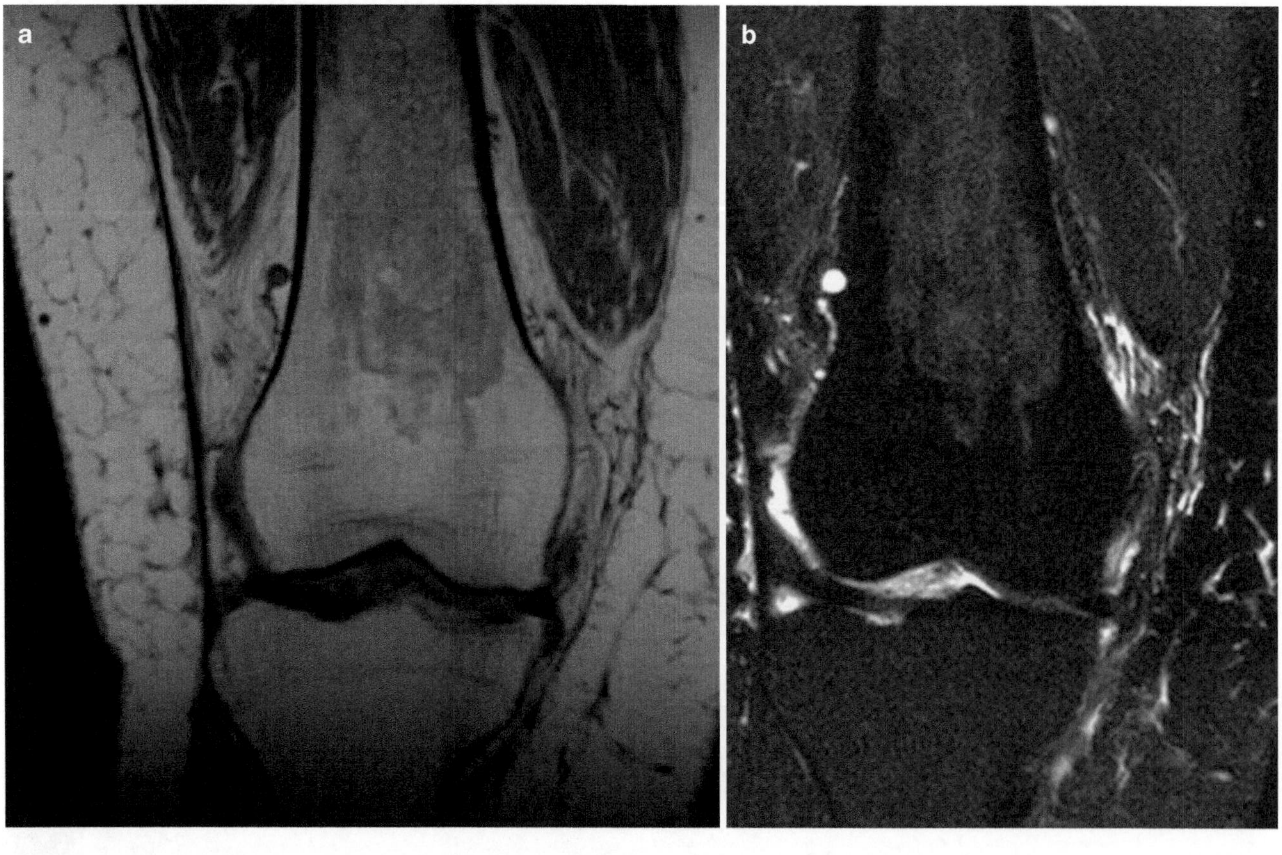

Fig. 4.2 A 42-year-old female with a body mass index of 36. Coronal T1-weighted (**a**) image demonstrates prominent red marrow in the distal femur with hyperintense signal compared to skeletal muscle. T2-weighted (**b**) fat-saturated coronal image demonstrates mildly hyperintense signal of red marrow

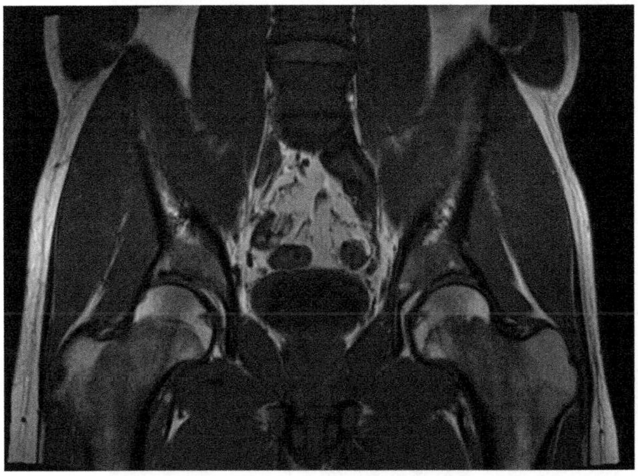

Fig. 4.3 A 32-year-old professional basketball player. Coronal T1-weighted image demonstrates prominent red marrow in the lower lumbar spine, pelvis, and proximal femurs

4.3 Bone Marrow Failure

The bone marrow failure syndromes include a heterogeneous group of disorders than can be either inherited or acquired. These disorders of the hematopoietic stem cell can involve either one cell line or all of the cell lines (erythroid; myeloid for megakaryocytic). The lymphocytes are not involved in these disorders. The etiology of bone marrow failure can be congenital or acquired. Fanconi anemia is the most frequently reported inherited bone marrow failure syndrome. Fanconi anemia typically manifests in young adults and children with hypoplastic or aplastic anemia. In addition, Fanconi anemia patients may present with cytopenia, unexplained macrocytosis, myelodysplastic syndrome (Fig. 4.4), acute myelogenous leukemia, epithelial malignancies, and certain physical anomalies [3]. Acquired causes of bone marrow failure include toxins, chemicals, drugs, radiation, viral infection, vitamin deficiencies, and myelodysplastic syndrome [3].

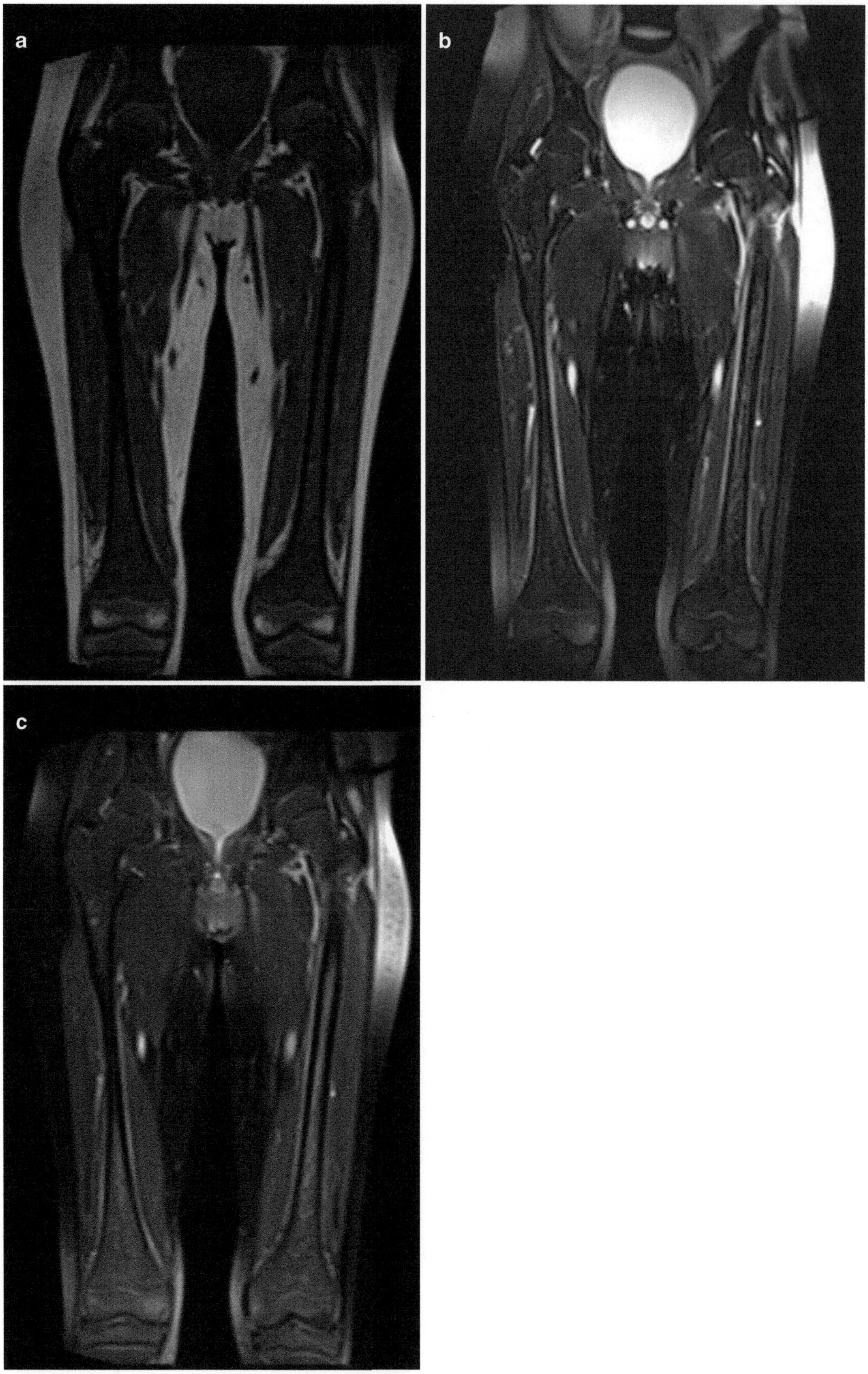

Fig. 4.4 A 13-year-old male with Fanconi anemia and myelodysplastic syndrome. Coronal T1-weighted (**a**) and T2-weighted fat-suppressed (**b**) images of bilateral femurs demonstrate diffuse hypointense signal. Mild patchy enhancement is noted in postcontrast T1-weighted fat-saturated coronal image (**c**)

4.4 Hemoglobinopathies and Thalassemias

Hemoglobinopathies are a group of blood disorders characterized by reduced or abnormal production of a hemoglobin protein. The underlying etiology is a genetic defect that results in an abnormal structure of one of the globin chains of the hemoglobin molecule. Unlike hemoglobinopathies, thalassemias typically result in underproduction of normal globin proteins, often through mutations in regulatory genes. The two conditions may overlap, however, as some conditions that cause abnormalities in globin proteins (hemoglobinopathy) also affect their production.

Hemoglobinopathies are most frequently seen in Africa, the Mediterranean basin, and Southeast Asia [4]. The most common hemoglobinopathy is sickle cell disease. Approximately 7 % of the world's population are carriers of this trait [4]. Sickle cell disease results from a mutation in a gene coding for the beta chain of the hemoglobin molecule, called HbS. Sickle cell disease occurs when two abnormal beta chains are present together. Individuals with one HbS beta chain and one normal beta chain are said to have the "sickle cell trait." Sickle cell trait patients are usually asymptomatic. Increased red blood cell destruction and consequent anemia are the main stimuli for the persistence and subsequent expansion of hematopoietic bone marrow in patients with sickle cell anemia. Bone marrow expansion is typically manifested in the skull as widening of the diploic space with thinning of the inner and outer tables. In the appendicular skeleton, bone marrow expansion may not be as obvious as in the skull but hematopoietic marrow can be seen in unusual locations such as the epiphyses (Fig. 4.5) or hand and feet (Fig. 4.6). Osteonecrosis is a debilitating complication of sickle cell disease. Infarcts result directly from destruction of the red blood cells in the bone marrow, which slows blood flow with sequestration of cells and leads to tissue hypoxia and eventual cell death. Although this can occur in any bone of the body, in infants and young children, small tubular bones in the hands and feet are most frequently involved. This entity is called sickle cell dactylitis or hand–foot syndrome. The long bones are also frequently involved in both pediatric and adult patients with sickle cell disease (Fig. 4.6). Flat bone involvement with osteonecrosis is less frequently seen (Fig. 4.7). Epiphyseal avascular necrosis is common, resulting in eventual collapse of the articular surfaces in the humeral and femoral heads (Fig. 4.8). Hypoplastic vertebral endplates, or H-shaped deformities, are typically seen on spine MRI in sickle cell patients (Fig. 4.9). Sickle cell disease patients are prone to have severe infections frequently as a result of impaired immune function and functional asplenia. Osteomyelitis can be acute or a chronic in these patients, and the most common organism responsible for osteomyelitis is *Salmonella* [5]. Diagnosing osteomyelitis in children with sickle cell disease can be difficult due to overlapping clinical findings between osteomyelitis and vascular occlusion. On MRI, the diagnosis of osteomyelitis is considered when there is infiltration of the fatty bone marrow. When there is diffuse hypertrophy of the hematopoietic red marrow, fatty marrow signal may not be present to delineate the focus of infection which creates challenges in diagnosing osteomyelitis in sickle cell patients. Cortical destruction and sinus tracts, when present, can be helpful in these patients to diagnose osteomyelitis differentiating from osteonecrosis (Fig. 4.10). Unlike in other hemoglobinopathies, extramedullary hematopoiesis is not a typical feature of sickle cell anemia.

The beta-thalassemias are a group of autosomal recessive disorders characterized by reduced or absent synthesis of the red blood cell beta-globin chains. The beta-thalassemias are the most common single-gene disorder in the world and are found at high frequencies in many populations worldwide [6]. Mild anemia caused by the alpha-thalassemia trait might be mistaken for iron-deficiency anemia clinically and on imaging. These patients may not be diagnosed until later in adulthood. Patients with hemoglobin H disease or beta-thalassemia major have a severe form of thalassemia. The signs and symptoms of this disease usually arise early, within the first year of life. Thalassemia intermedia may not present until later in childhood and is associated with a less severe disease course [6]. Hematopoietic bone marrow expansion is a typical feature of severe thalassemia. Findings are dramatic in the skull, with expansion of the diploic space (Fig. 4.11), and less pronounced in the appendicular skeleton. After repeated transfusions, hemosiderin deposition in the bone marrow can be seen on MRI (Fig. 4.12). An overall increase in the amount of hematopoietic marrow is also seen in these patients (Fig. 4.13). In addition, hematopoietic bone marrow signal may be seen in unexpected locations, such as the epiphyses (Fig. 4.13) and bones of the hands and feet, where fatty marrow signal is normally seen. It is not unusual to find areas of extramedullary hematopoiesis in these patients, particularly in the paravertebral soft tissues, although many body sites may be involved, including the liver, spleen, and lymph nodes [7].

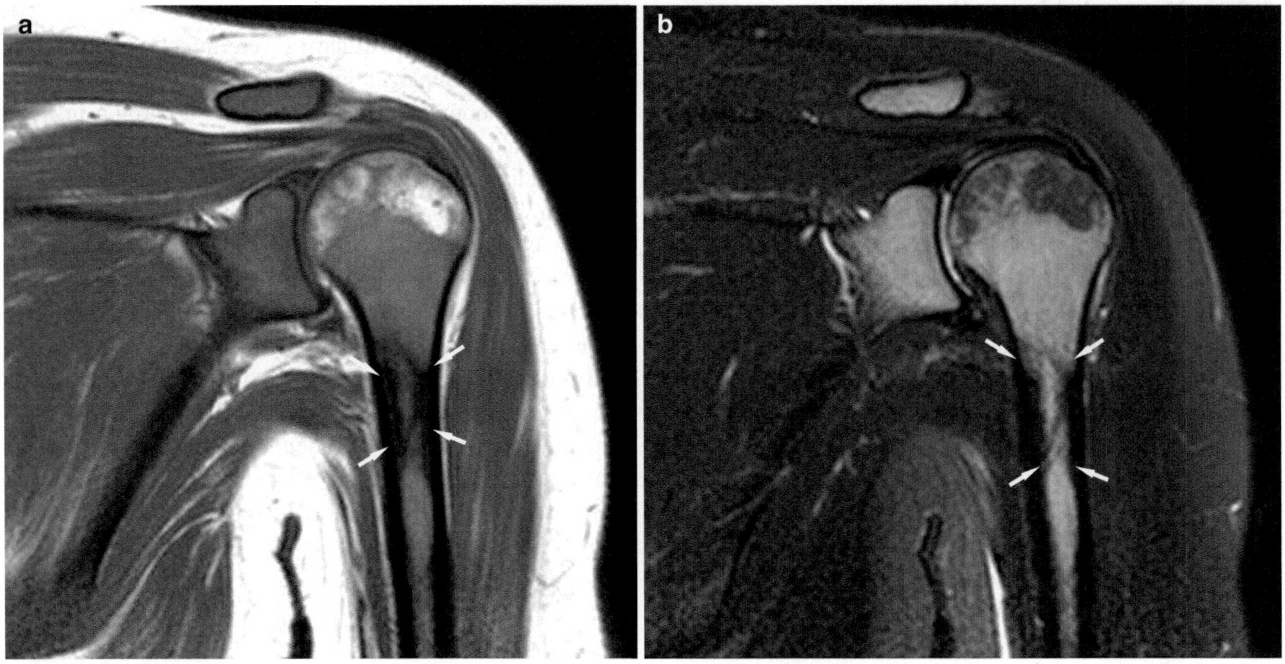

Fig. 4.5 A 16-year-old male with sickle cell disease. Coronal T1-weighted (**a**) and T2-weighted fat-suppressed (**b**) images of the left shoulder demonstrate diffuse prominent red marrow signal extending into the proximal humeral epiphysis and apophysis (*arrows*). Subtle areas of bone marrow signal changes in the proximal humeral diaphysis likely related to osteonecrosis

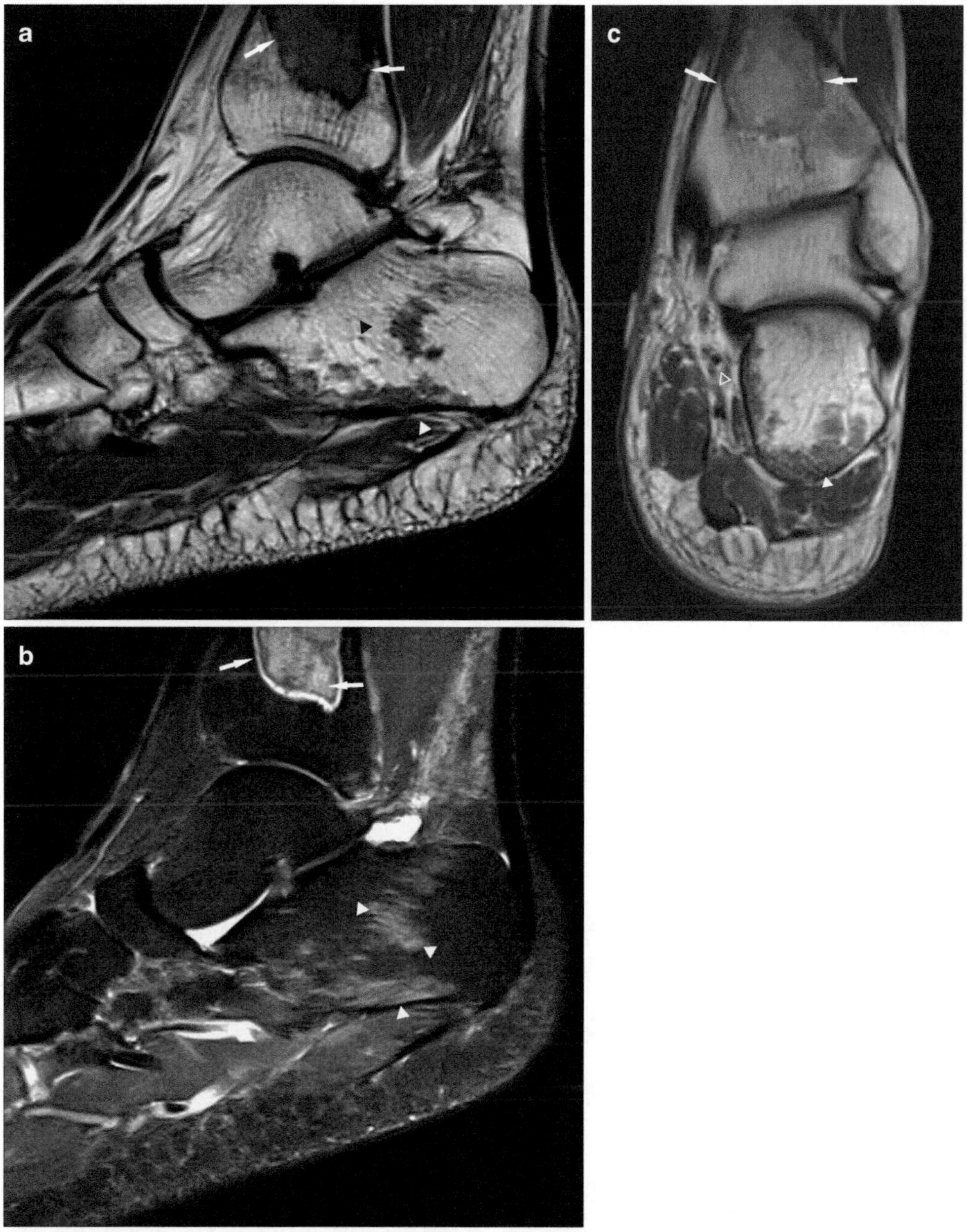

Fig. 4.6 A 29-year-old male with sickle cell disease. Sagittal T1-weighted (**a**), T2-weighted fat-suppressed (**b**), and T2-weighted coronal (**c**) images of the left ankle demonstrate a partially visualized large distal tibial osteonecrosis (*arrows*) and foci of red bone marrow signal in the calcaneus (*arrowheads*)

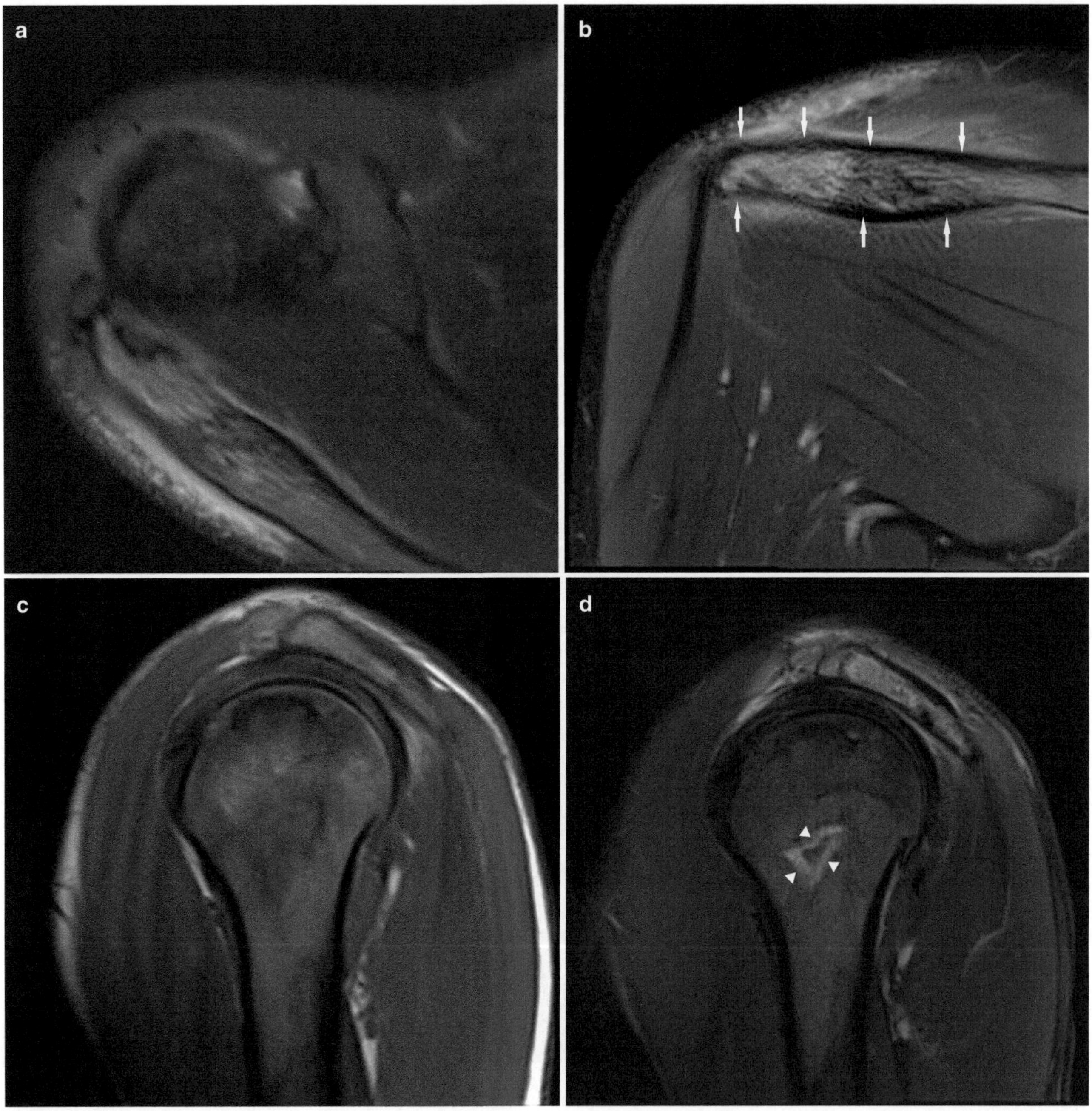

Fig. 4.7 A 26-year-old male with sickle cell disease and right shoulder pain. T2-weighted fat-suppressed axial (**a**) and coronal (**b**) images demonstrate abnormal marrow signal and periostitis along the coracoid process of the scapula consistent with an acute osteonecrosis (*arrows*). Sagittal T1-weighted (**c**) and T2-weighted fat-suppressed (**d**) images also demonstrate proximal humeral osteonecrosis (*arrowheads*)

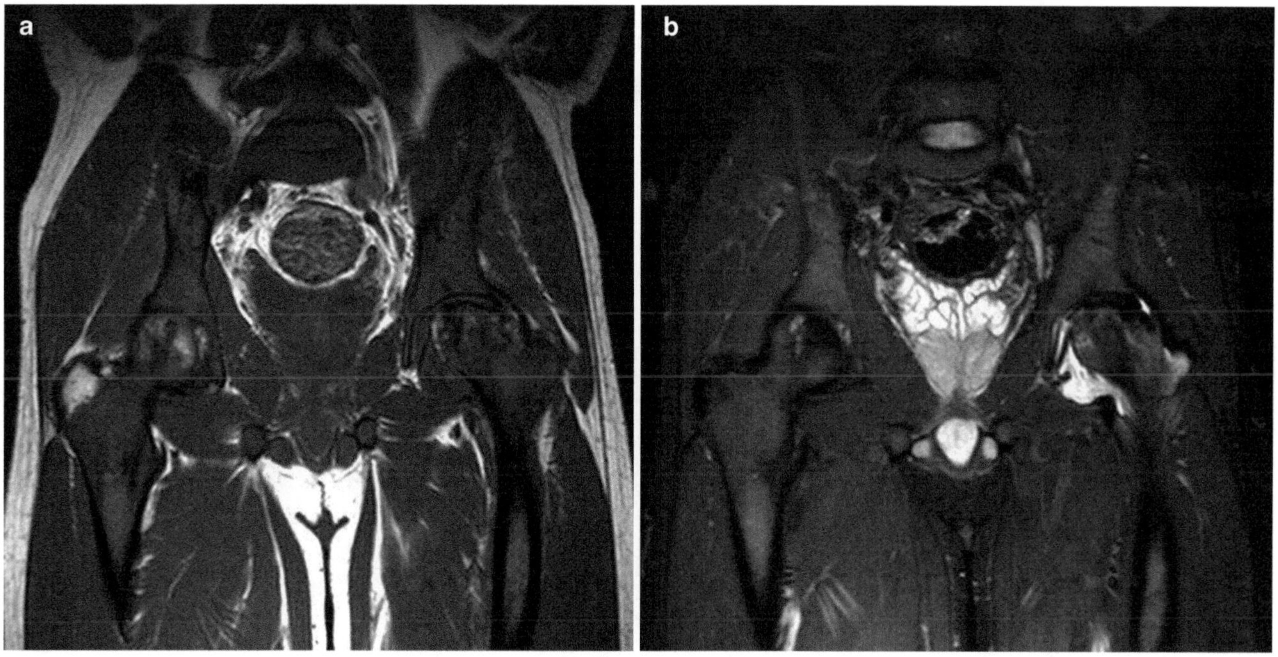

Fig. 4.8 A 24-year old male with sickle cell disease and gradually worsening left hip pain. Coronal T1-weighted (**a**) and STIR (**b**) images of the pelvis demonstrate avascular necrosis of bilateral femoral heads, more severe on the left with subarticular collapse and large joint effusion. Please note the diffuse red marrow signal throughout the pelvis, lower lumbar spine, and proximal femurs

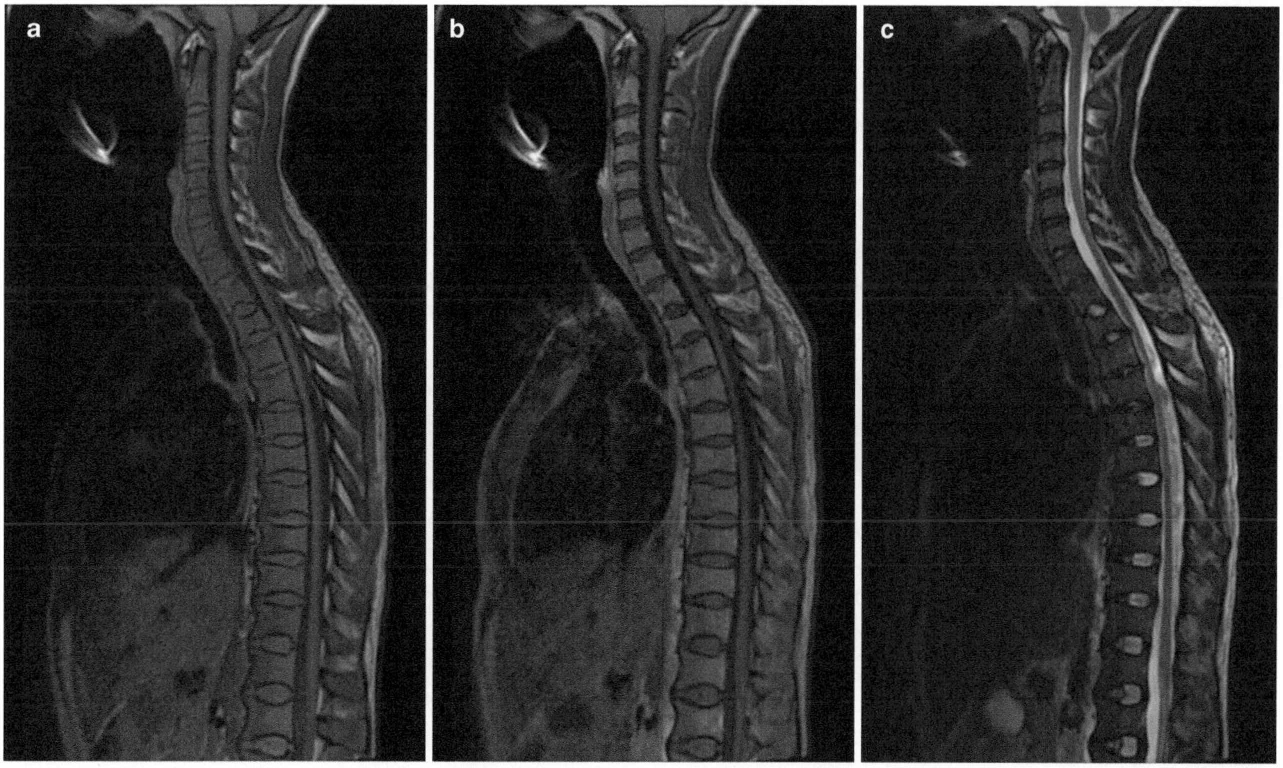

Fig. 4.9 A 25-year-old patient with known sickle cell disease. Sagittal T1-weighted (**a**), T1-weighted postcontrast images (**b**) and sagittal T2-weighted fat-suppressed (**c**) images of the spine demonstrate characteristic hypoplastic endplate changes of thoracic spine. Please note the diffuse red marrow signal with mild enhancement on postcontrast images

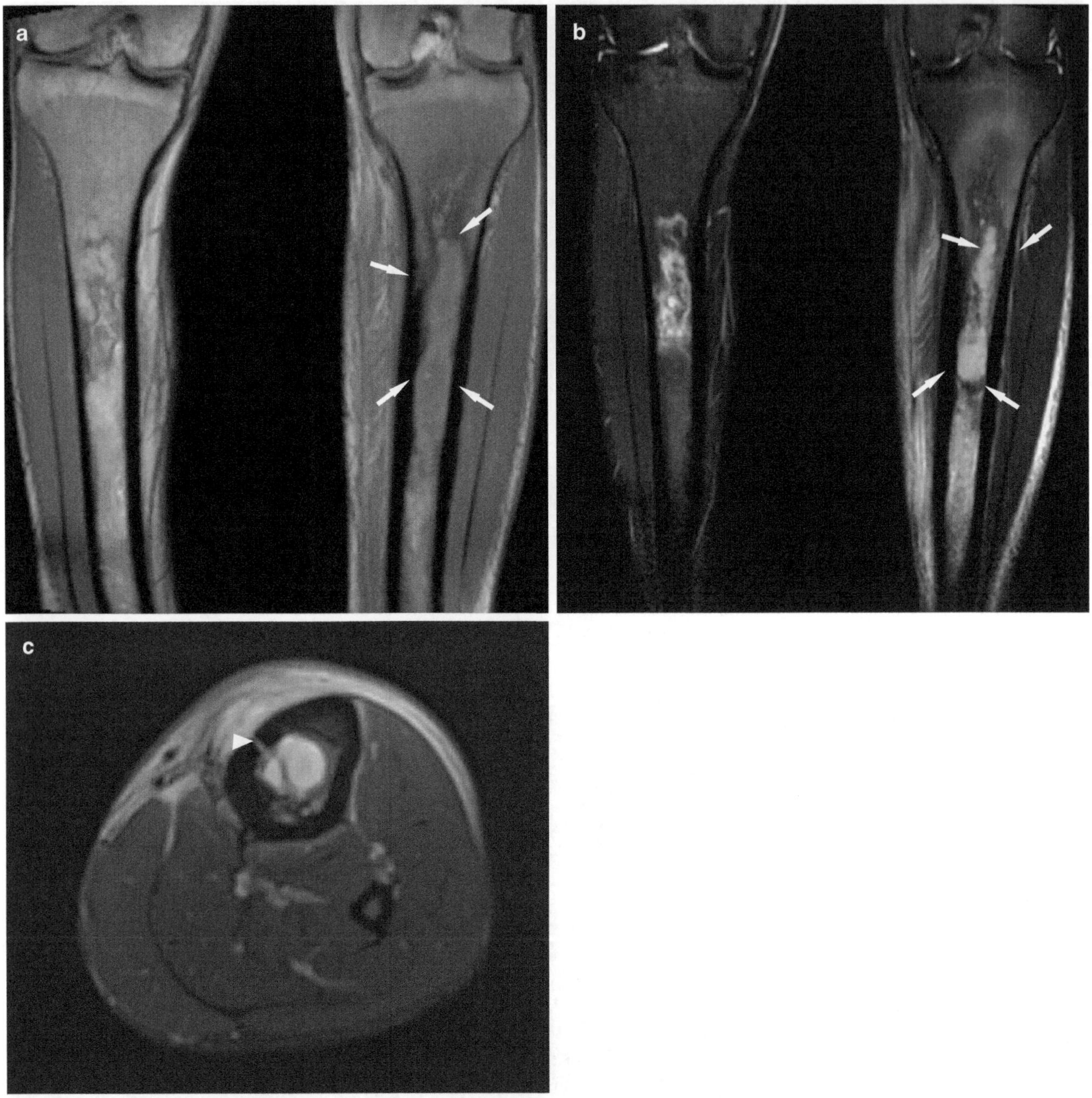

Fig. 4.10 A 23-year-old patient with sickle cell disease. Coronal T1-weighted (**a**) and T2-weighted images (**b**) of bilateral tibias demonstrate a large intraosseous abscess (*arrows*) in the left tibial diaphysis with marked surrounding bone marrow edema. Axial T2-weighted fat-suppressed image (**c**) demonstrates a sinus tract (*arrowhead*) through the anteromedial cortex with overlying soft tissue abscess. Serpiginous area of abnormal signal in the right tibial diaphysis consistent with osteonecrosis

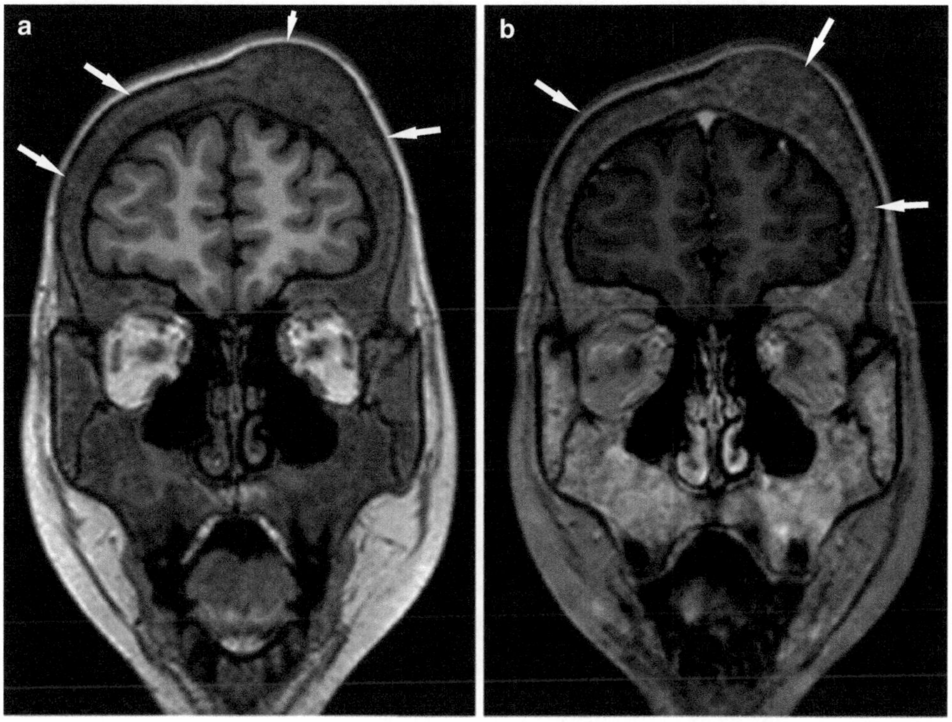

Fig. 4.11 A 9-year-old boy with history of thalassemia. T1-weighted precontrast (**a**) and postcontrast (**b**) coronal images of the skull before and following the contrast administration show markedly expanded marrow space (*arrows*). Please note the hypoplastic maxillary sinuses bilaterally due to marrow expansion

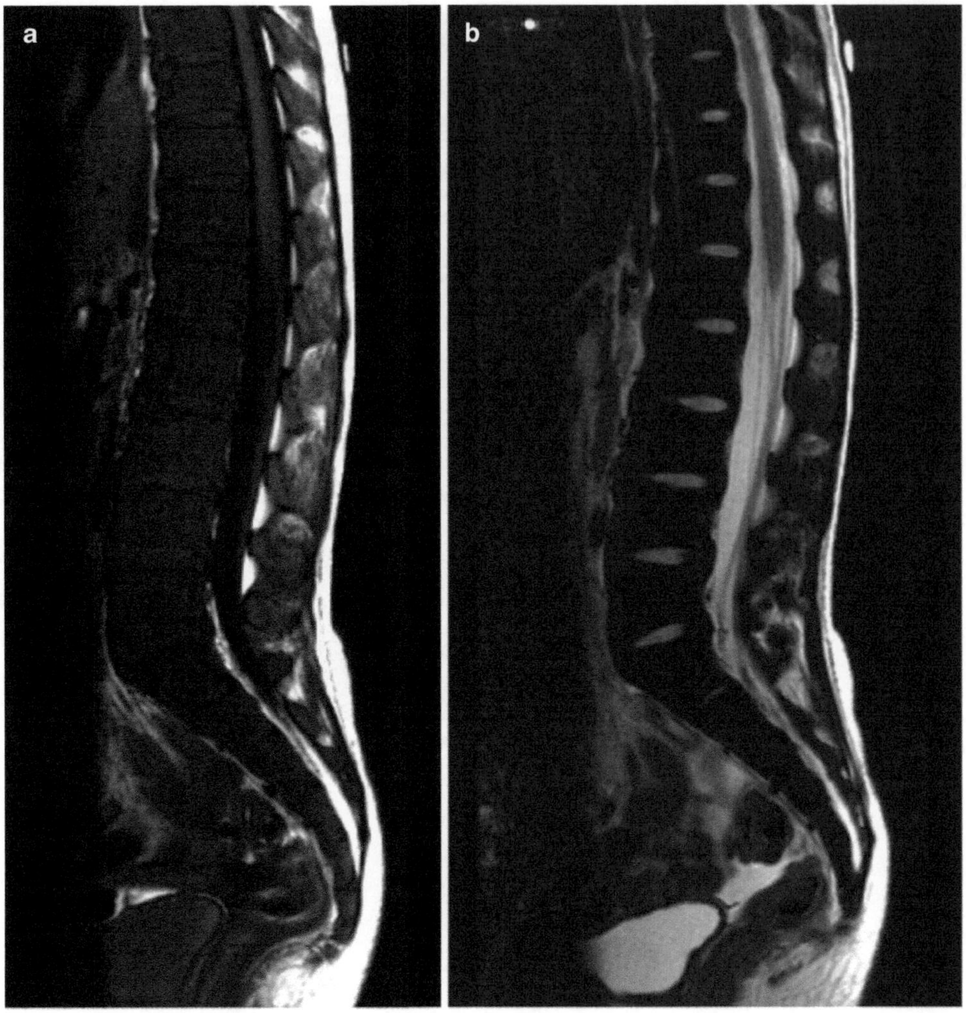

Fig. 4.12 A 19-year-old male with history of thalassemia. Coronal T1-weighted (**a**) and T2-weighted (**b**) images of the left knee spine show demonstrate diffuse hypointense bone marrow signal throughout likely due to hemosiderin deposition secondary to repeated transfusions

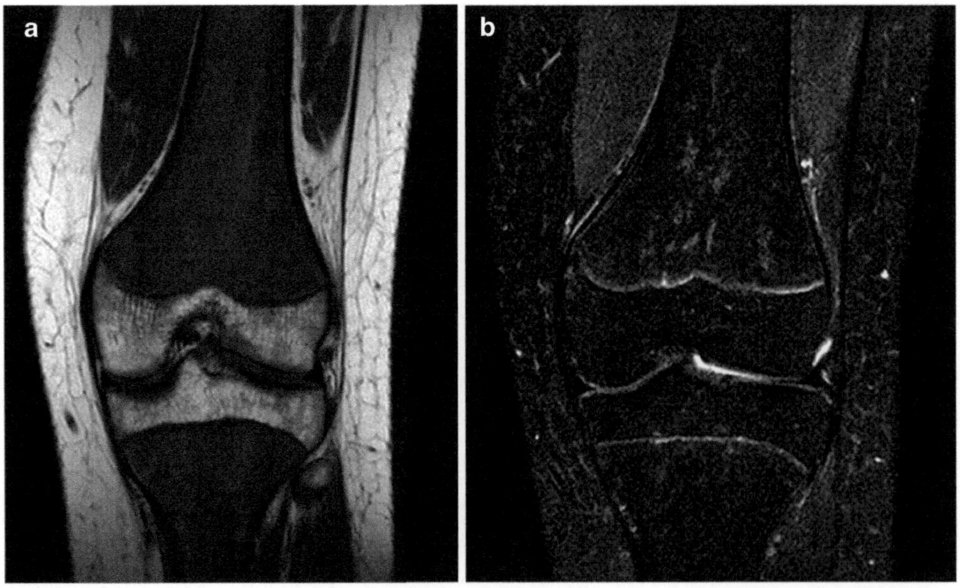

Fig. 4.13 A 14-year-old female with history of thalassemia. Coronal T1-weighted (**a**) and T2-weighted images (**b**) images of the left knee spine show prominent red marrow signal which appears to involve epiphyses

References

1. Terashima T, Wiggs B, English D, Hogg JC, van Eeden SF. The effect of cigarette smoking on the bone marrow. Am J Respir Crit Care Med. 1997;155:1021–6.
2. Shellock FG, Morris E, Deutsch AL, Mink JH, Kerr R, Boden SD. Hematopoietic bone marrow hyperplasia: high prevalence on MR images of the knee in asymptomatic marathon runners. AJR Am J Roentgenol. 1992;158(2):335–8.
3. Alter BP. Bone marrow failure: a child is not just a small adult (but an adult can have a childhood disease). Hematology Am Soc Hematol Educ Program. 2005;96–103.
4. Weatherall DJ, Clegg JB. Inherited haemoglobin disorders: an increasing global health problem. Bull World Health Organ. 2001;79(8):704–12.
5. Chambers JB, Forsythe DA, Bertrand SL, Iwinski HJ, Steflik DE. Retrospective review of osteoarticular infections in a pediatric sickle cell age group. J Pediatr Orthop. 2000;20(5):682–5. Pediatrics 1998;101(2):296–7.
6. Weatherall DJ, Clegg JB. The Thalassemia Syndromes. 4th ed. Oxford: Blackwell Scientific Publications; 2001.
7. Haidar R, Mhaidli H, Taher AT. Paraspinal extramedullary hematopoiesis in patients with thalassemia intermedia. Eur Spine J. 2010;19(6):871–8.

Miscellaneous Bone Marrow Disorders

5

Hakan Ilaslan and Murali Sundaram

5.1 Introduction

Bone marrow involvement is frequently seen in patients with systemic disorders. Some of these disorders have unique magnetic resonance imaging (MRI) appearance which may be sufficient to make a diagnosis of the particular entity while others require correlation with clinical history and extramedullary findings.

5.2 Renal Osteodystrophy

Renal osteodystrophy is an alteration of bone architecture and marrow morphology in patients with chronic kidney disease. The primary cause of anemia in patients with chronic renal failure is insufficient production of erythropoietin by the abnormal kidneys. In patients with chronic renal failure, the development of anemia is due not only to erythropoietin deficiency but also to other factors such as iron or folic acid/B12 deficiency, chronic blood loss, hyperparathyroidism, aluminum toxicity, malnutrition, inadequate hemodialysis, shortened erythrocyte survival time, and hemolysis [1]. In addition, these patients may have accumulation of aluminum or amyloid in the bone marrow (Fig. 5.1). These patients often require erythropoietin replacement therapy to improve red blood cell production. On (MRI) in these patients, hematopoietic red marrow hypertrophy is frequently seen (Fig. 5.2), in addition to evidence of complications from long-standing renal failure and dialysis such as brown tumors. In chronic renal disease, excessive urinary calcium excretion can lower serum calcium level and lead to a rise in parathyroid hormone secretion. This results in secondary hyperparathyroidism in which there is rapid bone loss and hemorrhage, and reparative granulation tissue may replace bone marrow with active, vascular, proliferating fibrous tissue called brown tumors. The MRI appearance depends on the age of the lesion and may appear solid, cystic, or mixed. Solid components are intermediate to low intensity on T1- and T2-weighted images (Fig. 5.3), while the cystic components are hyperintense on T2-weighted images and may have fluid–fluid levels, reflecting on active hemorrhage (Fig. 5.4).

H. Ilaslan, M. Sundaram, *Pediatric and Adult MRI Atlas of Bone Marrow: Normal Appearances, Variants and Diffuse Disease States*, DOI 10.1007/978-3-642-02740-6_5

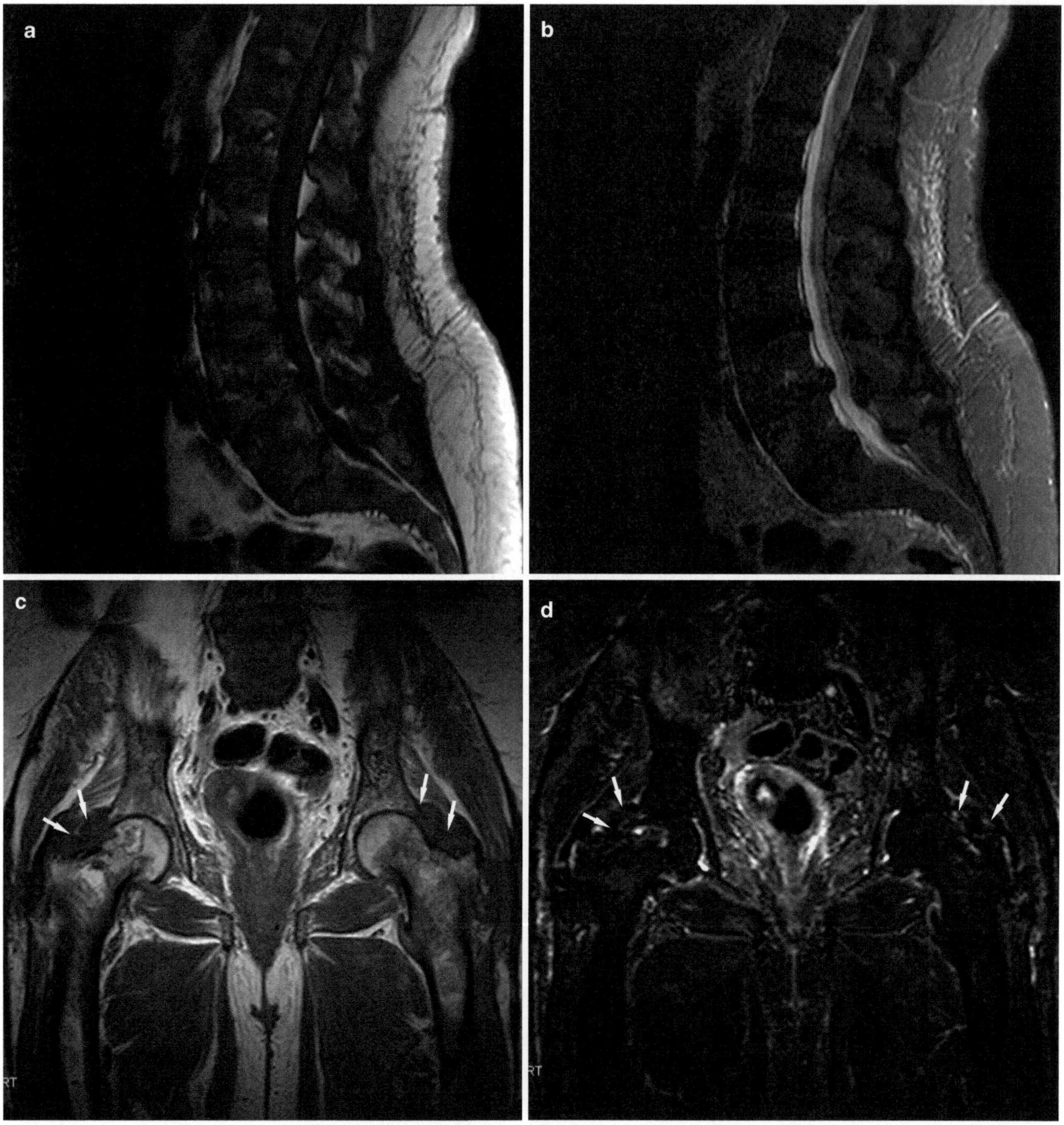

Fig. 5.1 A 61-year-old female with long history of dialysis-dependent chronic renal failure. Sagittal T1-weighted (**a**) and T2-weighted fat-saturated (**b**) images of the lumbar spine demonstrate diffuse hypointense signal with minimal preservation of fat throughout the visualized spine. There is hypointense bone marrow signal about the pelvis and proximal femora on coronal T1-weighted (**c**) and STIR (**d**) sequences. Hypointense synovial masses in bilateral hip joints (*arrows*) have been shown to be amyloid deposition

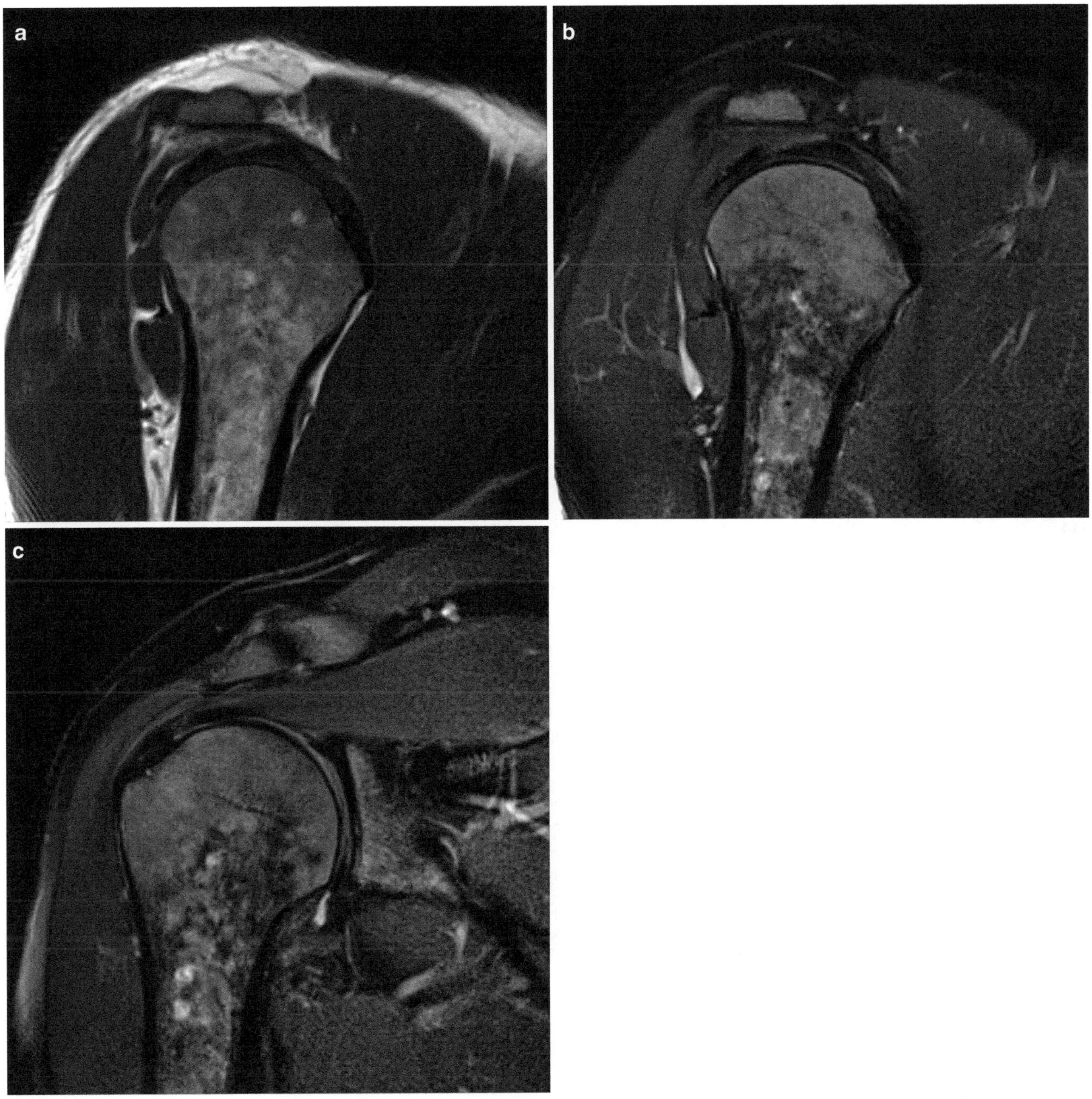

Fig. 5.2 A 53-year-old man with history of chronic renal failure and treated with erythropoietin for anemia. Sagittal T1-weighted (**a**), coronal (**b**), and sagittal (**c**) T2-weighted fat-suppressed images of the right shoulder demonstrate diffuse red marrow including proximal humeral epiphysis and apophysis

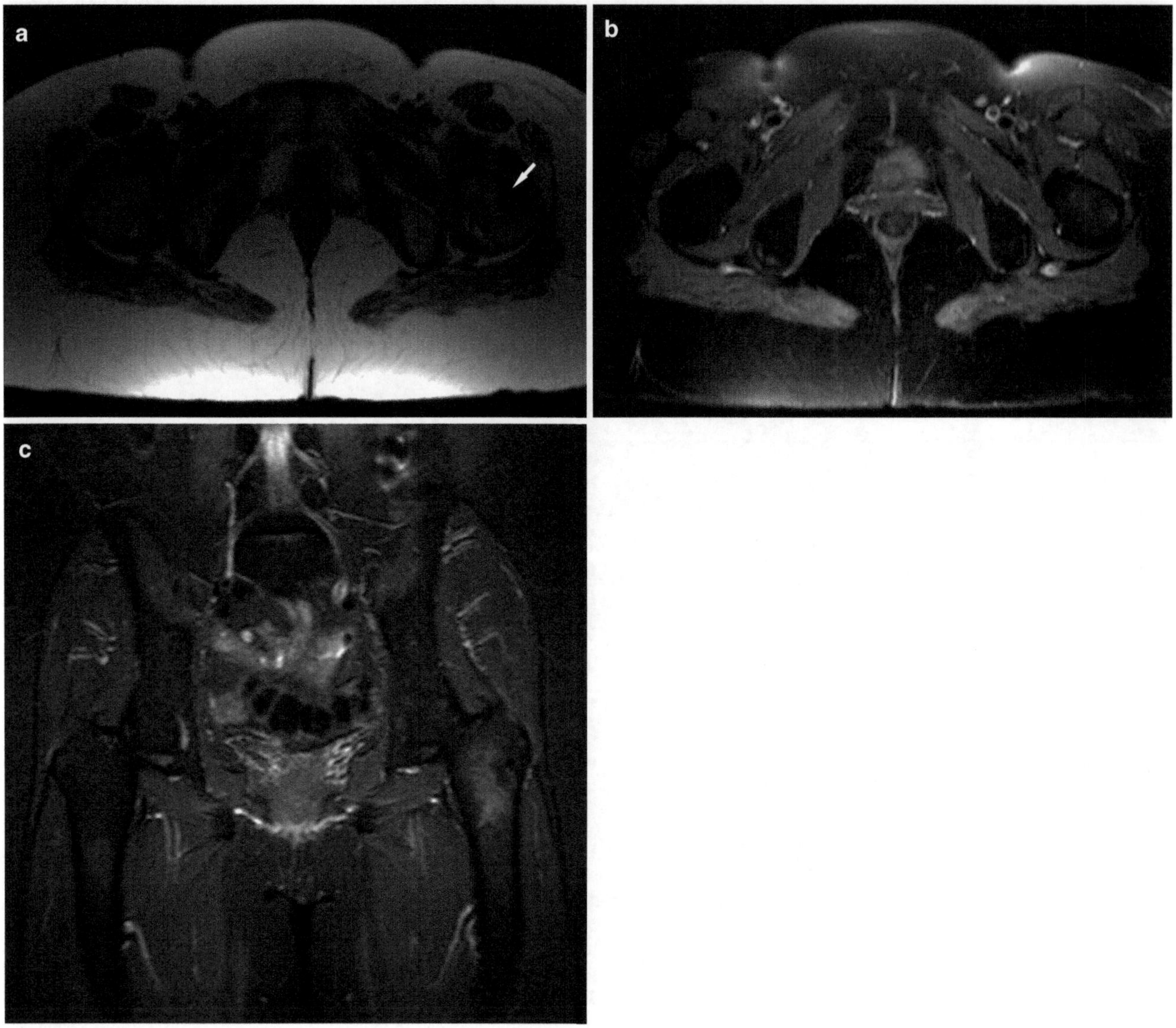

Fig. 5.3 A 48-year-old female with recent renal transplantation for chronic kidney failure. Axial T1-weighted image (**a**) of the left proximal femur demonstrates a marrow-infiltrating hypointense lesion (*arrow*). This lesion appears hypointense on coronal STIR (**b**) and axial T2-weighted fat-suppressed (**c**) images with surrounding bone marrow edema. An image-guided biopsy revealed a healing Brown tumor

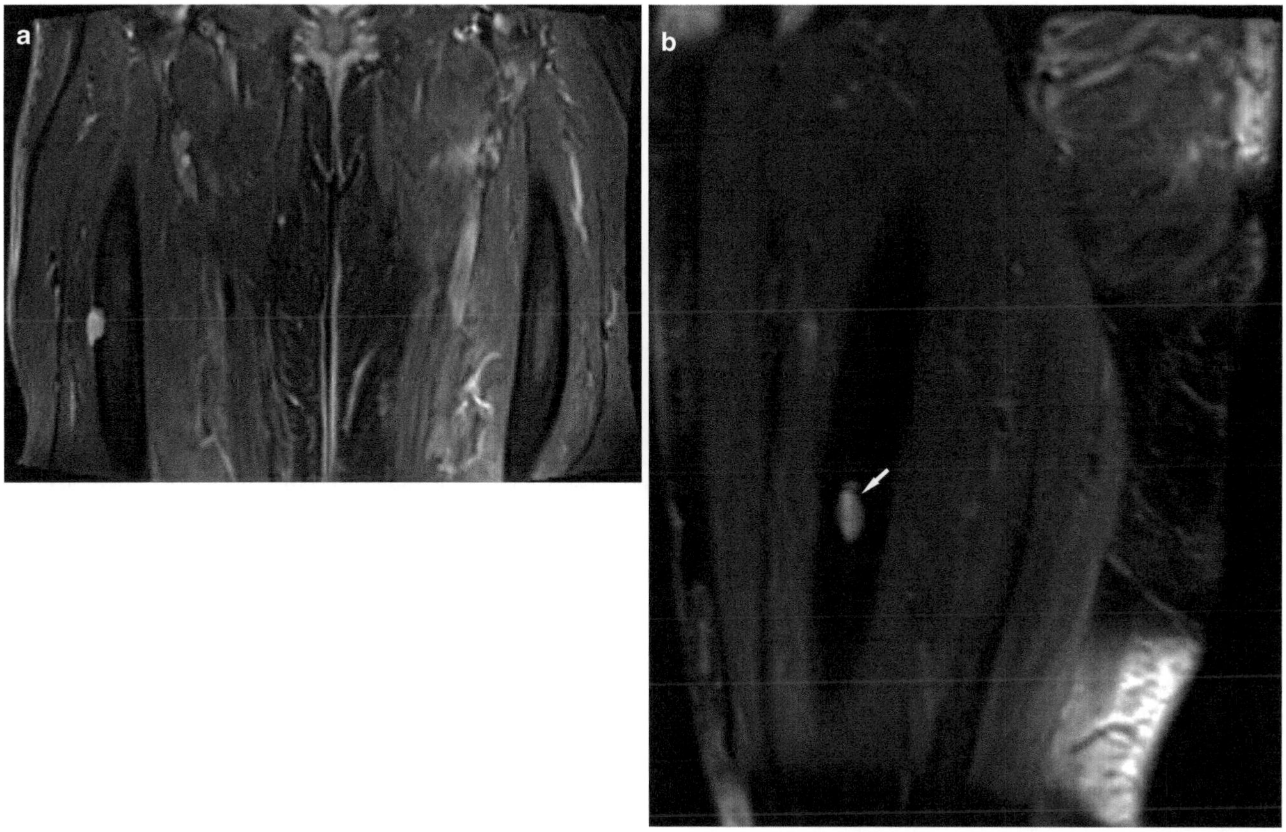

Fig. 5.4 A 50-year-old woman with history of chronic renal failure and secondary hyperparathyroidism. Coronal (**a**) and sagittal (**b**) T2-weighted fat-suppressed images of the right femur demonstrate an eccentric marrow infiltrating lesion of the femoral diaphysis laterally with fluid levels (*arrows*)

5.3 Histiocytosis

Histiocytosis is a general name for a group of disorders or syndromes that involve an abnormal increase in the number of histiocytes. Histiocytosis group disorders are often classified into Langerhans cell histiocytosis (LCH), non-Langerhans cell histiocytosis, and malignant histiocytosis.

LCH is a rare systemic disease with a wide and heterogeneous clinical spectrum and variable extent of involvement due to uncontrolled monoclonal proliferation of monocyte–macrophage lineage cells called Langerhans cells. The pathogenesis of LCH remains unknown. The most widely accepted etiology of this disease is a reactive rather than neoplastic condition. Arguments supporting the reactive nature of the disease include the occurrence of spontaneous remissions, a lack of consistent genetic abnormalities, and a high survival rate in patients without organ dysfunction. Although this disease may be seen at any age, Langerhans cell histiocytosis is typically found in pediatric patients, with incidence peaking at 1–3 years of age. Whole-body MRI has been reported to be an excellent diagnostic method for the evaluation of disseminated musculoskeletal disease in patients with this disorder [2]. The skull is the most frequently involved bone (50 %) followed by pelvic bones (22 %) [3]. Skull lesions often show double contour or beveled-edge appearance due to greater involvement of the inner than the outer table (Figs. 5.5 and 5.6). Fluid levels (Fig. 5.6) due to intralesional hemorrhage or bony sequestrum (Fig. 5.5) may occasionally be seen in LCH lesions. The femur is the most frequently involved long bone followed by the humerus. Spine involvement is usual, presenting with typical severe compression deformity termed "vertebra plana," nearly pathognomonic for this disease (Fig. 5.7). On MRI, LCH lesions demonstrate focal areas of bone marrow infiltration on T1-weighted images with hyperintense T2-weighted and short tau inversion recovery (STIR) signal. Extensive bone marrow edema is typically seen around these lesions. The MRI appearance of LCH, especially outside the skull and vertebra is often aggressive and could simulate the appearance of osteomyelitis or a primary bone neoplasm (Fig. 5.8).

Erdheim–Chester disease is a rare non-Langerhans histiocytic disease that is typically characterized by bone marrow infiltration and multifocal osteosclerotic lesions of the long bones. Biopsy in patients with this disease will demonstrate sheets of foamy histiocytes with or without histiocytic infiltration of extraskeletal tissues. On MRI, there is often diffuse infiltration of the bone marrow on T1-weighted images that is hypointense to skeletal muscle and involves the lower extremities, particularly the tibia (Fig. 5.9). Radiographic or computed tomography (CT) correlation typically shows sclerosis of the involved skeletal structures.

Malignant histiocytosis is a very rare disease of the bone marrow in which patients present with systemic symptoms including lymphadenopathy, splenomegaly, and hepatomegaly. These patients typically have severe thrombocytopenia and anemia [4].

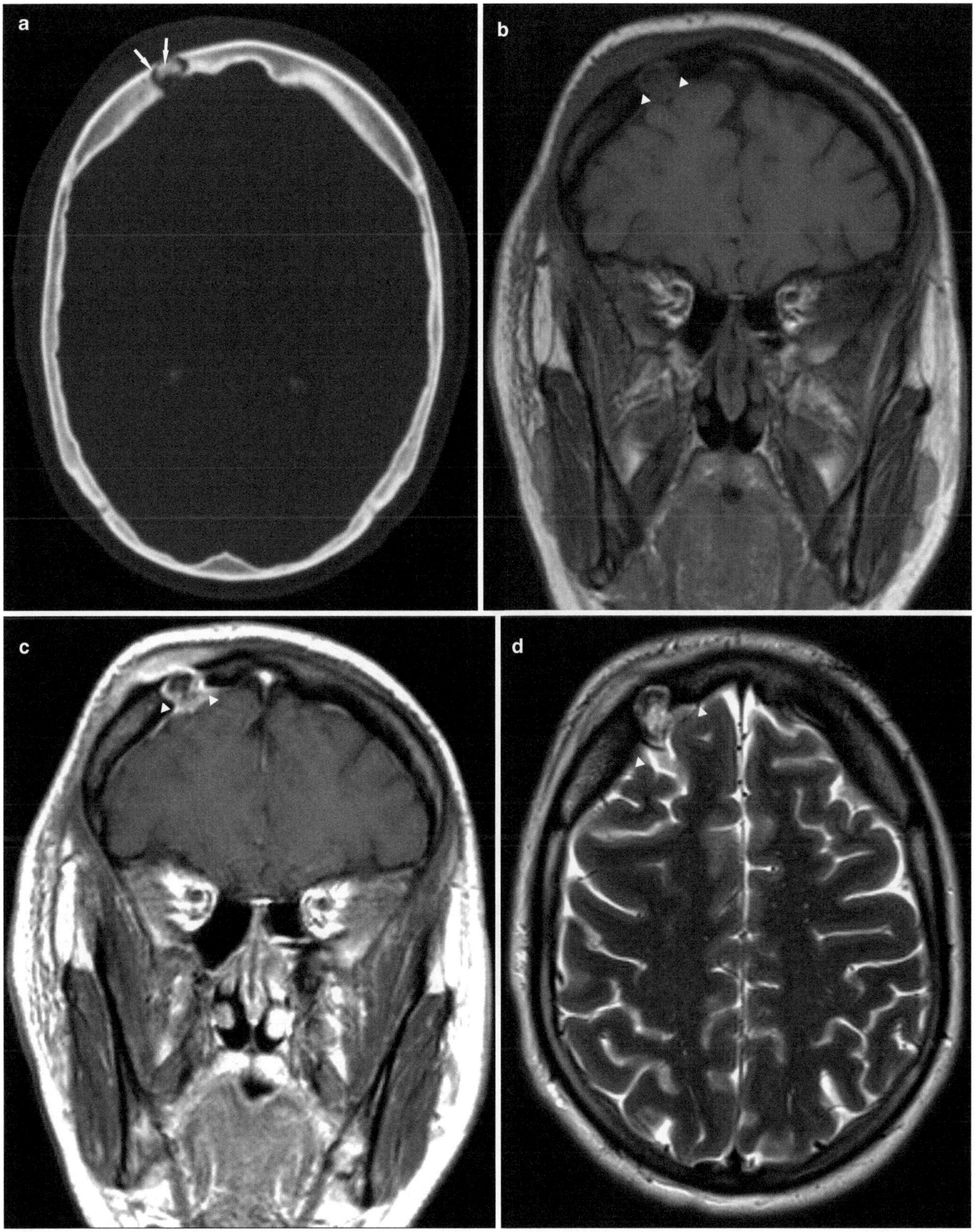

Fig. 5.5 A 27-year-old male with soft tissue swelling and pain in the forehead. Axial CT image (**a**) demonstrates a lytic lesion with central bony sequestrum (*arrows*). Coronal T1-weighted precontrast (**b**) and postcontrast (**c**) and axial T2-weighted (**d**) MR images demonstrate a right frontal destructive bony lesion with predominantly peripheral enhancement. Both CT and MR images demonstrate greater involvement of the inner table (*arrowheads*). Surgical curettage demonstrated Langerhans cell histiocytosis

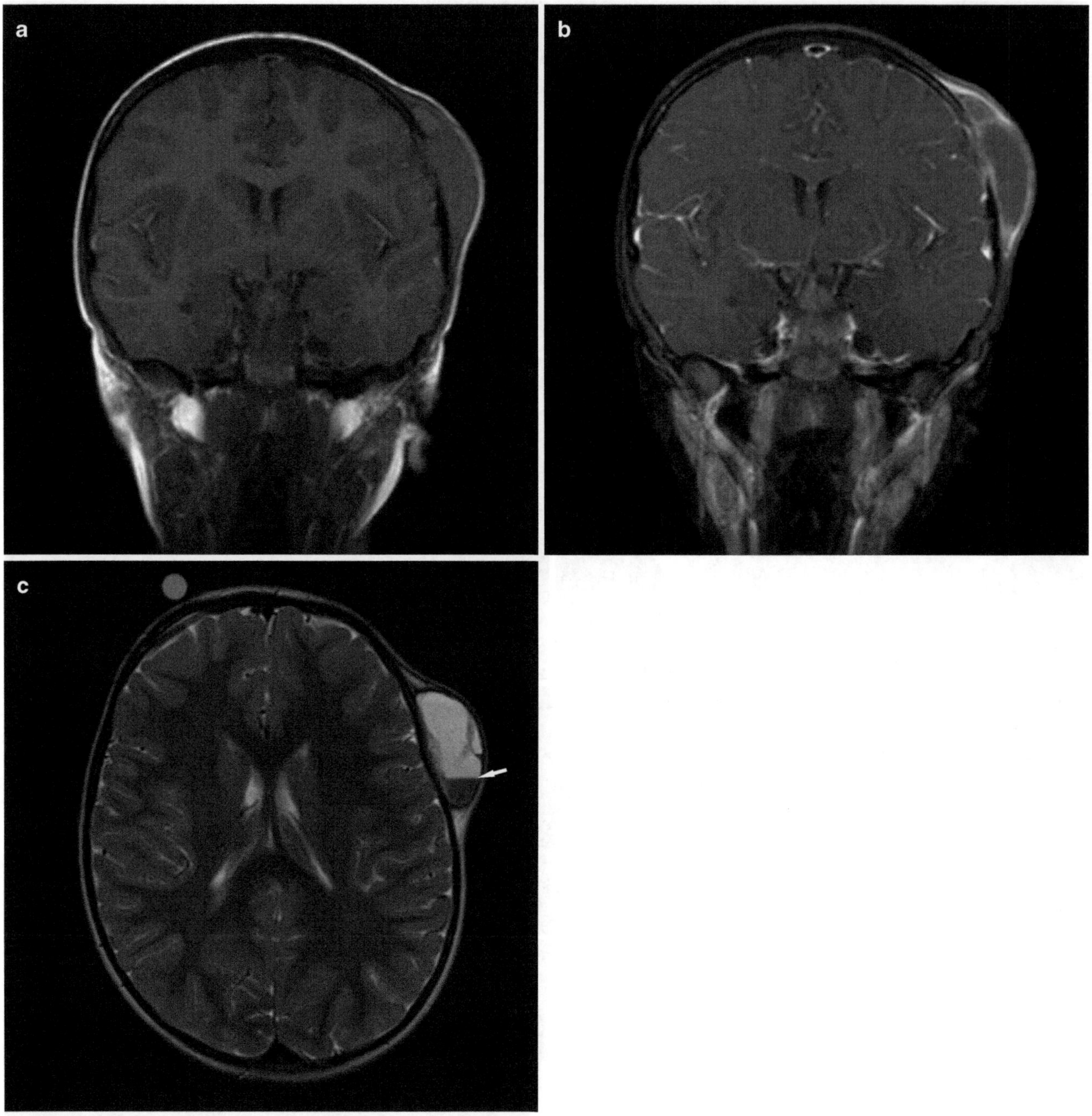

Fig. 5.6 A 4-year-old boy with palpable skull mass. Coronal T1-weighted precontrast (**a**) and postcontrast (**b**) and axial T2-weighted (**c**) MR images demonstrate a large destructive bony lesion with peripheral enhancement. There is fluid level (*arrow*) on axial T2-weighted image suggestive of intralesional hemorrhage. Coronal MR images reveal greater involvement of the inner table. Surgical curettage demonstrated Langerhans cell histiocytosis

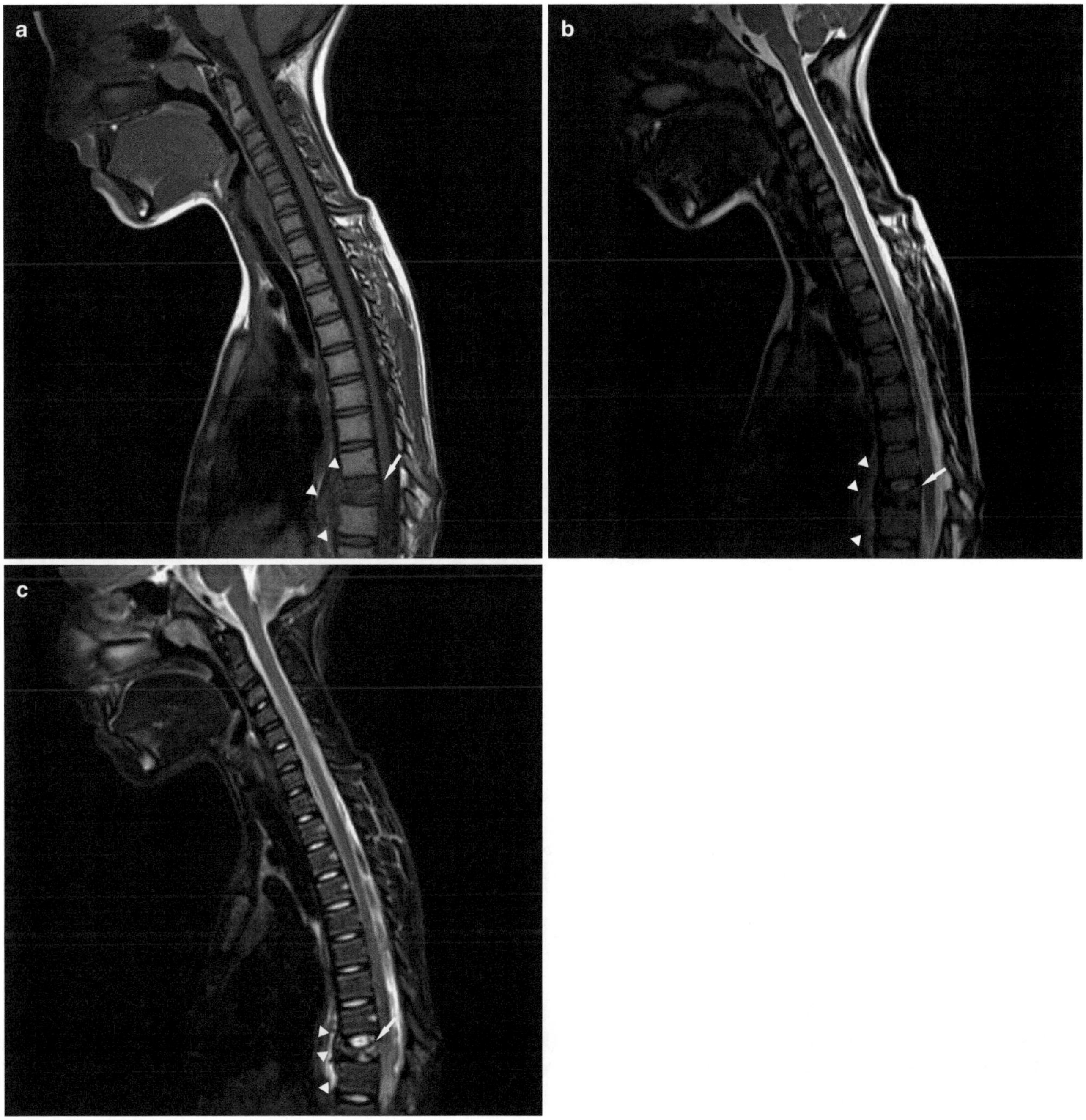

Fig. 5.7 A 10-year-old girl with thoracic back pain. Sagittal T1-weighted (**a**), T2-weighted (**b**), and STIR (**c**) images of thoracic spine demonstrate severe compression deformity of T9 vertebral body (*arrow*) and inflammatory soft tissue changes anteriorly (*arrowheads*)

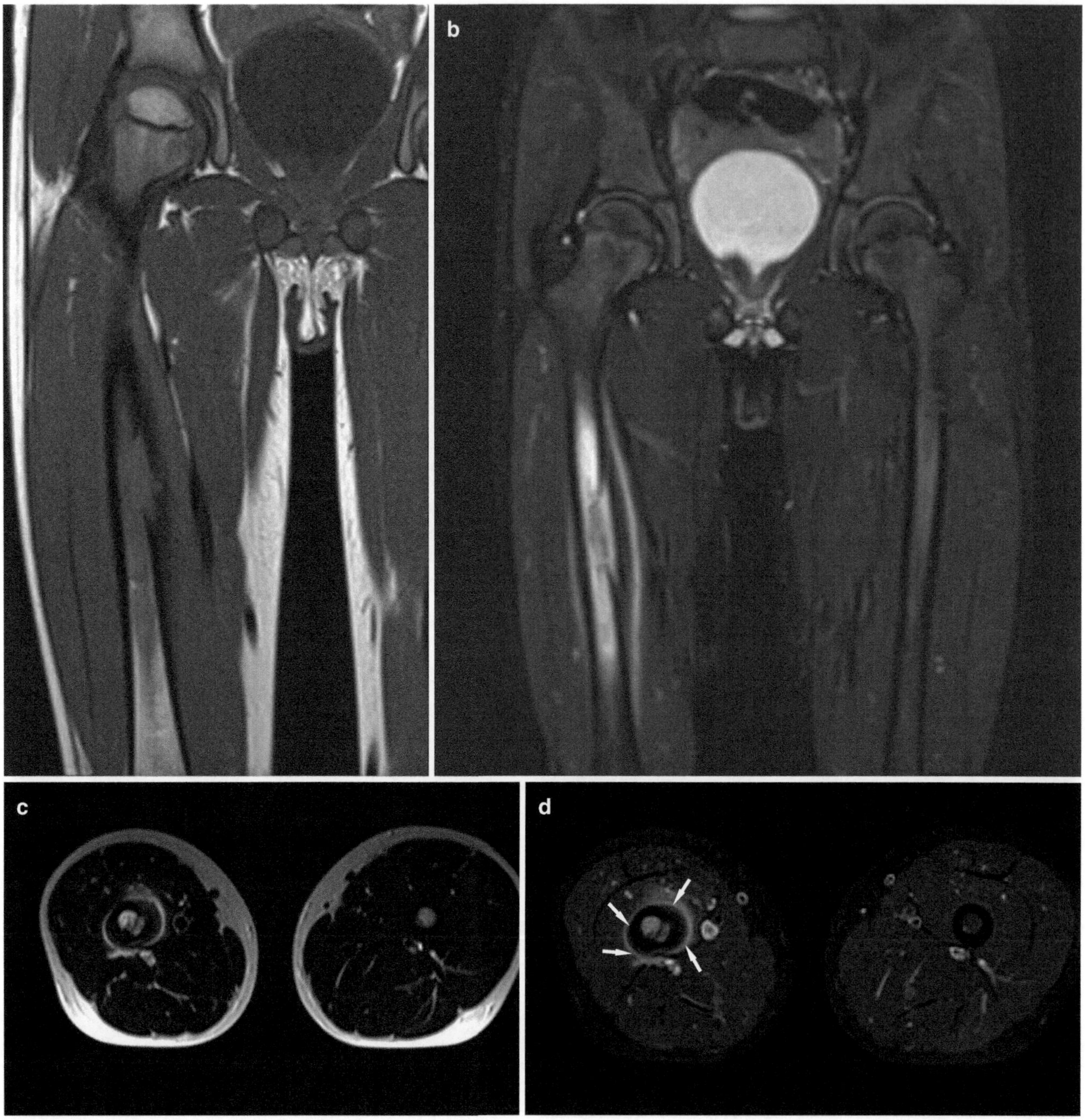

Fig. 5.8 5-year-old boy with leg pain and difficulty walking. Coronal T1-weighted (**a**), STIR (**b**), and axial T2-weighted (**c**) images of the right femur demonstrate an aggressive diaphyseal lesion with subperiosteal extension and marked surrounding bone marrow edema. Postcontrast axial T1-weighted image (**d**) demonstrates circumferential periosteal enhancement (*arrows*). A biopsy revealed Langerhans cell histiocytosis

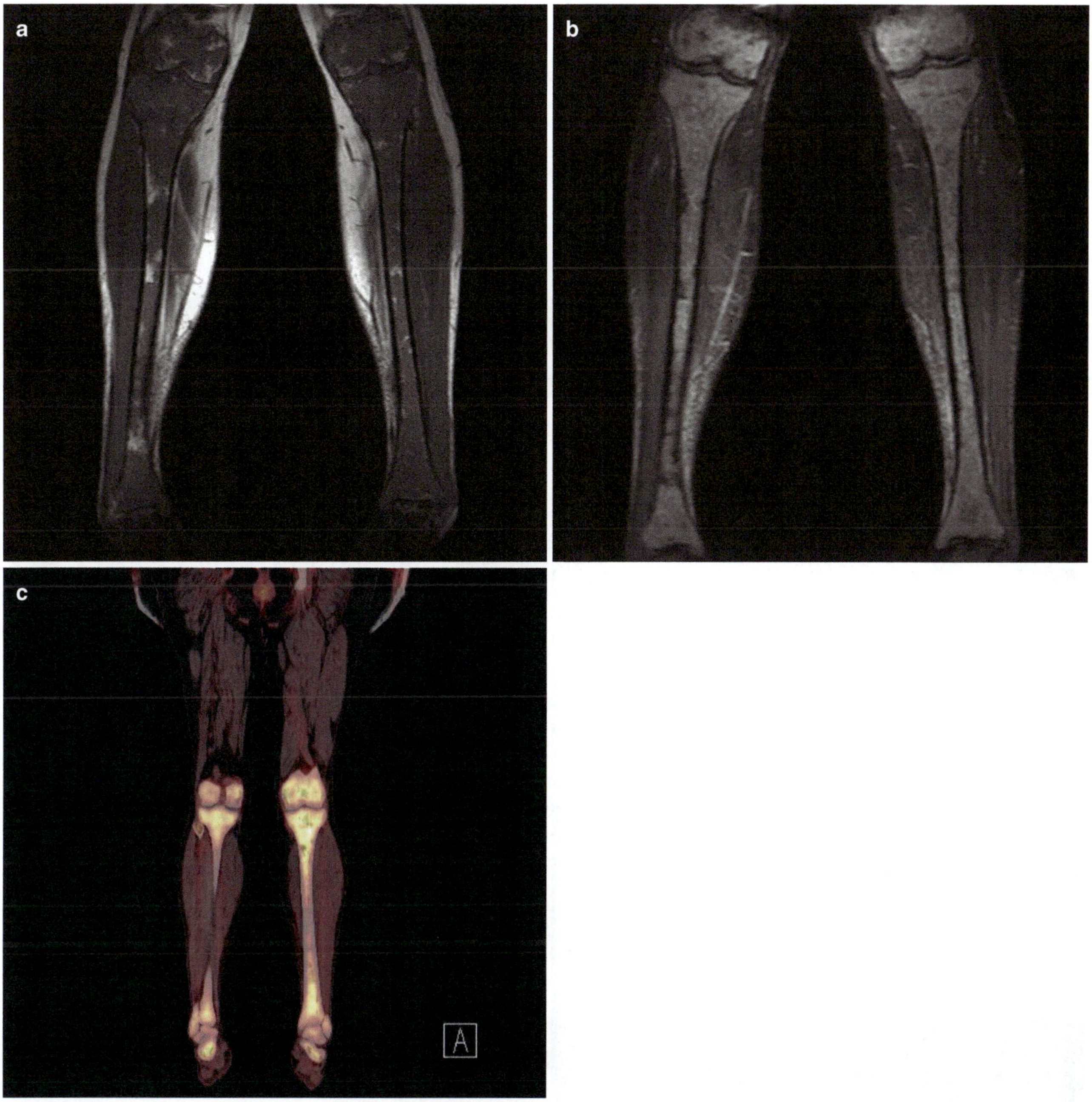

Fig. 5.9 A 57-year-old female with history of uterine cancer and melanoma. Coronal T1-weighted (**a**) and T2-weighted fat-saturated (**b**) images of bilateral legs demonstrate a symmetric diffuse marrow-infiltrating process bilaterally. Coronal positron emission tomography PET/CT image (**c**) demonstrates increased bone marrow metabolic activity. CT-guided biopsy of the left tibia showed foamy histiocytes consistent with Erdheim–Chester disease

5.4 Mastocytosis

Mastocytosis is a heterogeneous group of disorders characterized by mast cell proliferation in different organs, including the skin. These disorders can be localized or systemic. Systemic mastocytosis is a rare form of the disease that typically affects adults. Bone marrow involvement is seen in 70 % of systemic mastocytosis cases, with clinical symptoms similar to those of lymphoma or leukemia [5]. In addition to bone marrow, many other organs can be involved, including the skin, liver, spleen, and lymph nodes. Mast cell proliferation in bone marrow stimulates fibroblastic activity and granulomatous reaction, which leads to trabecular destruction and fractures, especially when the spine is involved. The bone marrow infiltration in systemic mastocytosis had been shown to be homogeneously or heterogeneously diffuse with mottled areas on MRI [3] (Fig. 5.10).

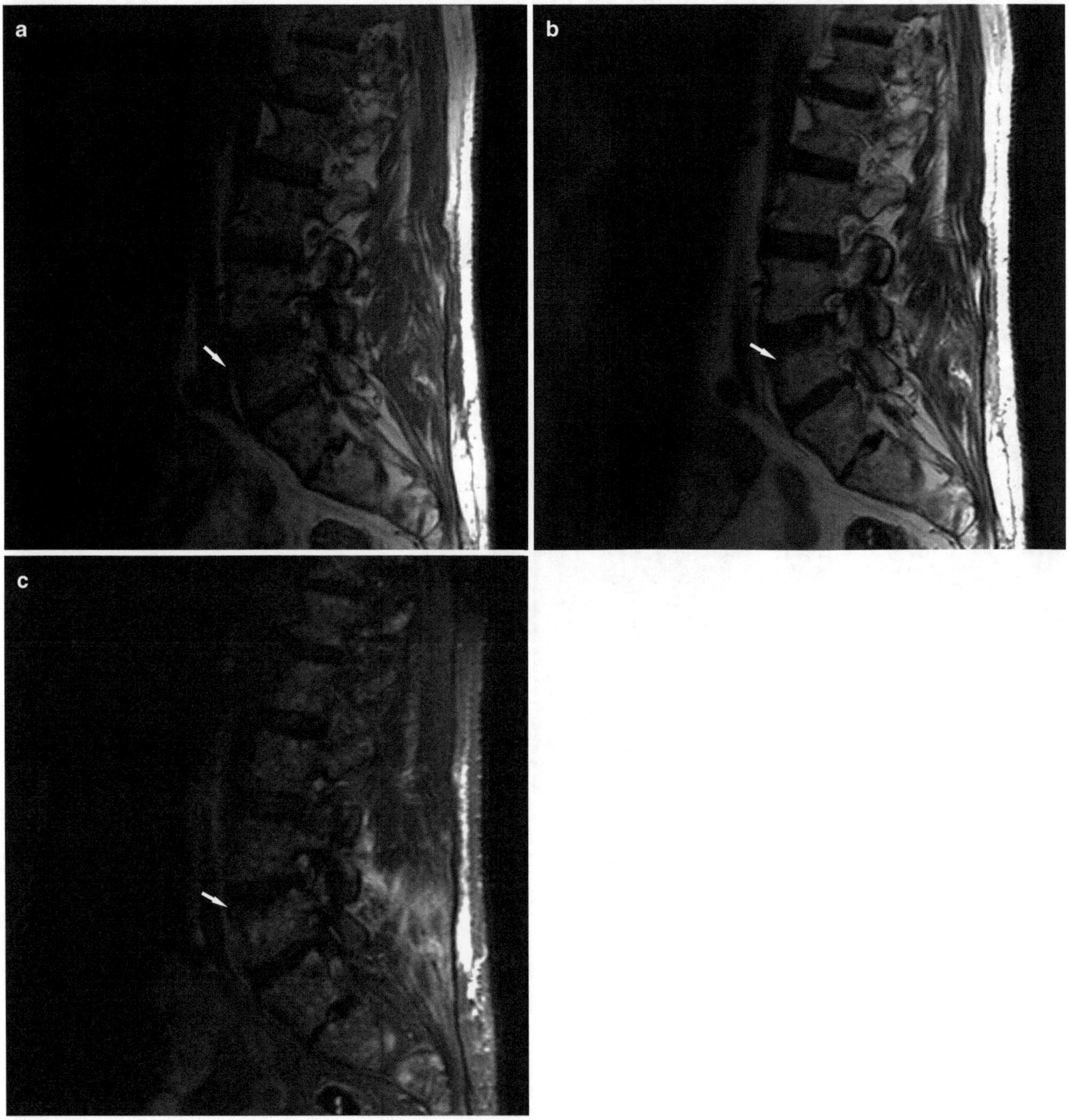

Fig. 5.10 A 63-year-old female with back pain. Sagittal T1-weighted (**a**), T2-weighted (**b**), and STIR (**c**) images of the lumbar spine demonstrate multiple foci of round lesions scattered in the visualized bone marrow and a mild compression deformity of L4 (*arrow*). A biopsy showed diffuse mast cell infiltration consistent with systemic mastocytosis

5.5 Paget Disease

Paget disease is a localized disorder of osseous remodeling that typically begins with excessive bone resorption and is followed by an increase in bone formation. Although the etiology of Paget disease is unclear, both genetic and environmental contributors have been suggested. The initial osteoclastic overactivity of Paget disease is followed by compensatory osteoblastic activity, which leads to a structurally disorganized mosaic of the bone. The bone affected by Paget disease is larger, more vascular, and mechanically weaker than the healthy bone. MRI findings in patients with Paget disease are often subtle, especially when compared to obvious radiographic or CT abnormalities. Preserved fatty bone marrow signal must be present for Paget disease in all phases. Prominent fatty marrow signal can simulate an intraosseous lipoma on MRI (Fig. 5.11) in the lytic or hot phase before cortical and trabecular thickening occurs. In the mixed lytic–blastic and blastic phases, thickening of the trabeculae and cortex is seen in the background of fatty bone marrow (Figs. 5.12 and 5.13). Fibrovascular tissue may be visualized inside pagetoid bone after the initial phase which should not be mistaken for bone lesions (Figs. 5.13 and 5.14). When lower extremity long bones are involved, bowing deformity is not uncommon. MRI detection of osseous enlargement in Paget disease may be difficult except in the spine where comparison with other vertebral bodies is possible (Fig. 5.15). MRI can also be used to diagnose various complications of Paget disease, including fractures and sarcomatous degeneration.

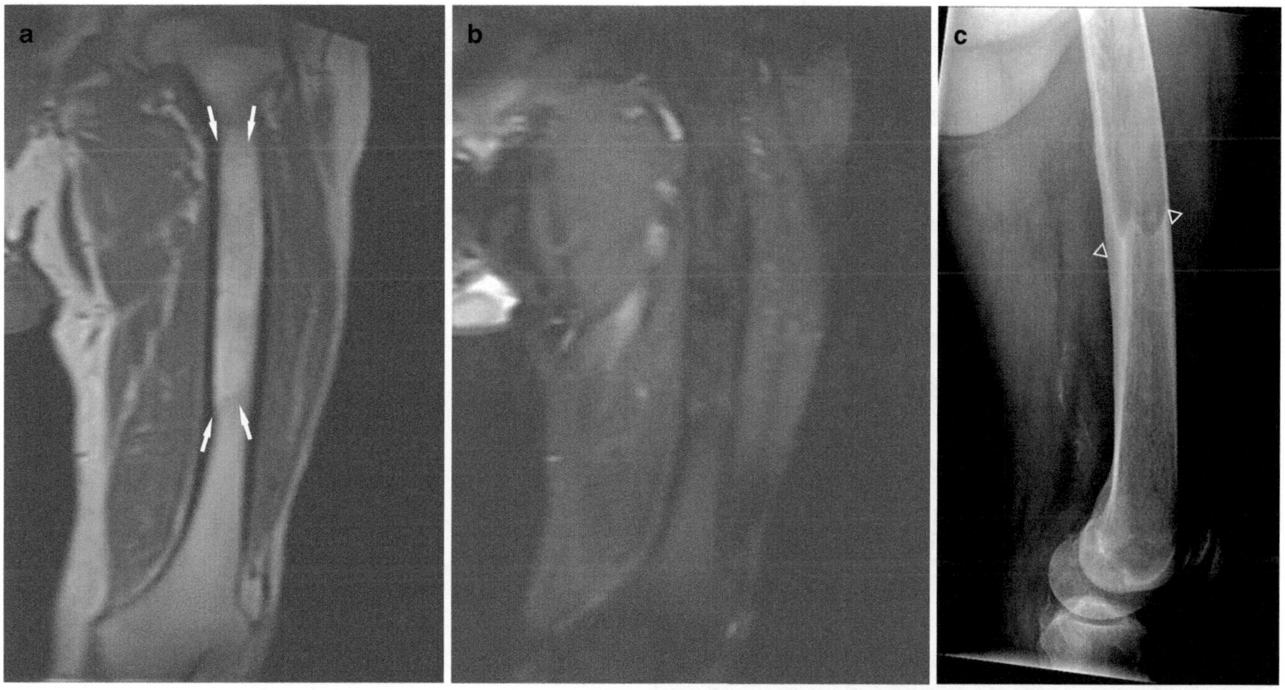

Fig. 5.11 An 81-year-old male with left hip pain. Coronal T1-weighted (**a**) and STIR (**b**) sequence from left femur MRI demonstrate a subtle cortical expansion involving the diaphysis with circumscribed fatty intralesional signal which can be separated from adjacent normal marrow signal both proximally and distally (*arrows*). Lateral radiograph of the femur (**c**) demonstrates lytic nature of the lesion with the blade of grass sign (*arrowhead*)

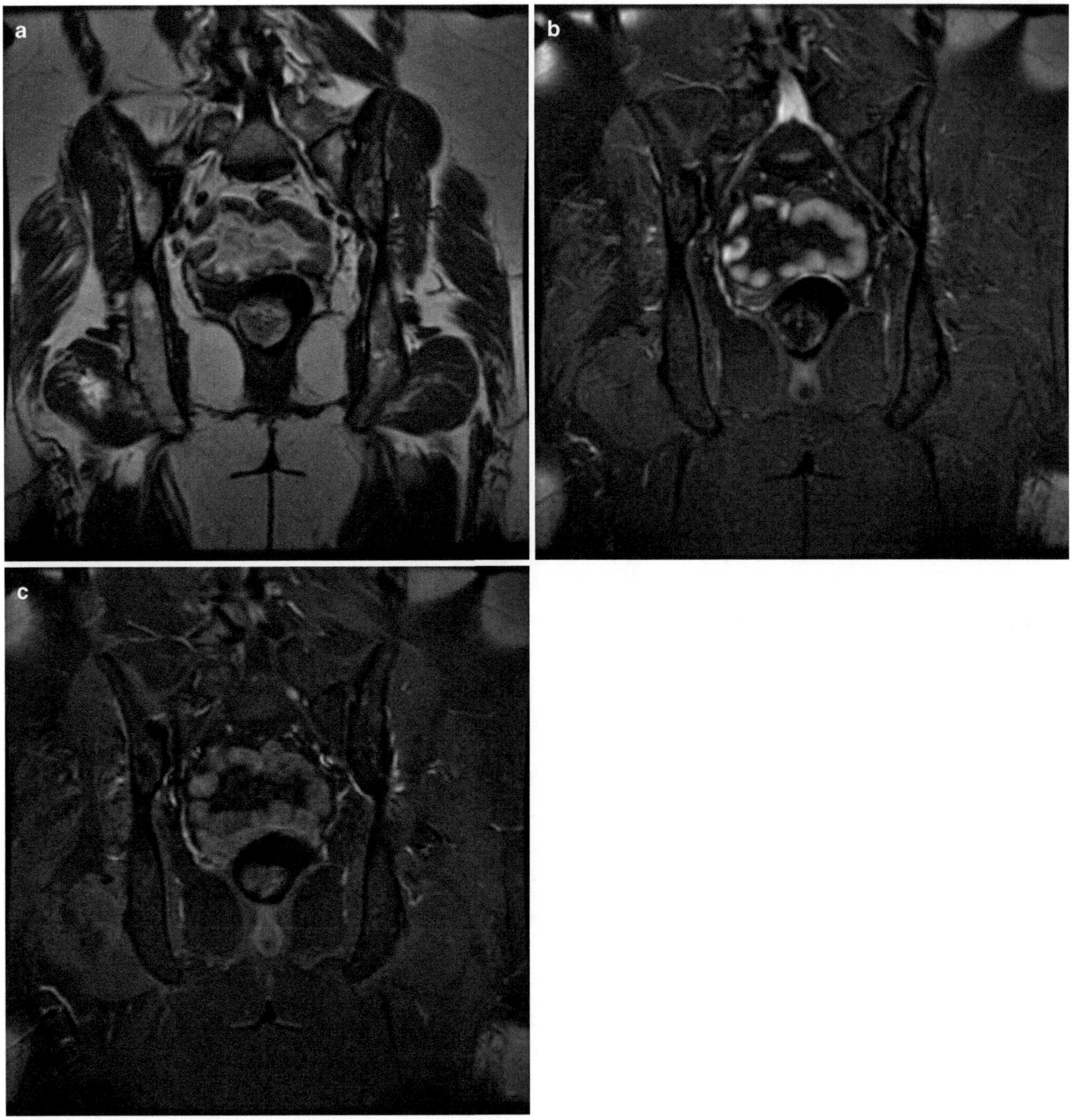

Fig. 5.12 A 50-year-old female with low back pain. Coronal T1-weighted (**a**) and coronal T2-weighted fat-suppressed (**b**) images of the pelvis demonstrate asymmetric bone marrow signal of left ilium and ischium with subtle cortical thickening. No significant enhancement is visualized on coronal T1-weighted fat-saturated postcontrast image (**c**). An image biopsy of the left iliac bone revealed mixed phase Paget disease

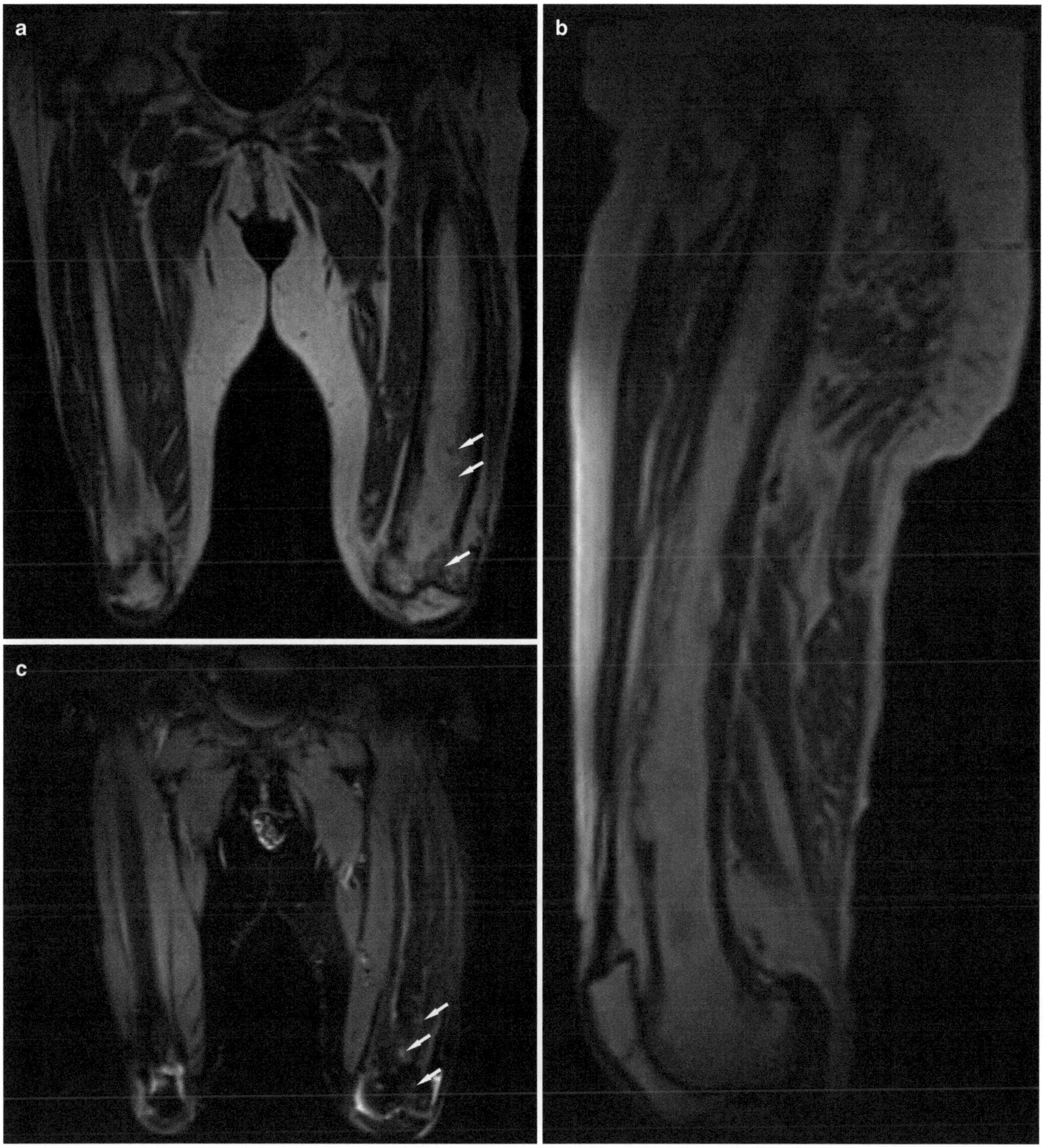

Fig. 5.13 A 91-year-old female. Coronal T1-weighted (**a**), sagittal T1-weighted (**b**), and coronal STIR (**c**) images of the left femur demonstrate diffuse, irregular cortical thickening and expansion with bowing deformity consistent with Paget disease. Punctate areas of hypointense T1 and hyperintense STIR signal underneath the cortex suggestive of fibrovascular tissue (*arrows*)

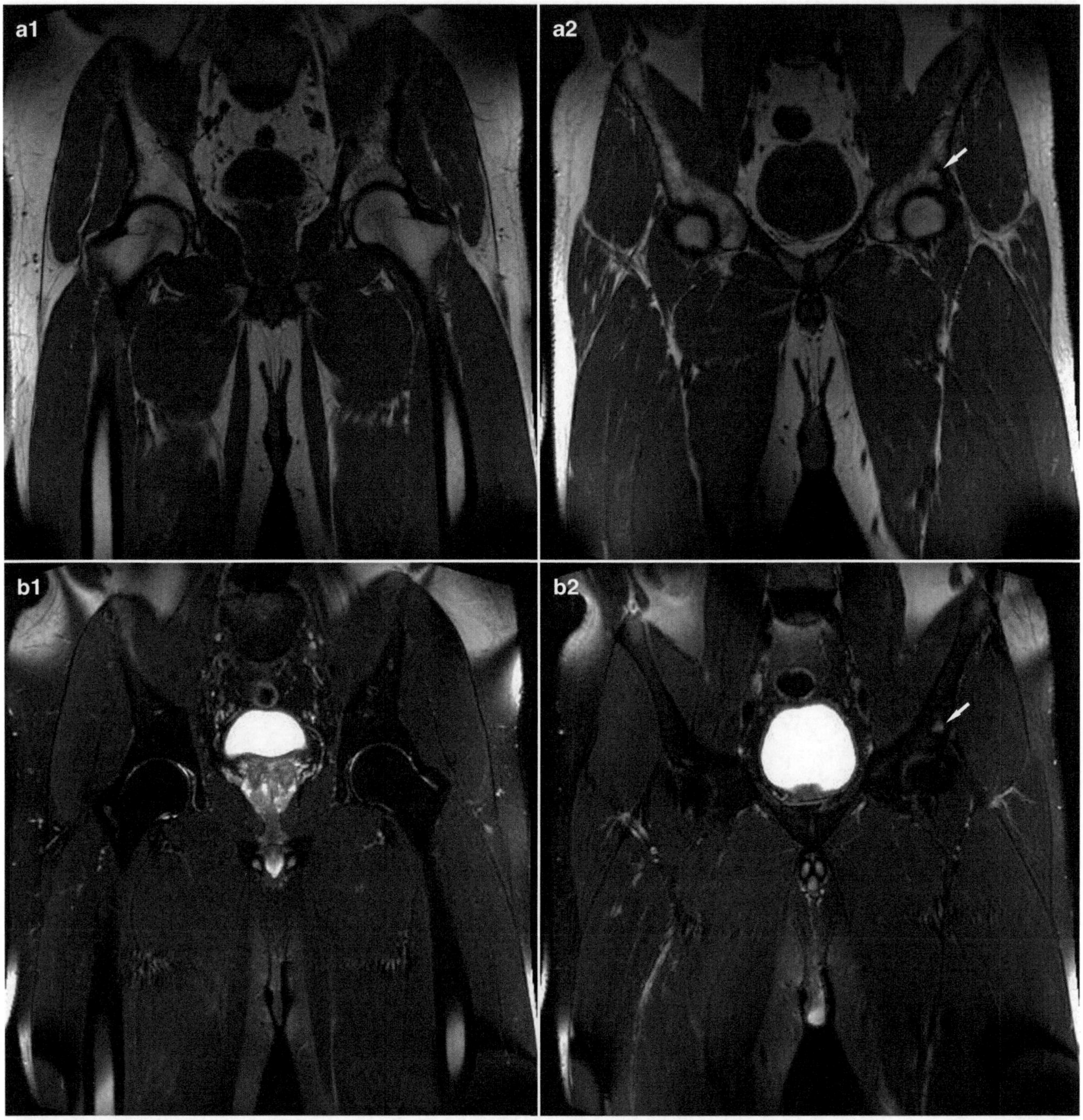

Fig. 5.14 A 50-year-old male. Coronal T1-weighted (**a**) and coronal STIR images of the pelvis demonstrate cortical thickening with prominent trabeculae along the left ilium consistent with Paget disease. Several foci of hypointense T1 and hyperintense STIR sequence involving the left ilium and ischium most prominent at the left acetabular region (*arrows*) consistent with fibrovascular tissue

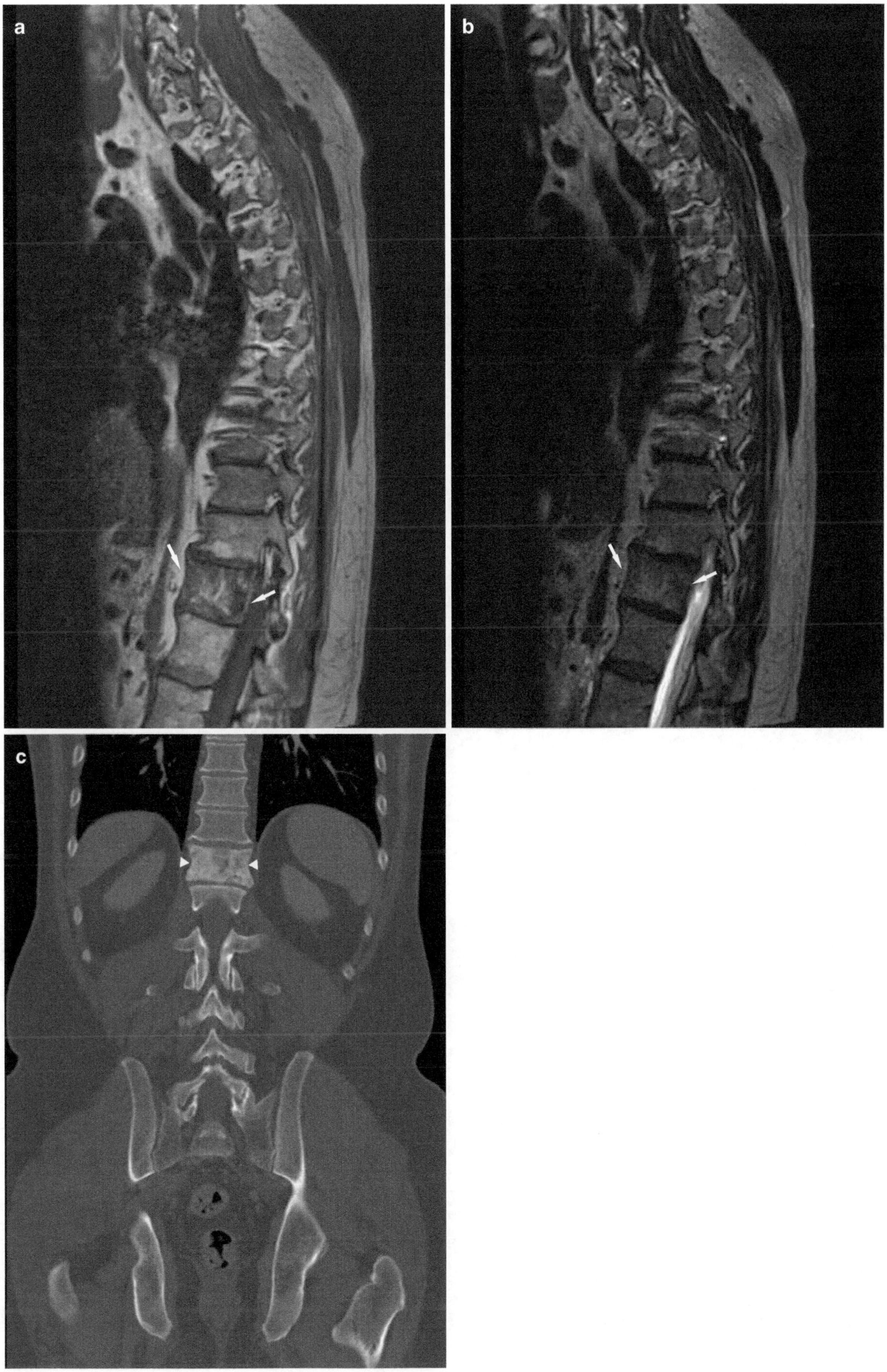

Fig. 5.15 A 57-year-old male with history of prostate cancer. Sagittal T1-weighted (**a**) and T2-weighted (**b**) images of the thoracolumbar spine demonstrate bony enlargement and prominent trabeculae at T11 with preservation of fatty marrow signal consistent with Paget disease (*arrows*). Coronal CT image (**c**) demonstrates sclerotic changes of T11 with bony enlargement compared to other levels (*arrowheads*)

5.6 Serous Atrophy of the Bone Marrow

Serous atrophy or gelatinous degeneration of the bone marrow is a rare bone marrow-replacing process in patients who are starved of carbohydrates and calories. In this condition, there is gradual reduction of adipose tissue in the bone marrow, and the adipose tissue is replaced by fluidlike gelatinous tissue. This is not a fibrotic process, however, and has been found to be reversible [6]. The most common underlying cause of this condition is anorexia nervosa, although other conditions such as starvation, HIV infection, malignancy, systemic lupus erythematosus, and post-chemotherapy bone marrow aplasia can result in serous atrophy of the bone marrow [7]. On MRI, this condition appears as typically hypointense signal compared to skeletal muscle on T1-weighted images and markedly hyperintense signal on T2-weighted and STIR sequences (Fig. 5.16). Near-complete absence of the overlying subcutaneous fat may also be observed. In less severe cases, patchy residual fatty bone marrow may be seen (Fig. 5.17).

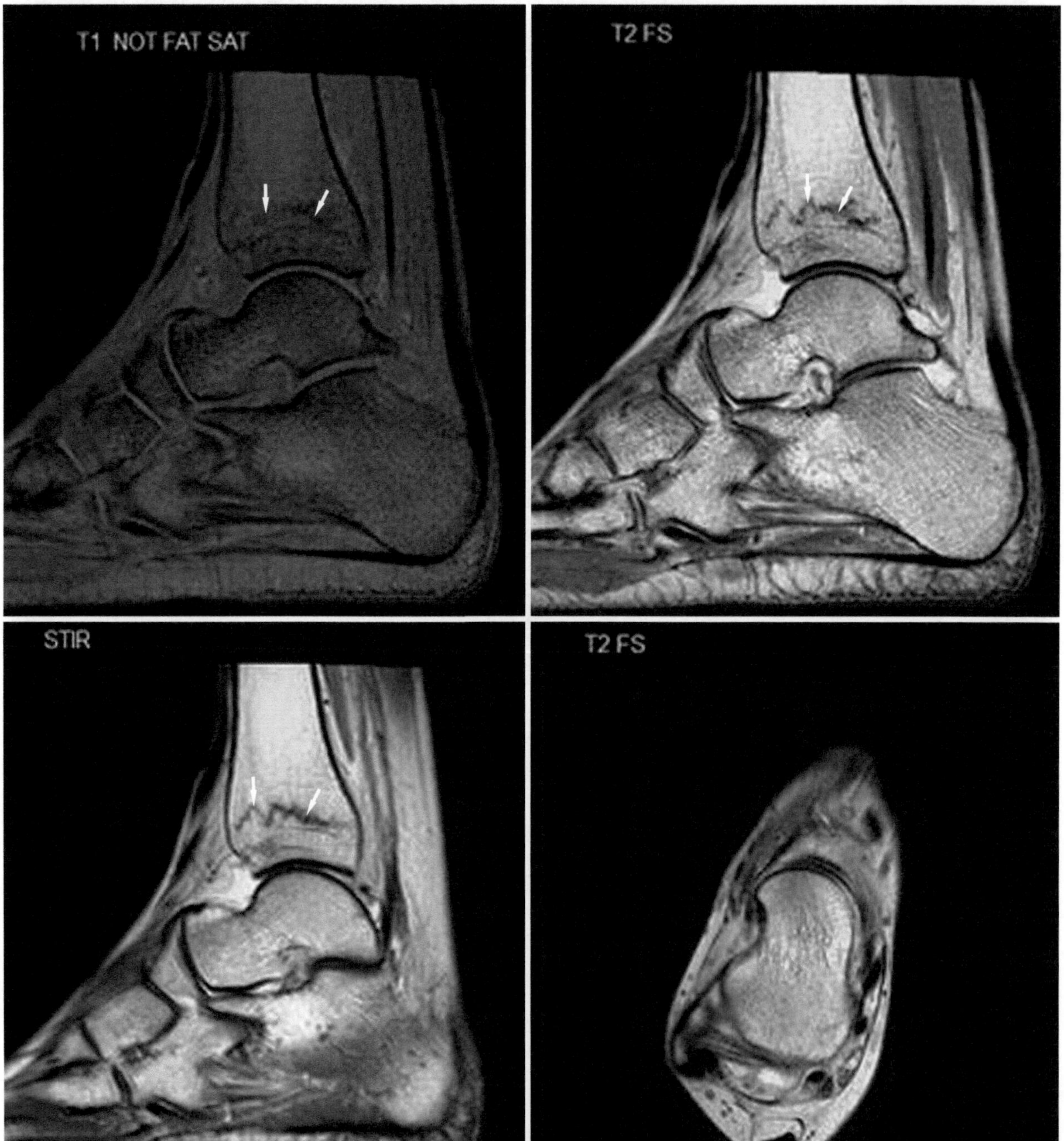

Fig. 5.16 A 17-year-old female with anorexia nervosa and right ankle pain. T1-weighted sagittal image of the right ankle without fat suppression demonstrates complete absence of bone marrow and subcutaneous fat. Sagittal STIR, sagittal T2-weighted fat-suppressed, and axial T2-weighted fat-suppressed images demonstrate diffuse hyperintense fluidlike signal. Findings are typical of serous bone marrow atrophy. Please note the insufficiency fracture in the distal tibia (*arrows*) (Image courtesy of Hilary Umans, MD)

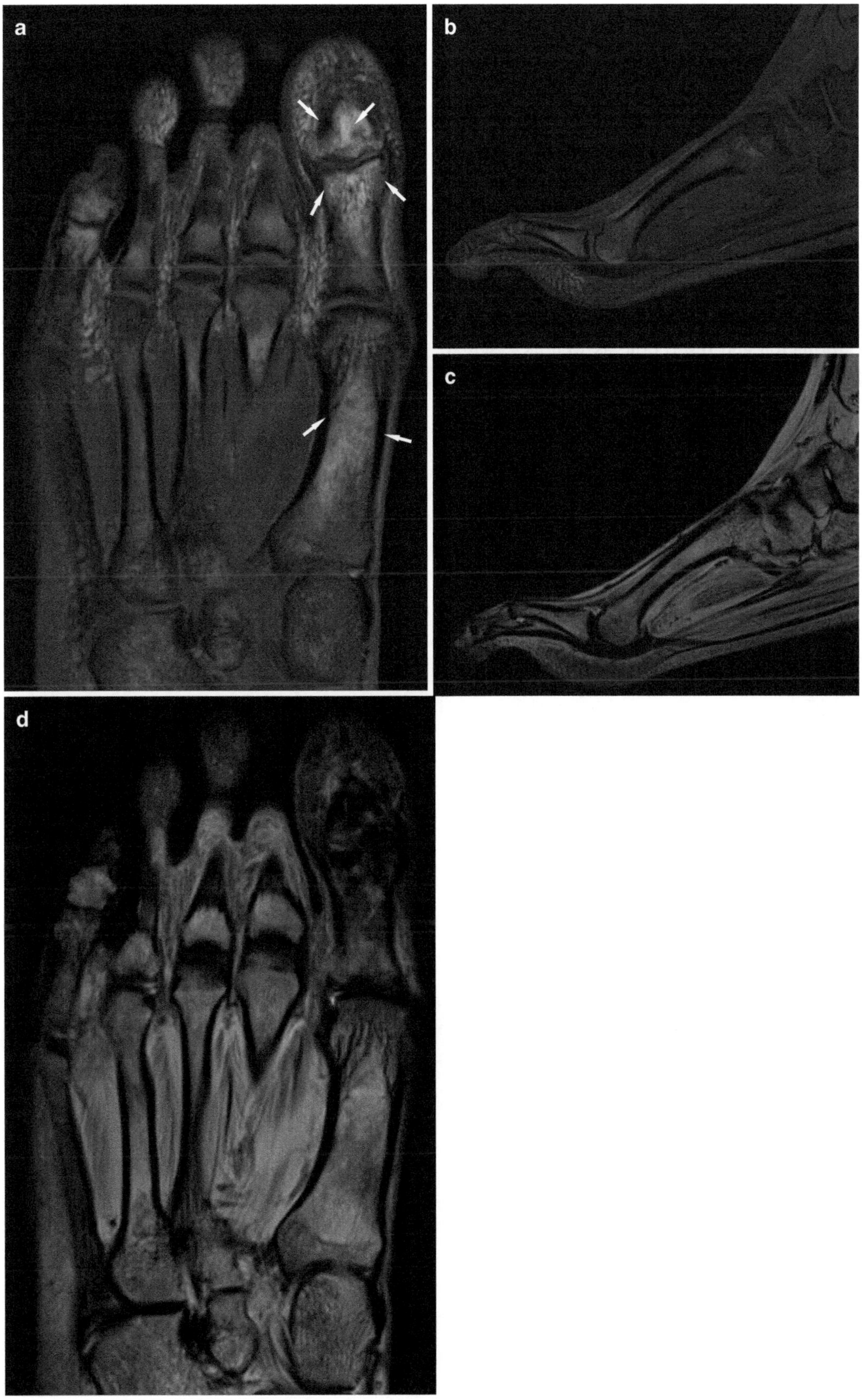

Fig. 5.17 Severely malnourished 42-year-old male with significant recent weight loss due to inflammatory bowel disease. T1-weighted axial (**a**) and sagittal (**b**) images of the right foot demonstrate near-complete absence of bone marrow fat with minimal residual fatty marrow signal particularly at the first redistribution (*arrows*). STIR sagittal (**c**) and axial (**d**) images demonstrate diffuse edema and fluidlike hyperintense signal in bone marrow and soft tissues. Findings suggest developing serous marrow atrophy

5.7 Gaucher Disease

Gaucher disease is the most common of the lysosomal storage diseases, resulting from accumulation of undegraded glucosylceramide in lysosomes within macrophages of the reticuloendothelial cell system due to a deficiency of the enzyme glucocerebrosidase [8]. These enlarged macrophages filled with glycolipids are called Gaucher cells and are most abundant in the bone marrow, spleen, and liver. The bone marrow involvement of Gaucher disease leads to the most debilitating complications of the disease. Proposed mechanisms for osseous changes in Gaucher disease include altered bone formation and resorption, as well as vascular occlusion resulting from increased intraosseous pressure secondary to marrow infiltration [9]. Vascular occlusion may result in osteonecrosis with typical imaging findings (Figs. 5.18 and 5.19). Marrow replacement with Gaucher cells often leads to expansion of the medullary cavity with thinning of the cortex and endosteal scalloping. In the distal femurs, this medullary expansion is called Erlenmeyer flask deformity (Fig. 5.20). MRI has been shown to be the most effective method for detecting bone marrow involvement in Gaucher disease and quantifying bone marrow burden (2 *Tables-spine and femora* by Maas et al. -Quantification of Bone Involvement in Gaucher Disease: MR Imaging Bone Marrow Burden Score as an Alternative to Dixon Quantitative Chemical Shift MR Imaging—Initial Experience). MRI also plays an important role in the follow-up of these patients to monitor bone marrow response during treatment [9]. Bone marrow invasion in Gaucher disease is similar to that of hematopoietic bone marrow, demonstrating similar distribution and signal characteristics.

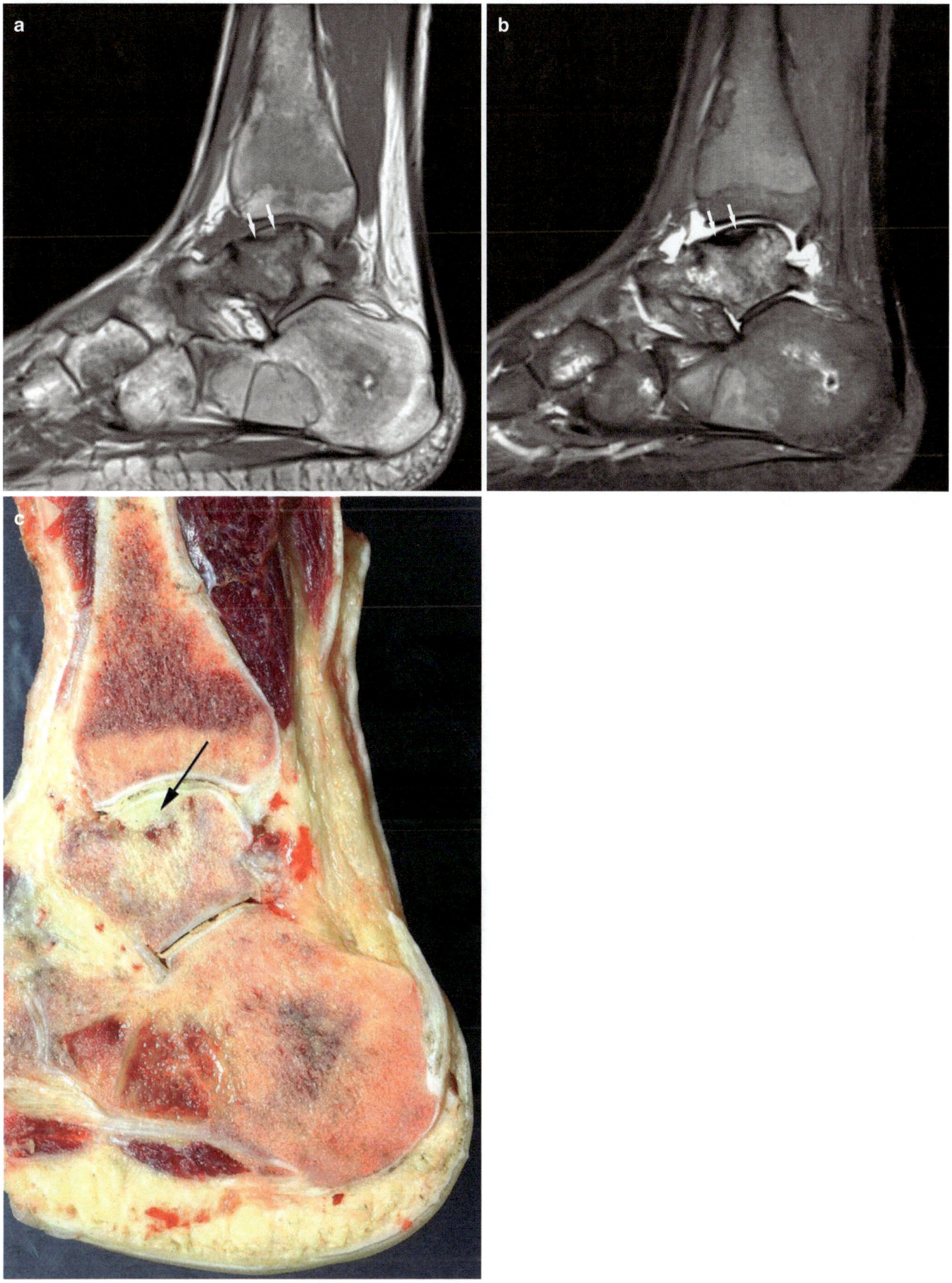

Fig. 5.18 A 21-year-old woman with known Gaucher disease. Sagittal T1-weighted (**a**) and STIR (**b**) images of the right ankle demonstrate several foci of osteonecrosis with talar head subchondral collapse (*short arrows*). Surgical specimen (**c**) after below-knee amputation showing talar dome osteonecrosis (*long arrow*). Please note prominent appearance of the bone marrow in distal tibia on both MRI and surgical specimens

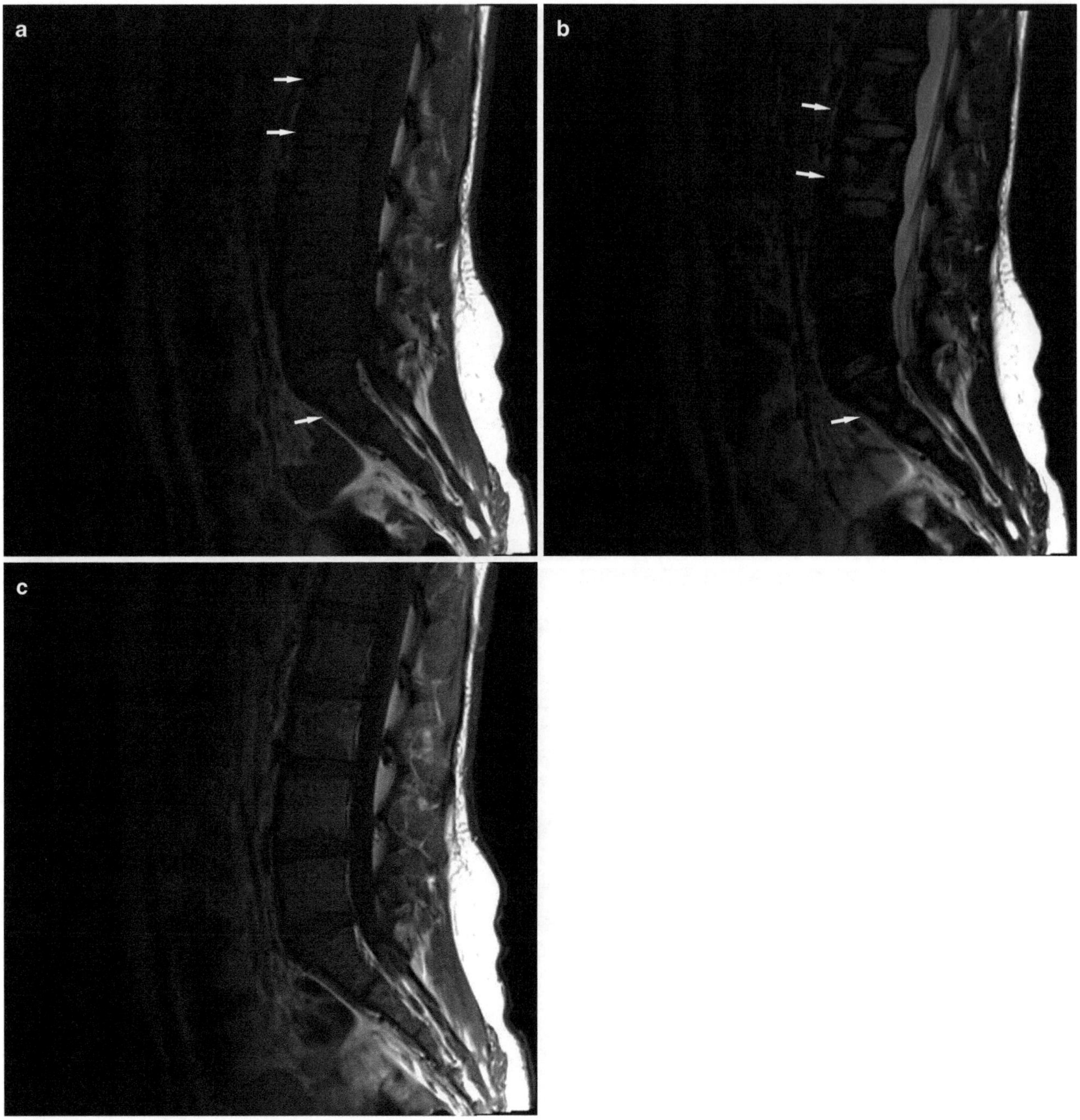

Fig. 5.19 19-year-old woman with Gaucher disease. Sagittal T1-weighted precontrast (**a**) and T2-weighted (**b**) images of the lumbar spine demonstrate diffuse bone marrow infiltration and serpentine areas of abnormal signal at L2, L3, and sacral segments suggestive of osteonecrosis (*arrows*). Postcontrast T1-weighted sagittal image (**c**) demonstrates peripheral enhancement around the foci of osteonecrosis

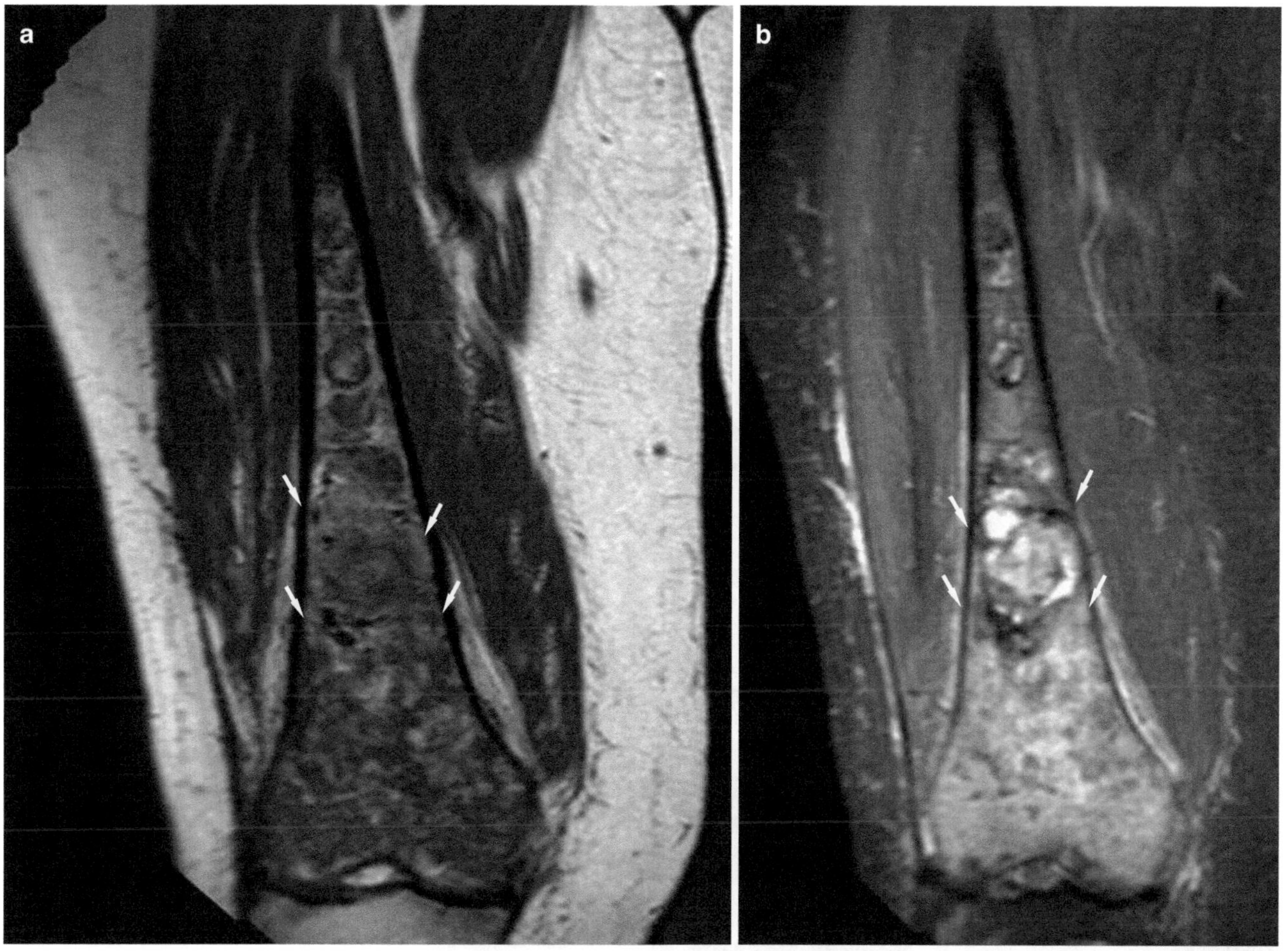

Fig. 5.20 A 69-year-old female with known Gaucher disease. Coronal T1-weighted (**a**) and STIR (**b**) images of the right femur demonstrate mild cortical expansion along the distal femur with cortical thinning (*arrows*). Extensive bone marrow signal abnormality consistent with Gaucher disease and associated osteonecrosis

5.8 Osteopetrosis

Osteopetrosis is a group of very rare bone disorders caused by defective osteoclast function. The autosomal dominant form is relatively benign and occurs most commonly in adults. The autosomal recessive type is usually more severe, with mortality resulting from infection or bone marrow failure during childhood. Markedly thickened cortices result in decreased medullary space available for bone marrow (Fig. 5.21). On MRI, different distribution of the hematopoietic bone marrow is often seen in patients with osteopetrosis due to narrowed medullary spaces.

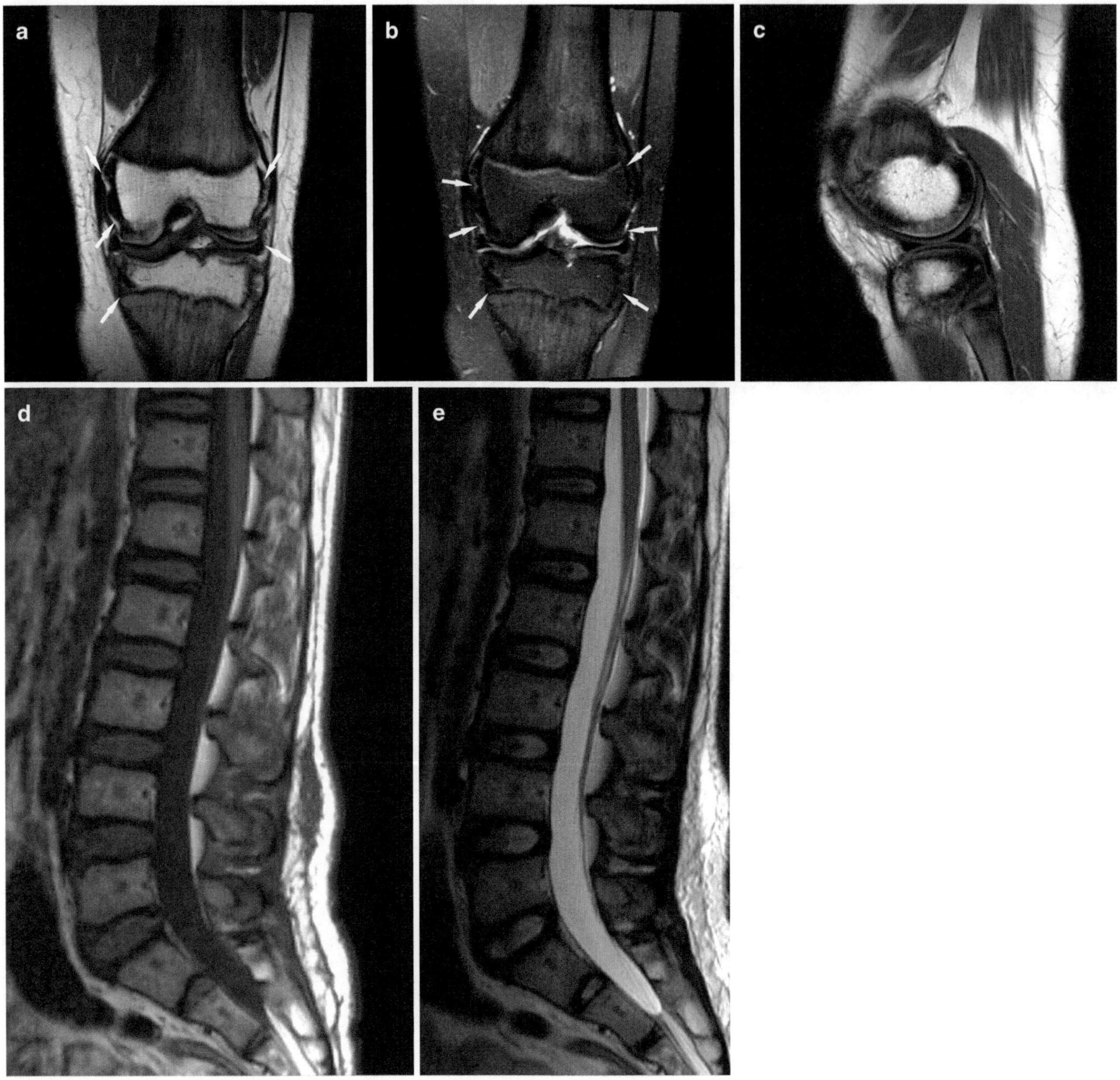

Fig. 5.21 A 31-year-old female with known osteopetrosis. Coronal T1-weighted (**a**), T2-weighted fat-suppressed (**b**), and sagittal proton-density-weighted (**c**) MR images of the left knee demonstrate prominent cortical thickening especially in the epiphyses (*arrows*). On lumbar spine MRI, hypointense thickening of the endplates is noted on T1-weighted sagittal (**d**) and T2-weighted sagittal (**e**) images

5.9 Sarcoidosis

Sarcoidosis is a systemic inflammatory disorder in which noncaseating granulomas infiltrate multiple organ systems, including the bone marrow. Most patients with sarcoidosis have underlying chest disease, although isolated bone marrow involvement has been encountered when MRI is performed for routine joint or spine evaluation (Fig. 5.22). Sarcoid bone marrow lesions are frequently multiple and in most cases contain intralesional macroscopic fat (Fig. 5.23), a sign of benignity differentiating these lesions from metastatic disease.

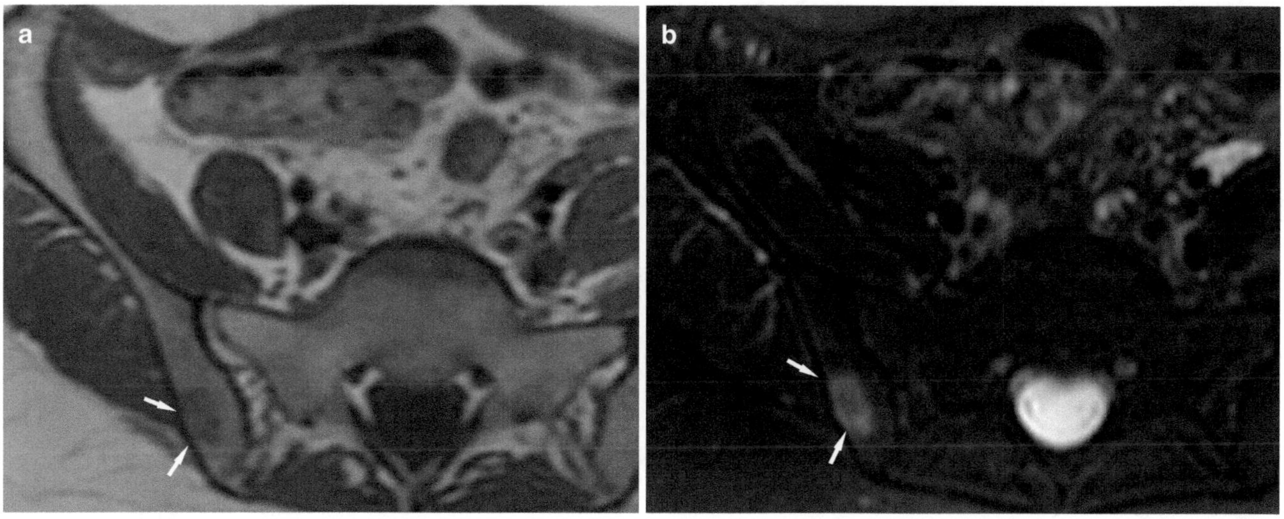

Fig. 5.22 A 37-year-old female with low back pain and no known malignancy or systemic disease. An MRI examination of the pelvis revealed several marrow-infiltrating lesions on T1-weighted axial (**a**) and STIR axial images (**b**). The largest lesion in the right ilium posteriorly (*arrows*) was biopsied under imaging guidance. Histologic evaluation revealed granulomas consistent with sarcoid

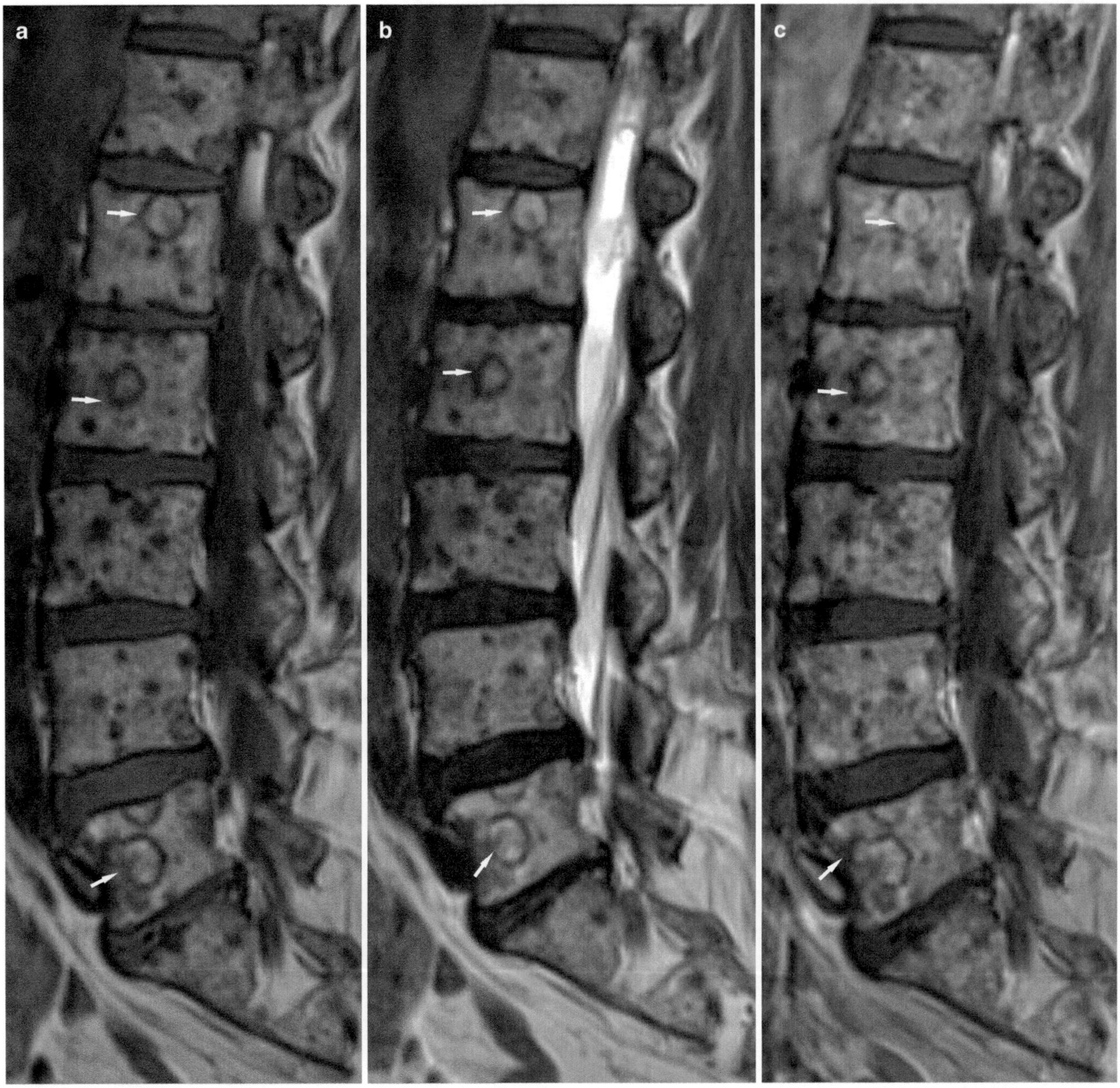

Fig. 5.23 A 48-year-old male with known sarcoid. Multiple lesions are seen throughout the visualized lumbar spine on sagittal T1-weighted precontrast (**a**) and T2-weighted (**b**) and T1-weighted postcontrast (**c**) images. Fatty signal is noted in larger lesions (*arrows*), a sign of benignity

5.10 Infection

Osteomyelitis is the infection of the bone and bone marrow. *Staphylococcus* is the most frequently implicated bacteria in both adults and pediatric patients with osteomyelitis. Unusual bacteria such as *Salmonella* may be seen in patients with underlying sickle cell disease. Fungal etiology is rare except in patients with underlying immunodeficiency. MRI is able to detect early bone marrow involvement in patients with suspected osteomyelitis (Fig. 5.24). MRI is also helpful in the detection of associated abscesses that may occur in the bone marrow, subperiosteal region, or overlying soft tissues (Fig. 5.25). On T1-weighted images, osteomyelitis shows hypointense signal compared to skeletal muscle. On T2-weighted and STIR images, a hyperintense signal corresponding to osteomyelitis with marked surrounding bone marrow edema can be seen. There is often surrounding soft tissue edema, as well. The penumbra sign [10] is an MRI feature of subacute osteomyelitis which refers to a discrete peripheral zone of hyperintense signal intensity on unenhanced T1-weighted images, surrounding the central bony abscess cavity with associated reactive new bone and edema (Fig. 5.25). Contrast-enhanced images are most helpful in demonstrating sinus tract and soft tissue changes, if present. In children osteomyelitis is common in the long bones of the appendicular skeleton such as the femur, tibia, and humerus. Metaphyseal involvement is typical especially in children with occasional extension through growth plate into the epiphysis. Distinguishing normal hematopoietic marrow from osteomyelitis can be challenging in certain situations because of the normal hematopoietic marrow that is often seen in the metaphyses in children, which appears similar to osteomyelitis. However, normal hematopoietic marrow T1 signal should be hyperintense relative to skeletal muscle without surrounding edema in the bone marrow or soft tissues. Osteomyelitis of axial skeleton is more frequently seen in adult patients likely due to hematogenous seeding. When spine osteomyelitis occurs, it is often due to progression of discitis. When multilevel spinal infection is encountered particularly with the presence of adjacent soft tissue abscess, tuberculosis should be considered in the differential.

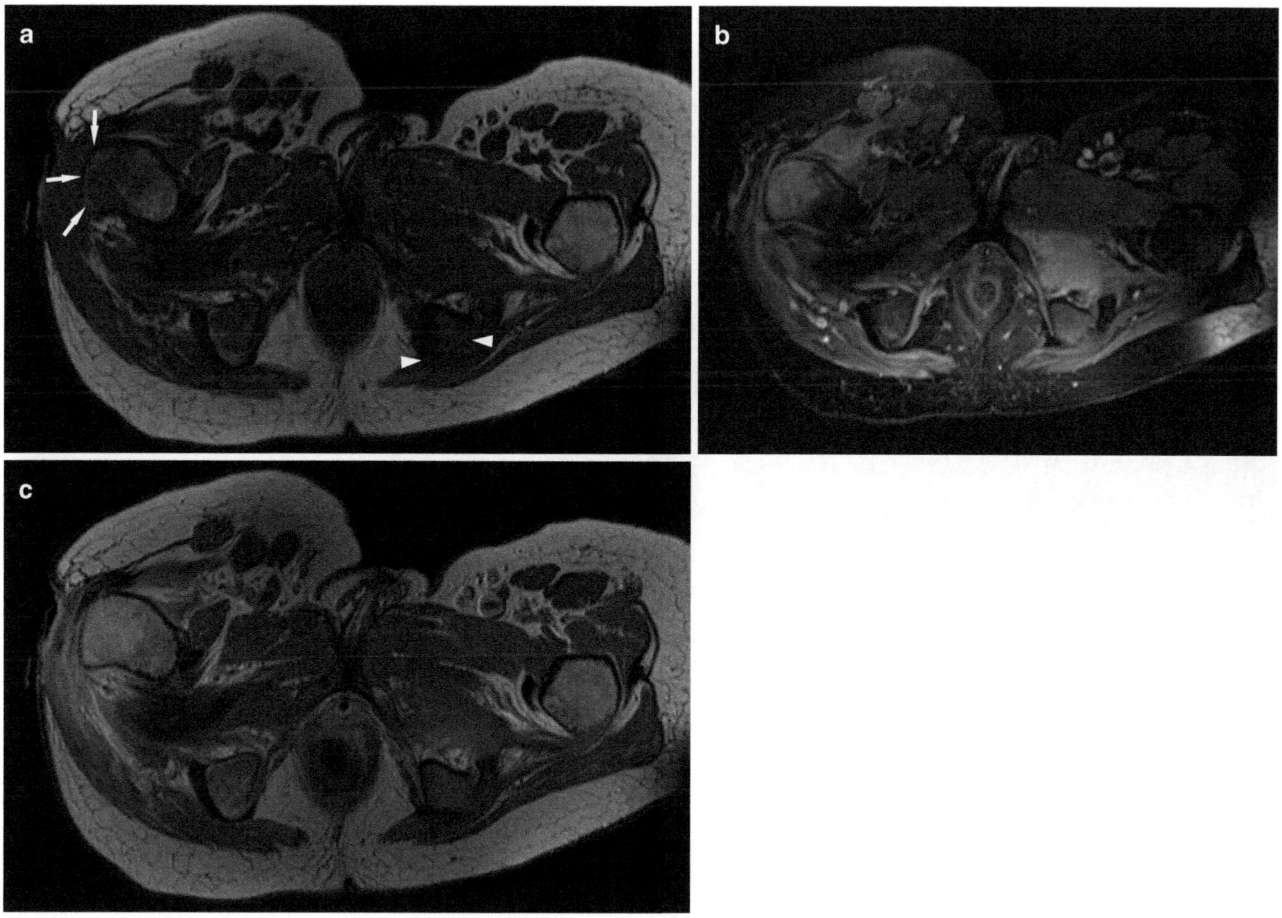

Fig. 5.24 A 39-year-old male with paraplegia and decubitus ulcers. Abnormal bone marrow infiltration of the right greater trochanter (*arrows*) and left ischial tuberosity (*arrowheads*) are noted on axial T1-weighted MR images of the pelvis (**a**). Associated soft tissue and bone marrow edema is present on T2-weighted fat-suppressed image (**b**). Enhancement of bone marrow and soft tissues is noted on the post-contrast T1-weighted image (**c**)

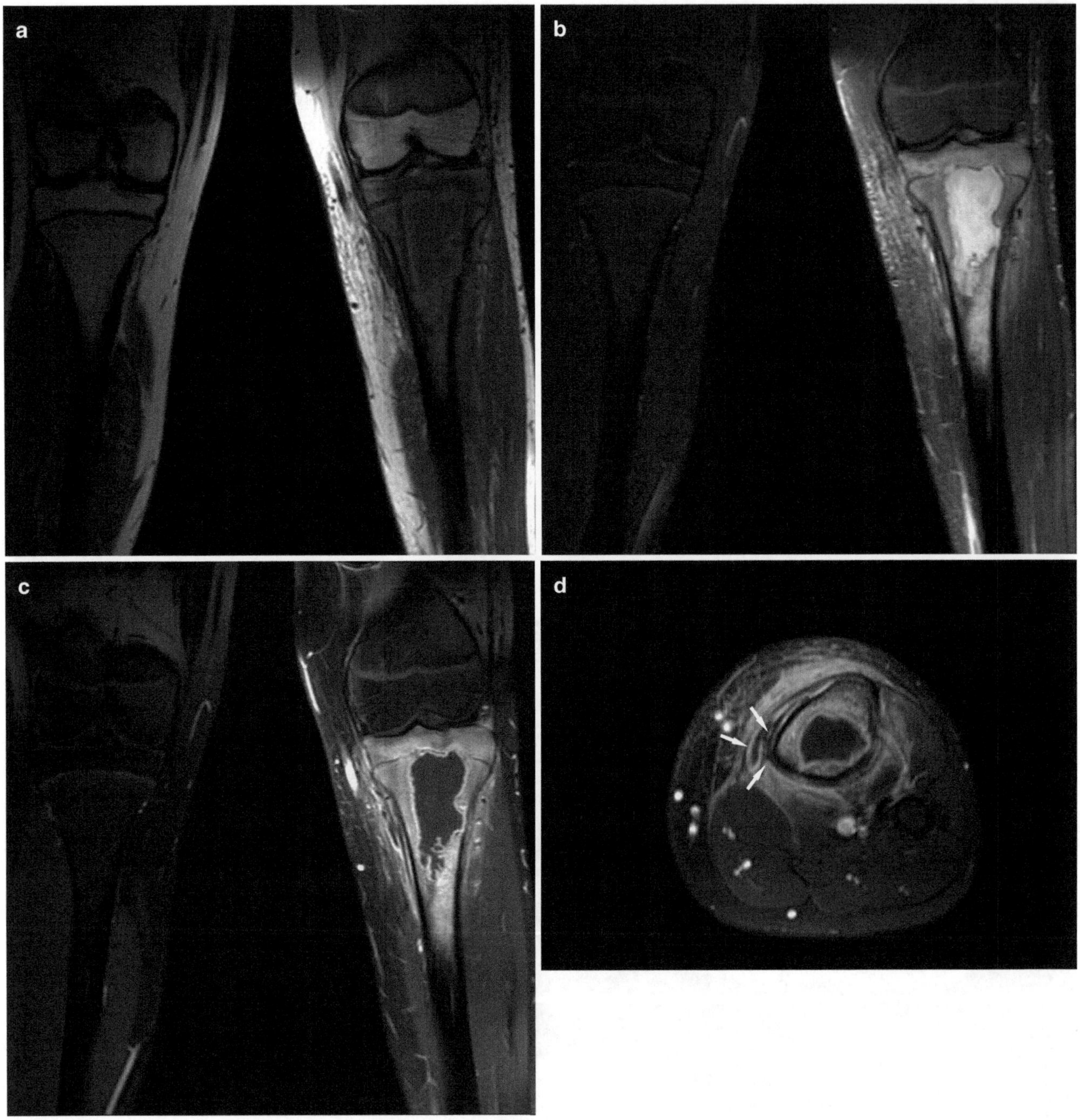

Fig. 5.25 An 18-year-old male with left leg pain and swelling. Coronal T1-weighted (**a**) and T2-weighted fat-suppressed (**b**) MR images demonstrate a large intraosseous abscess in the proximal tibia with marked surrounding bone marrow edema and subtle extension through the growth plate. Postcontrast T1-weighted fat-saturated coronal (**c**) and axial (**d**) images outline the intraosseous abscess and show extraosseous extension (*arrows*). On T1-weighted images, there is a hyperintense rim around the interosseous abscess consistent with "penumbra sign"

5.11 Chronic Recurrent Multifocal Osteomyelitis

Chronic recurrent multifocal osteomyelitis (CRMO) is a disorder of children and young adults that is characterized by nonbacterial osseous inflammation. The etiology of CRMO remains unclear, although the results of several studies have suggested that a genetic component may be involved [11]. Patients with this condition typically present with solitary or multifocal bone pain secondary to sterile osseous inflammation. CRMO most frequently involves the metaphyses of the long bones and the medial clavicles. Other common sites of disease are the vertebral bodies, pelvis, ribs, and mandible. CRMO is often bilateral and multifocal at presentation. MRI findings are similar to those seen with osteomyelitis (Fig. 5.26) but without associated soft tissue abscess or sinus tracts. Because there is no certain diagnostic test for this condition, CRMO remains a diagnosis of exclusion. When this disease is suspected, whole-body MRI or bone scan may be helpful to detect subtle lesions. CRMO should be suspected when its characteristic imaging appearance and distribution of disease are seen (Fig. 5.27). Although generally a self-limiting disease, CRMO can have a prolonged course and may result in significant morbidity requiring treatment.

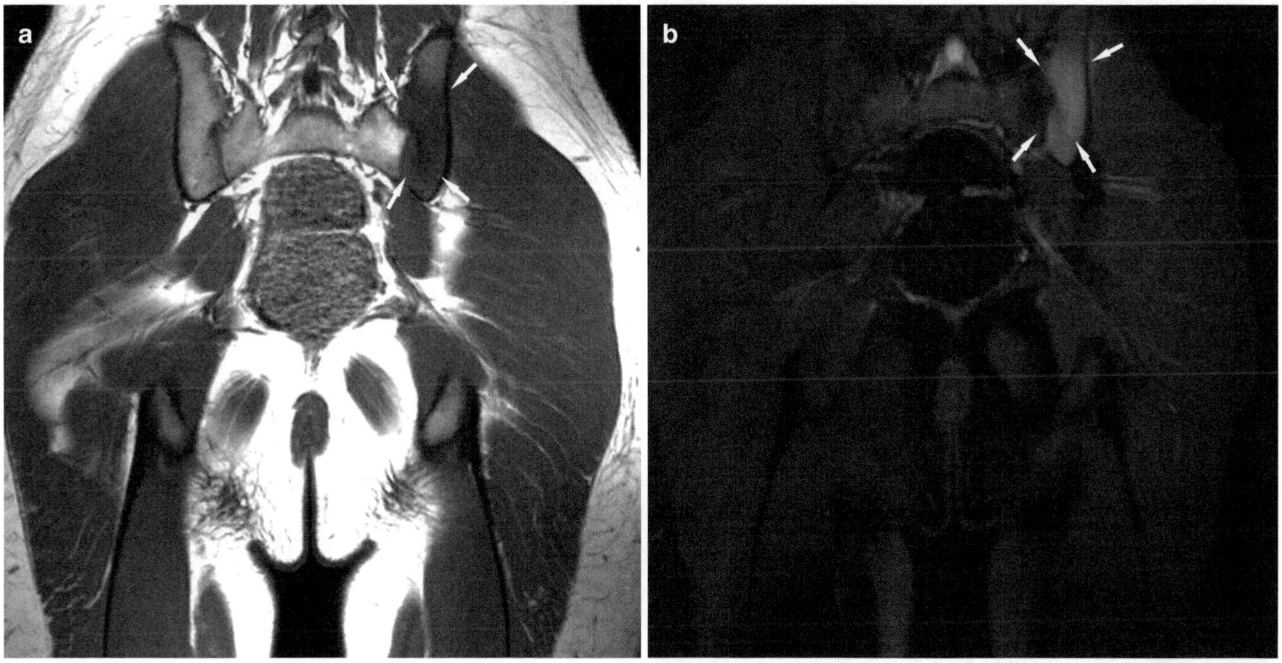

Fig. 5.26 An 18-year-old male with two-month history of lateral left hip pain. Coronal T1-weighted (**a**) and T2-weighted fat-suppressed (**b**) images of the pelvis demonstrate a marrow-infiltrating process in the left ilium abutting the SI joint (*arrows*). A CT-guided biopsy revealed changes of a nonbacterial osteomyelitis

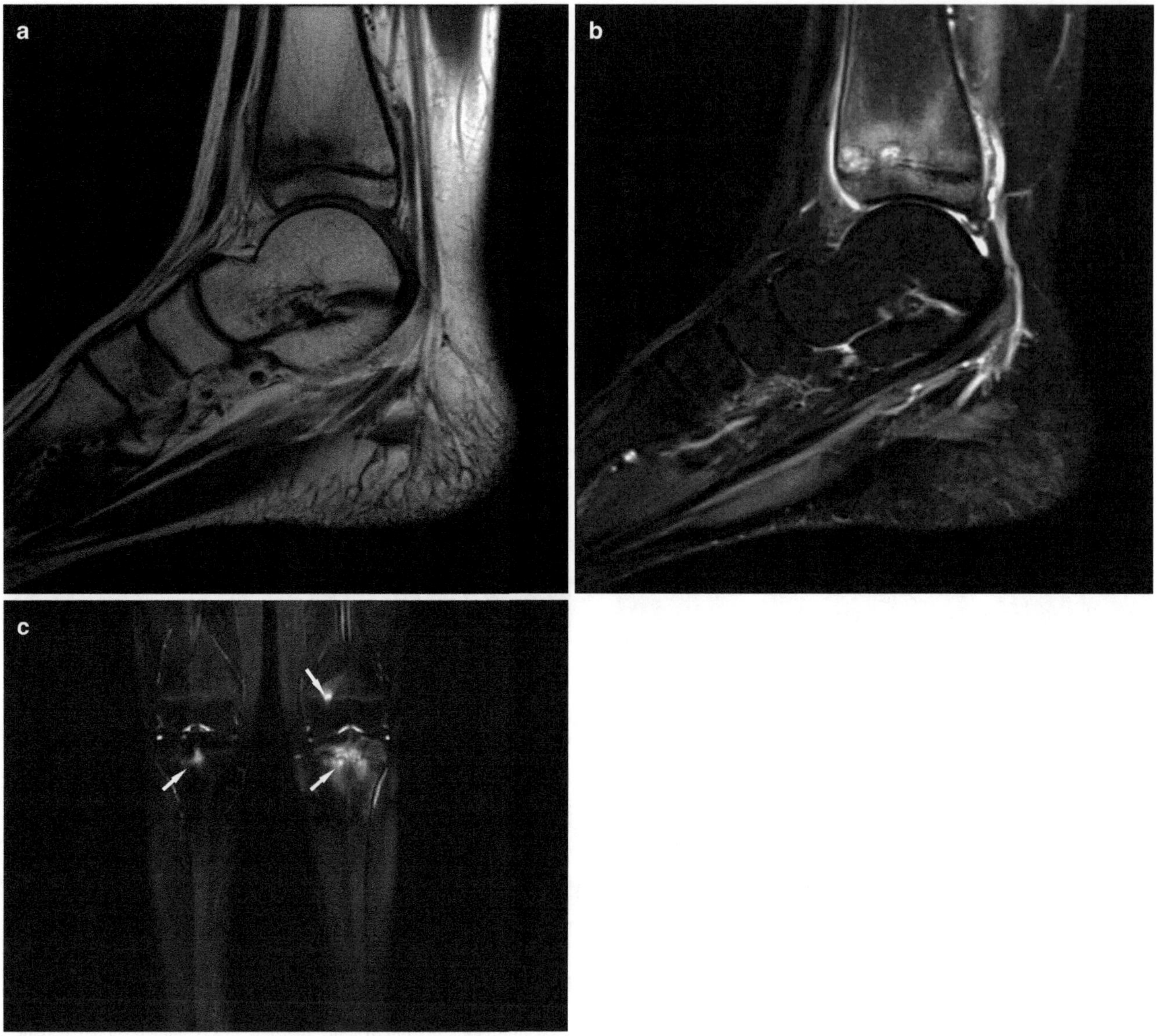

Fig. 5.27 A 13-year-old girl with left ankle pain. Sagittal T1-weighted (**a**) and T2-weighted fat-suppressed (**b**) images demonstrate a lobulated area of marrow infiltration with surrounding bone marrow edema in the metaphysis abutting the growth plate. Whole-body MR imaging evaluation of the patient (**c**) demonstrated similar lesions about the proximal tibia bilaterally and distal femur on the left on STIR coronal image (*arrows*)

5.12 Osteonecrosis

Osteonecrosis, also called avascular necrosis, bone infarction, or ischemic bone necrosis, is a condition that occurs when there is absence of blood supply to the bone.

Osteonecrosis can be seen in patients on long-term corticosteroid use, alcohol abuse, or trauma causing any obstruction of the blood supply. Other less frequently seen conditions causing osteonecrosis include Gaucher disease, sickle cell disease, pancreatitis, HIV infection, radiation treatment, autoimmune diseases, and decompression sickness. MRI is the most sensitive imaging modality and demonstrates osteonecrosis changes well before the radiographic changes are visible. A focal area of serpentine low-signal line with prominent fatty marrow signal centrally is the most typical MRI appearance [12] (Fig. 5.28). Double-line sign had been described on T2-weighted images showing hypointense and hyperintense line MRI around the area of osteonecrosis (Fig. 5.29). Bone marrow edema surrounding the osteonecrosis line is seen early in the disease. Recent development of bone marrow edema surrounding subacute or chronic osteonecrosis is usually seen when subarticular collapse occurs which is associated with significant pain (Fig. 5.30). When articular collapse and fragmentation occurs, secondary degenerative changes develop which is considered to be the final stage of the disease. Sarcoma arising from preexisting osteonecrosis is a rare phenomenon. These sarcomas are high-grade tumors with an aggressive MRI appearance (Fig. 5.31).

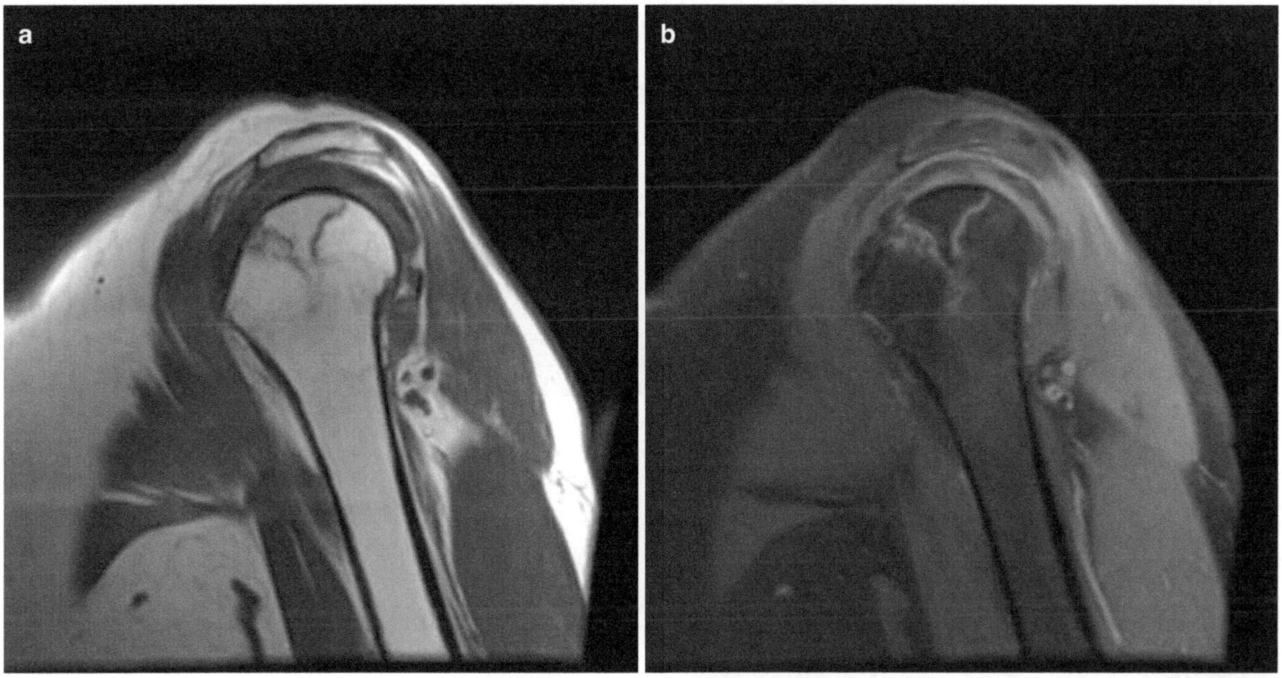

Fig. 5.28 A 52-year-old female with shoulder pain. Sagittal T1-weighted (**a**) and proton-density T2-weighted fat-suppressed (**b**) images of the right shoulder demonstrate serpiginous areas of abnormal signal with central fatty marrow signal in the humeral head consistent with osteonecrosis

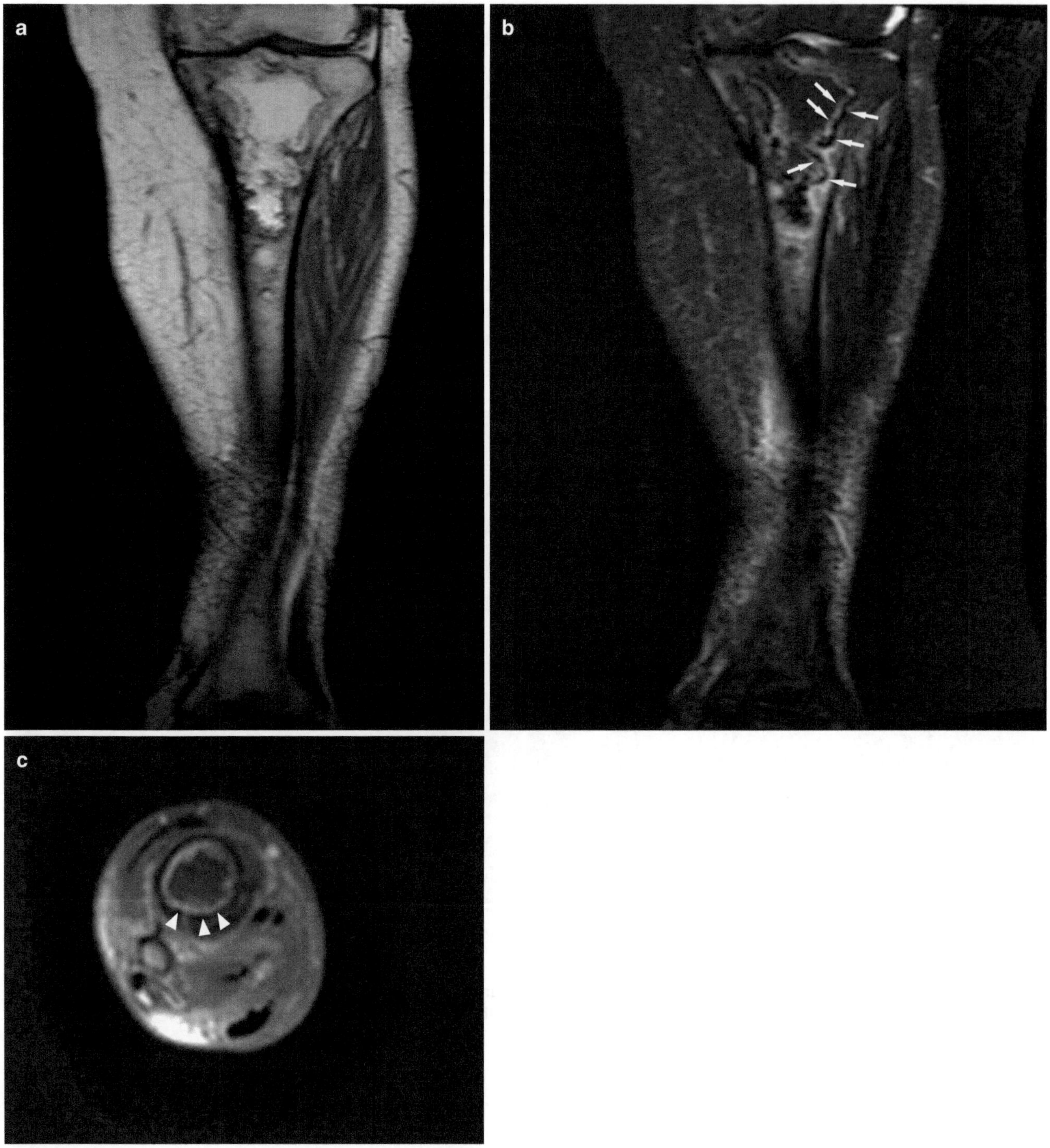

Fig. 5.29 67-year-old female with left leg pain. Coronal T1-weighted (**a**) and T2-weighted fat-suppressed (**b**) images of the left tibia demonstrate a large osteonecrosis. Please note "double-line" sign on T2-weighted fat-suppressed image (*arrows*). Postcontrast T1-weighted fat-suppressed axial image (**c**) demonstrates endosteal enhancement around the osteonecrosis (*arrowheads*)

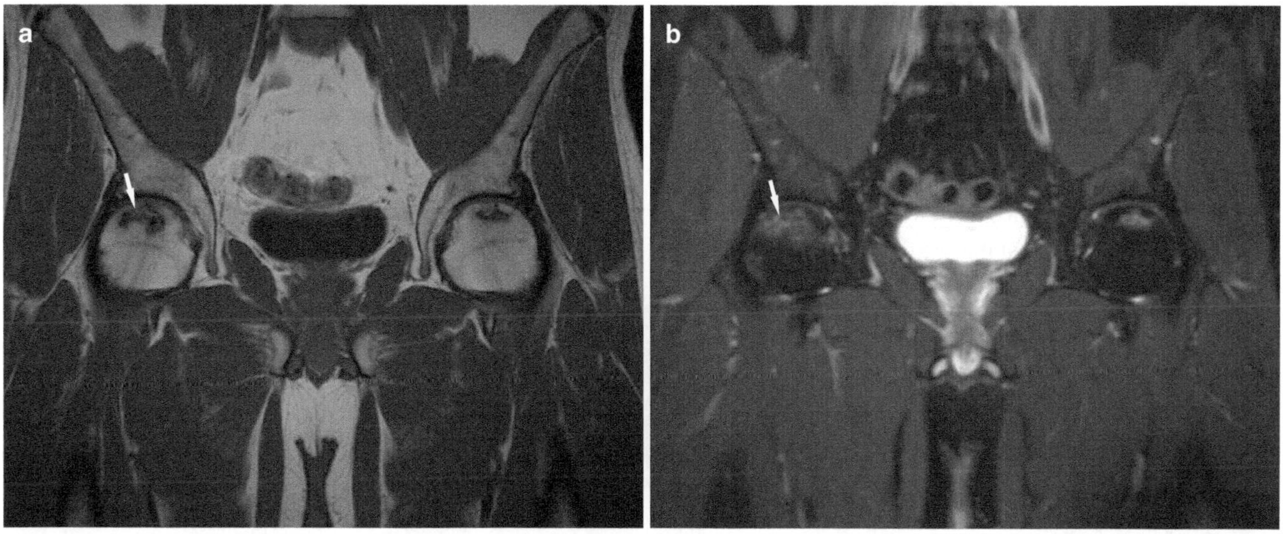

Fig. 5.30 A 31-year-old male with recent onset of worsening right hip pain. Coronal T1-weighted (**a**) and STIR (**b**) images of the pelvis demonstrate osteonecrosis of the femoral heads bilaterally. There is bone marrow edema surrounding right femoral head osteonecrosis with mild overlying subchondral collapse (*arrows*)

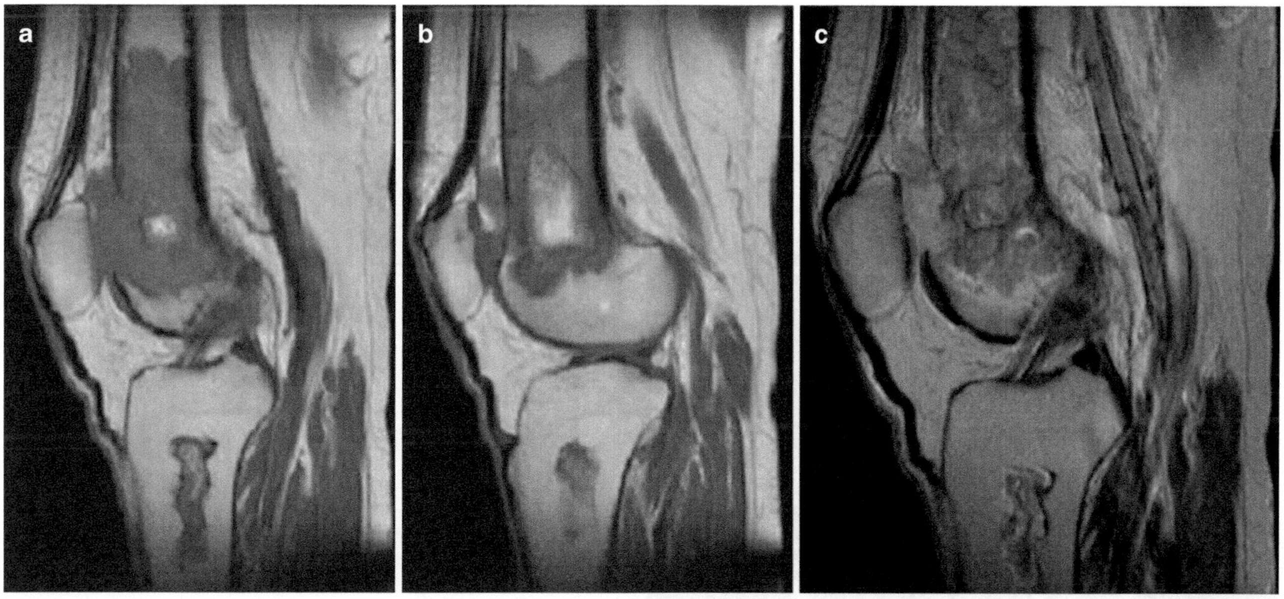

Fig. 5.31 An 80-year-old woman with a high-grade sarcoma of the distal femur arising from preexisting osteonecrosis on sagittal T1-weighted (**a** and **b**) and T2-weighted (**c**) images. Please note area of proximal tibial osteonecrosis without a complication. (Used with permission from editor Springer-Imaging findings journal and year-Skeletal Radiology, prevalence and outcome of de novo and secondary malignant fibrous histiocytoma of bone. Koplas MC, Lefkowitz RA, Bauer TW, Joyce MJ, Ilaslan H, Landa J, Sundaram M)

5.13 Rheumatological Conditions

Inflammatory arthritis typically involves the synovium and bony involvement is secondary from erosions or enthesitis. Seronegative spondyloarthropathies may present with significant bone marrow edema due to enthesitis (Fig. 5.32). The Romanus lesion (Fig. 5.33) represents an early finding in inflammatory spondyloarthropathies, such as ankylosing spondylitis and inflammatory bowel disease-related arthritis, and appears as a bone marrow edema and later erosion involving the anterior and posterior edges of the vertebral endplates [13]. Patient's history and location of bone marrow edema can help making the diagnosis of a spondyloarthropathy when widespread bone marrow edema around joints and disc spaces is encountered.

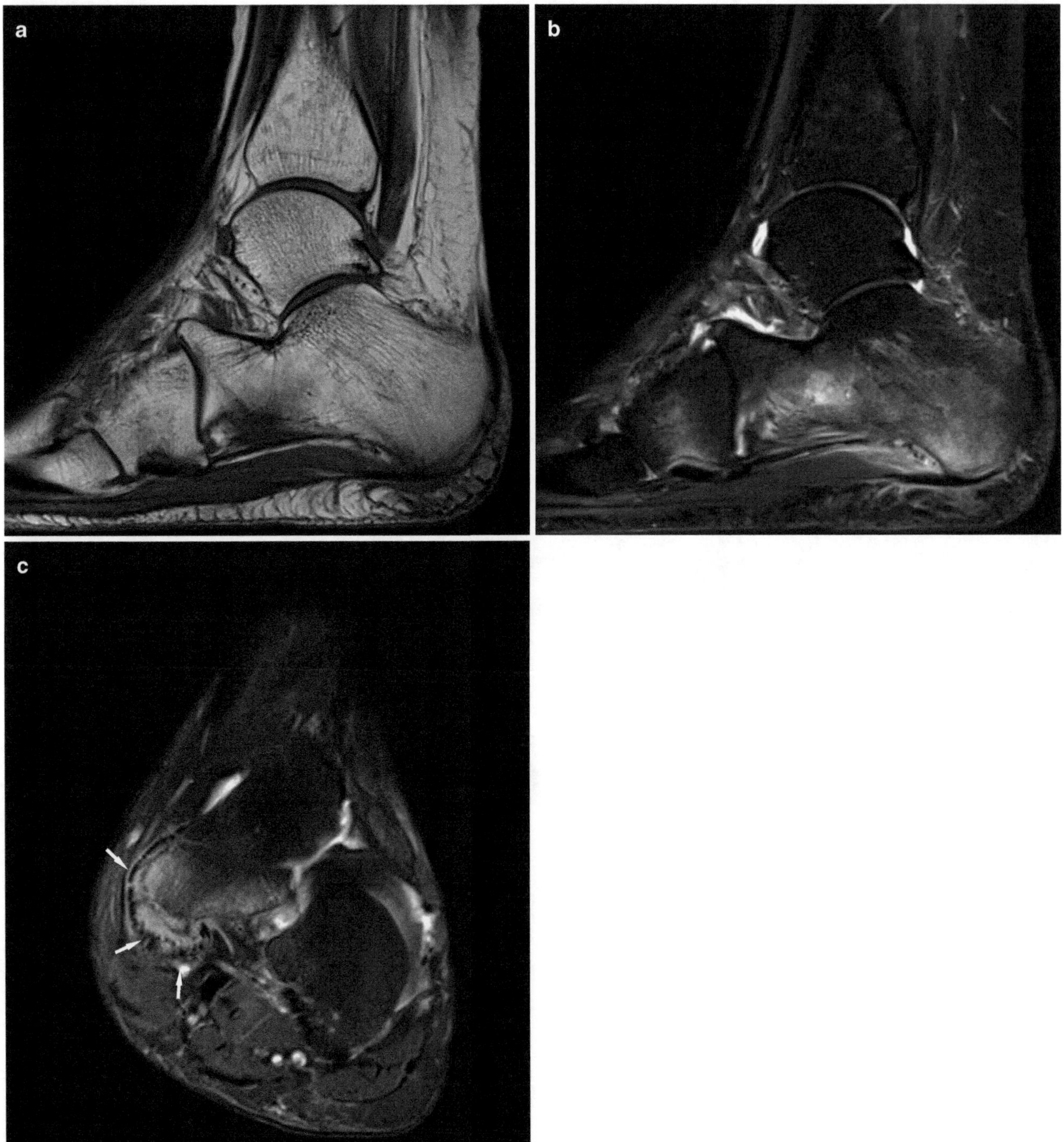

Fig. 5.32 A 36-year-old female with known seronegative spondyloarthropathy. Sagittal T1-weighted (**a**) and T2-weighted (**b**) images demonstrate bone marrow edema involving calcaneus and cuboid most marked around the plantar fascial insertion consistent with enthesitis. Marked bone marrow edema is also noted at the posterior tibial tendon insertion (*arrows*) on the T2-weighted coronal image (**c**)

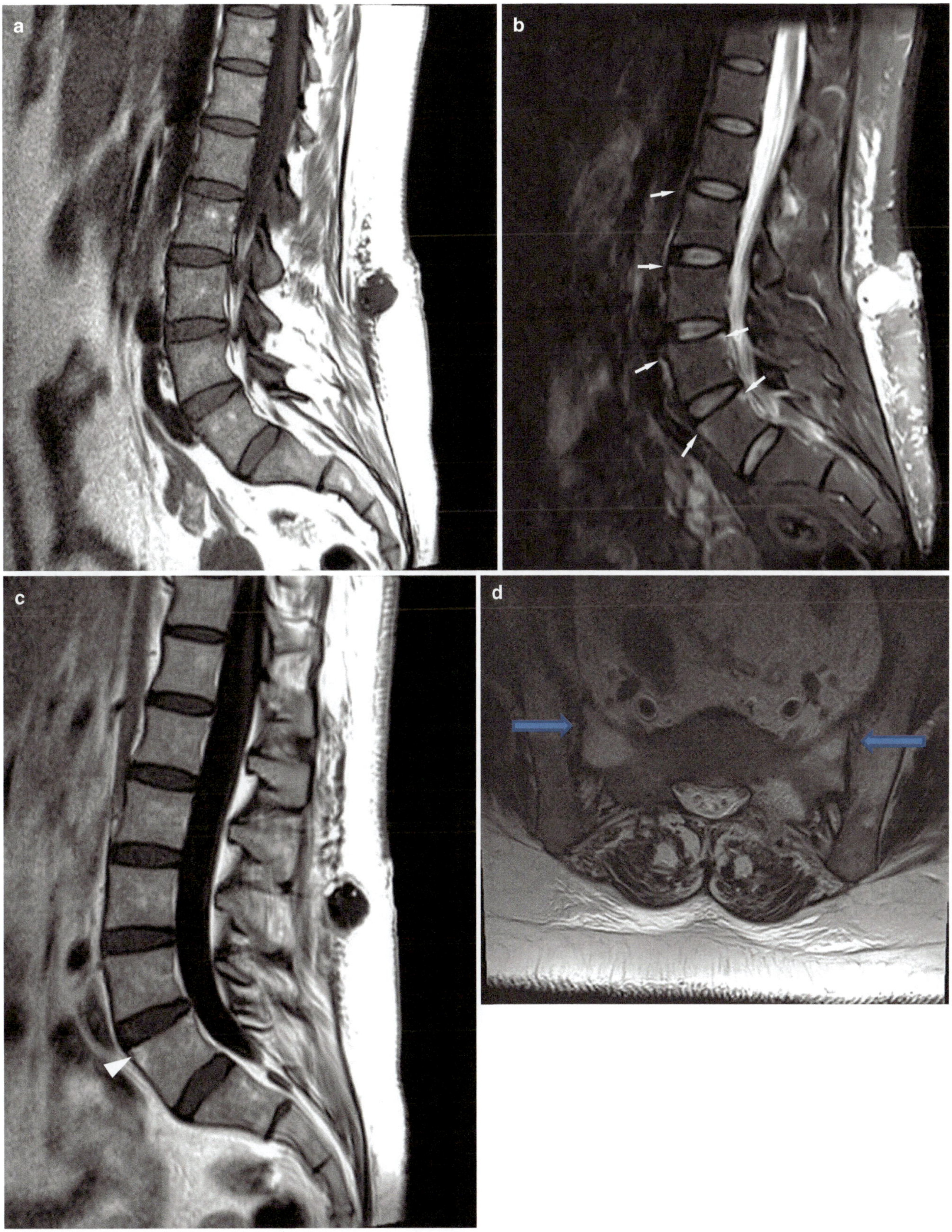

Fig. 5.33 A 42-year-old male with recently diagnosed ankylosing spondylitis. Sagittal T1-weighted (**a**) and STIR (**b**) images of the lumbar spine demonstrate multilevel anterior and posterior corner endplate bone marrow edema (*arrows*) consistent with Romanus lesions. Sagittal postcontrast T1-weighted image (**c**) demonstrates subtle enhancement of the lesion most marked at L5 level (*arrowhead*). (**d**) Axial T2-weighted image shows surrounding SI joint erosions (*arrows*) and surrounding edema

5.14 Transient Bone Marrow Edema Syndrome

Transient bone marrow edema syndrome (TBMS) is an uncommon clinical entity characterized by the spontaneous appearance and resolution over time of joint pain and the associated delayed appearance of osteoporosis on radiographs. This syndrome is most frequently seen in femoral head although other locations have been described [14]. Although initially described in pregnant woman, TBMS most frequently affects middle-aged men [14, 15]. On MRI, the diagnosis is made when subarticular bone marrow edema is visualized with hypointense T1 and hyperintense T2-weighted or STIR sequence is present (Fig. 5.34). When these findings are seen on MRI, a number of other conditions should be ruled out [15]. Osteoarthritis frequently presents with subarticular bone marrow edema, although associated cartilage defects and subchondral cyst formation are often present. Other entities that may cause bone marrow edema particularly in the femoral head include osteonecrosis and subchondral insufficiency fractures where the linear fracture line or serpiginous lines could be seen in subarticular location with or without articular surface deformity. In general, the diagnosis of transient osteoporosis of the femoral head remains presumptive, until demonstration of complete resolution of clinical and imaging findings. Transient osteoporosis does not recur in the same bone but may involve another location, a situation called migratory transient osteoporosis (Fig. 5.35).

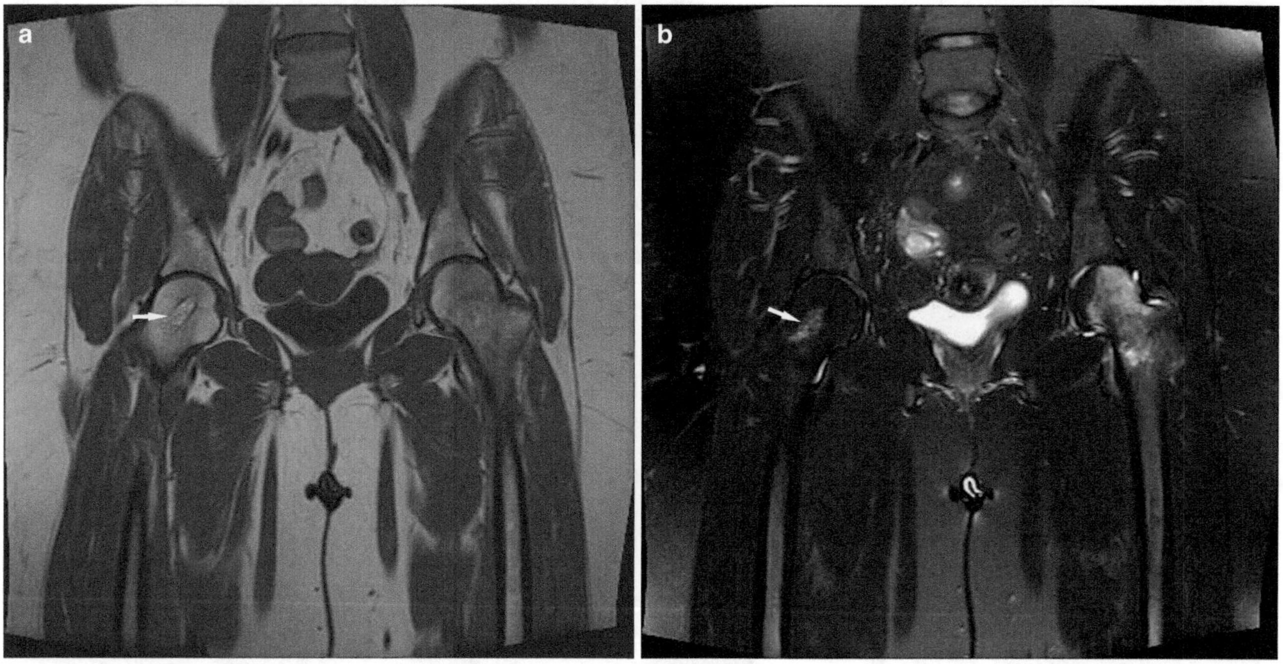

Fig. 5.34 A 34-year-old female with left hip pain. Coronal T1-weighted (**a**) and STIR (**b**) images of the pelvis demonstrate marked edema-like signal in the femoral head extending into the neck without discrete fracture line or subchondral collapse consistent with transient bone marrow edema syndrome. Please note residual susceptibility artifacts from post-operative changes of core compression in the right femoral head and neck (*arrow*) 6 months earlier for presumed early avascular necrosis which was likely due to migratory transient bone marrow edema syndrome

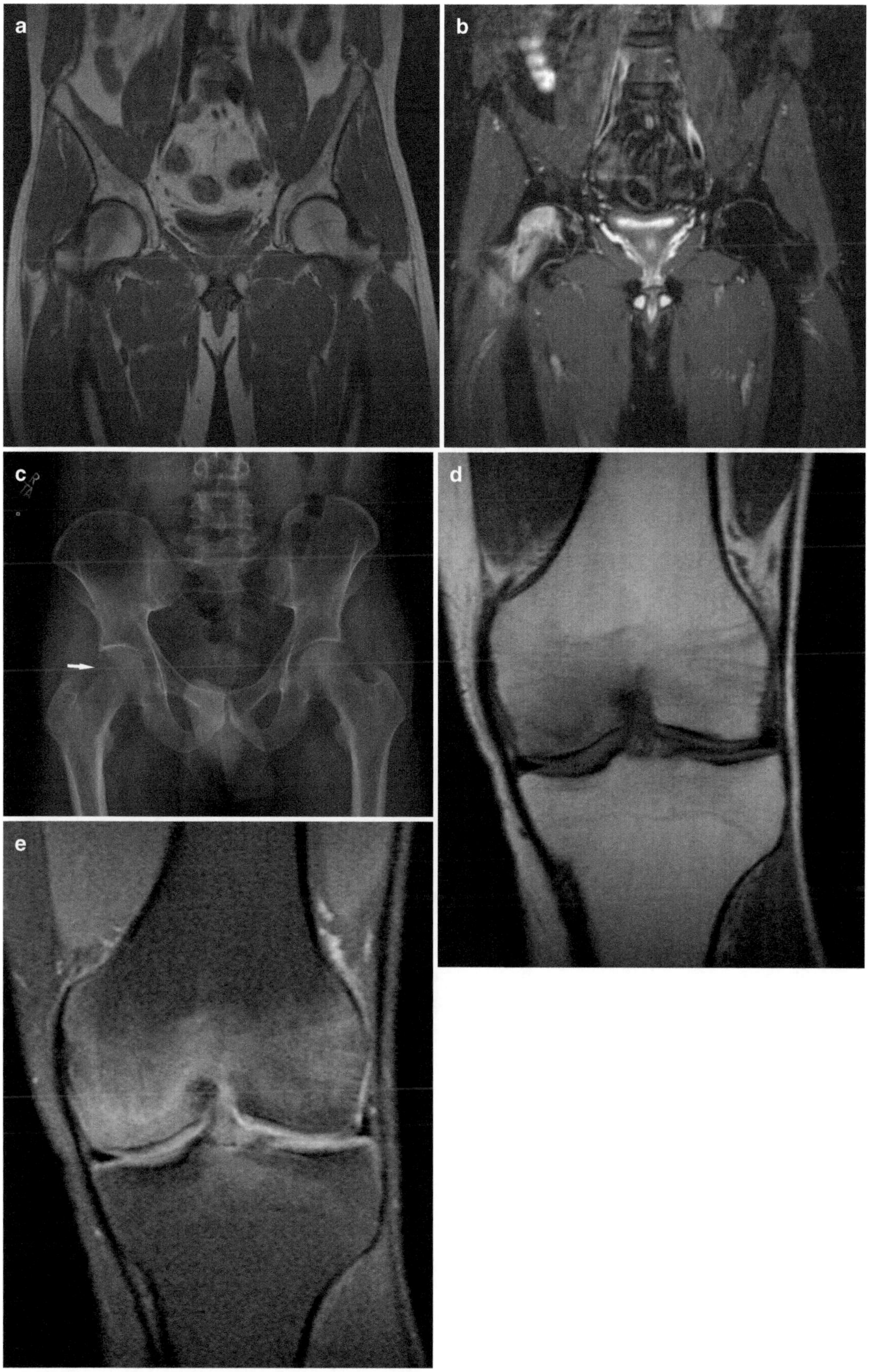

Fig. 5.35 A 38-year-old male with right hip pain. Coronal T1-weighted (**a**) and STIR (**b**) images of the pelvis demonstrate severe bone marrow edema in the right femoral head extending into the femoral neck without discrete fracture line or articular surface depression. Patient was treated conservatively; 1-month follow-up radiograph (**c**) demonstrates localized osteoporosis of the right femoral head (*arrow*). The patient came back with left knee pain 1 year later, MRI demonstrating bone marrow edema about the femoral condyle on coronal T1-weighted (**d**) and T2-weighted fat-suppressed (**e**) images greater medially without cartilage defects or fracture lines. A diagnosis of migratory transient bone marrow edema syndrome was made

References

1. Eschbach JW, Adamson JW. Anemia of end-stage renal disease (ESRD). Kidney Int. 1985;28:1–5.
2. Goo HW, Yang DH, Ra YS, et al. Whole-body MRI of Langerhans cell histiocytosis: comparison with radiography and bone scintigraphy. Pediatr Radiol. 2006;36(10):1019–31.
3. Stull MA, Kransdorf MJ, Devaney KO. Langerhans cell histiocytosis of bone. Radiographics. 1992;12(4):801–23.
4. Sonneveld P, van Lom K, Kappers-Klunne M, et al. Clinicopathological diagnosis and treatment of malignant histiocytosis. Br J Haematol. 1990;75(4):511–6.
5. Roca M, Mota J, Giraldo P, Garcia Erce JA. Systemic mastocytosis: MRI of bone marrow involvement. Eur Radiol. 1999;9(6):1094–7.
6. Steinberg SE, Nasraway S, Peterson L. Reversal of severe serous atrophy of bone marrow in anorexia nervosa. JPEN J Parenter Enteral Nutr. 1987;11(4):422–3.
7. Vande Berg BC, Malghem J, Devuyst O, et al. Anorexia nervosa: correlation between MR appearance of bone marrow and severity of disease. Radiology. 1994;193(3):859–64.
8. Maas M, van Kuijk C, Stoker J, et al. Quantification of bone involvement in Gaucher disease: MR imaging bone marrow burden score as an alternative to Dixon quantitative chemical shift MR imaging—initial experience. Radiology. 2003;229(2):554–61.
9. Wenstrup RJ, Roca-Espiau M, Weinreb NJ, Bembi B. Skeletal aspects of Gaucher disease: a review. Br J Radiol. 2002;75 Suppl 1: A2–12.
10. Davies AM, Grimer R. The penumbra sign in subacute osteomyelitis. Eur Radiol. 2005;15(6):1268–70.
11. Khanna G, Sato TS, Ferguson P. Imaging of chronic recurrent multifocal osteomyelitis. Radiographics. 2009;29(4):1159–77.
12. Glickstein MF, Burk DL, Schiebler ML, et al. Avascular necrosis versus other diseases of the hip: sensitivity of MR imaging. Radiology. 1988;169(1):213–5.
13. Hermann KG, Althoff CE, Schneider U, et al. Spinal changes in patients with spondyloarthritis: comparison of MR imaging and radiographic appearances. Radiographics. 2005;25(3):559–69.
14. Hayes CW, Conway WF, Daniel WW. MR imaging of bone marrow edema pattern: transient osteoporosis, transient bone marrow edema syndrome, or osteonecrosis. Radiographics. 1993;13(5): 1001–11.
15. Vande Berg BC, Lecouvet FE, Koutaissoff S, et al. Bone marrow edema of the femoral head and transient osteoporosis of the hip. Eur J Radiol. 2008;67(1):68–77.

Index

H. Ilaslan, M. Sundaram, *Pediatric and Adult MRI Atlas of Bone Marrow: Normal Appearances, Variants and Diffuse Disease States*, DOI 10.1007/978-3-642-02740-6

GPSR Compliance

The European Union's (EU) General Product Safety Regulation (GPSR) is a set of rules that requires consumer products to be safe and our obligations to ensure this.

If you have any concerns about our products, you can contact us on ProductSafety@springernature.com

In case Publisher is established outside the EU, the EU authorized representative is:

Springer Nature Customer Service Center GmbH
Europaplatz 3
69115 Heidelberg, Germany

Batch number: 10732819

Printed by Printforce, the Netherlands